Dermoscopy

Editors

GIUSEPPE ARGENZIANO
IRIS ZALAUDEK
JASON GIACOMEL

DERMATOLOGIC CLINICS

www.derm.theclinics.com

Consulting Editor
BRUCE H. THIERS

October 2013 • Volume 31 • Number 4

ELSEVIER

1600 John F. Kennedy Boulevard • Suite 1800 • Philadelphia, Pennsylvania, 19103-2899

http://www.theclinics.com

DERMATOLOGIC CLINICS Volume 31, Number 4
October 2013 ISSN 0733-8635, ISBN-13: 978-0-323-22748-3

Editor: Stephanie Donley

Dermatologic Clinics (ISSN 0733-8635) is published quarterly by Elsevier Inc., 360 Park Avenue South, New York, NY 10010-1710. Months of publication are January, April, July, and October. Business and editorial offices: 1600 John F. Kennedy Blvd., Suite 1800, Philadelphia, PA 19103-2899. Customer service office: 11830 Westline Drive, St. Louis, MO 63146. Periodicals postage paid at New York, NY, and additional mailing offices. Subscription prices are USD 346.00 per year for US individuals, USD 532.00 per year for US institutions, USD 404.00 per year for Canadian individuals, USD 636.00 per year for Canadian institutions, USD 473.00 per year for international individuals, USD 636.00 per year for international institutions, USD 159.00 per year for US students/residents, and USD 230.00 per year for Canadian and international students/residents. International air speed delivery is included in all *Clinics* subscription prices. All prices are subject to change without notice. **POSTMASTER:** Send address changes to *Dermatologic Clinics*, Elsevier Health Sciences Division, Subscription Customer Service, 3251 Riverport Lane, Maryland Heights, MO 63043. **Customer Service: 1-800-654-2452 (U.S. and Canada); 314-447-8871 (outside U.S. and Canada). Fax: 314-447-8029. E-mail: journalscustomerservice-usa@elsevier.com (for print support); journalsonlinesupport-usa@elsevier.com (for online support).**

Reprints. For copies of 100 or more, of articles in this publication, please contact the Commercial Reprints Department, Elsevier Inc., 360 Park Avenue South, New York, New York 10010-1710. Tel.: 212-633-3874; Fax: 212-633-3820; Email: repritns@elsevier.com.

The *Dermatologic Clinics* is covered in *MEDLINE/PubMed (Index Medicus)*, *Current Contents/Clinical Medicine*, *Excerpta Medica*, *Chemical Abstracts*, and *ISI/BIOMED*.

Printed and bound by CPI Group (UK) Ltd, Croydon, CR0 4YY

Transferred to digital print 2012

Contributors

CONSULTING EDITOR

BRUCE H. THIERS, MD
Professor and Chairman, Department of
Dermatology and Dermatologic Surgery,
Medical University of South Carolina,
Charleston, South Carolina

EDITORS

GIUSEPPE ARGENZIANO, MD
Professor of Dermatology, Dermatology and
Skin Cancer Unit, First Medical Department,
Arcispedale Santa Maria Nuova, Istituto
di Ricovero e Cura a Carattere
Scientifico-IRCCS, Reggio Emilia, Italy

IRIS ZALAUDEK, MD
Professor of Dermatology, Department of
Dermatology, Medical University of Graz, Graz,
Austria; Dermatology and Skin Cancer Unit,
Department of Dermatology, Arcispedale
Santa Maria Nuova, IRCCS, Reggio Emilia,
Italy

JASON GIACOMEL, MBBS
Skin Spectrum Medical Services, Como, Perth,
Western Australia, Australia

AUTHORS

GIUSEPPE ALBERTINI, MD
Dermatology and Skin Cancer Unit,
Arcispedale Santa Maria Nuova, Istituto di
Ricovero e Cura a Carattere Scientifico-
IRCCS, Reggio Emilia, Italy

SAMER AL JALBOUT, MD
Department of Dermatology and Venereology,
Medical University of Modena and Reggio
Emilia, Reggio Emilia, Italy

ZOE APALLA, MD
State Clinic of Dermatology, Hospital of Skin
and Venereal Diseases, Thessaloniki, Greece

GIUSEPPE ARGENZIANO, MD
Dermatology and Skin Cancer Unit, First
Medical Department, Arcispedale Santa Maria
Nuova, Istituto di Ricovero e Cura a Carattere
Scientifico-IRCCS, Reggio Emilia, Italy

ANDREAS BLUM, MD
Public, Private and Teaching Practice of
Dermatology, Konstanz, Germany

RALPH P. BRAUN, MD
Department of Dermatology, University
Hospital Geneva, Geneva, Switzerland

HORACIO CABO, MD
Deparment of Dermatology, Instituto de
Investigaciones Médicas A. Lanari, University
of Buenos Aires, Buenos Aires, Argentina

FABIO CASTAGNETTI, MD
Skin Cancer Unit, First Medical Department,
Arcispedale Santa Maria Nuova, Istituto
di Ricovero e Cura a Carattere
Scientifico-IRCCS, Reggio Emilia, Italy

STEFANO CAVICCHINI, MD
Dermatology Unit, Fondazione IRCCS Ca'
Granda Ospedale Maggiore Policlinico, Milan,
Italy

STÉPHANE DALLE, MD, PhD
Department of Dermatology, Centre
Hospitalier Lyon Sud, Université Claude
Bernard Lyon 1, Piere Bénite Cedex, France

SÉBASTIEN DEBARBIEUX, MD
Department of Dermatology, Centre
Hospitalier Lyon Sud, Université Claude
Bernard Lyon 1, Piere Bénite Cedex, France

VITO DI LERNIA, MD
Unit of Dermatology, Arcispedale Santa Maria
Nuova, Istituto di Ricovero e Cura a Carattere
Scientifico-IRCCS, Reggio Emilia, Italy

GERARDO FERRARA, MD
Anatomic Pathology Unit, Department of
Oncology, 'Gaetano Rummo' General
Hospital, Benevento, Italy

STEFANO GARDINI, MD
Skin cancer Unit, Arcispedale Santa Maria
Nuova, Istituto di Ricovero e Cura a Carattere
Scientifico-IRCCS, Reggio Emilia, Italy

JASON GIACOMEL, MBBS
Skin Spectrum Medical Services, Como, Perth,
Western Australia, Australia

RAFFAELE GIANOTTI, MD
Department of Pathophysiology and
Transplantation, University of Milan, Milan, Italy

ALLAN HALPERN, MD
Memorial Sloan-Kettering Cancer Centre,
New York, New York

RAINER HOFMANN-WELLENHOF, MD
Department of Dermatology, Medical
University of Graz, Graz, Austria

NATALIA JAIMES, MD
Dermatology Service, Aurora Skin Cancer
Center and Universidad Pontificia Bolivariana,
Medellín, Colombia

HARALD KITTLER, MD
Associate Professor of Dermatology,
Department of Dermatology, Medical
University of Vienna, Vienna, Austria

MARTA KURZEJA, MD
Department of Dermatology, CSK MSW,
Warsaw, Poland

AIMILIOS LALLAS, MD
Dermatology and Skin Cancer Unit, First
Medical Department, Arcispedale Santa Maria
Nuova, Istituto di Ricovero e Cura a Carattere
Scientifico-IRCCS, Reggio Emilia, Italy

CATERINA LONGO, MD, PhD
Dermatology and Skin Cancer Unit, First
Medical Department, Arcispedale Santa Maria
Nuova, Istituto di Ricovero e Cura a Carattere
Scientifico-IRCCS, Reggio Emilia, Italy

JOSEP MALVEHY, PhD
Melanoma Unit, Dermatology Department,
Hospital Clinic of Barcelona, Institut
d'Investigacions Biomèdiques August Pi i
Sunyer and U726 Centros de Investigacıon
Biomedica en Red de Enfermedades Raras,
Instituto de Salud Carlos III, Barcelona, Spain

ASHFAQ A. MARGHOOB, MD
Dermatology Service, Department of
Dermatology, Memorial Sloan-Kettering
Cancer Center, New York, New York

SCOTT W. MENZIES, MBBS, PhD
Professor, Sydney Medical School, Sydney
Melanoma Diagnostic Centre, Royal Prince
Alfred Hospital, Camper down; Discipline of
Dermatology, Sydney Medical School,
The University of Sydney, New South Wales,
Australia

ELVIRA MOSCARELLA, MD
Dermatology and Skin Cancer Unit, First
Medical Department, Arcispedale Santa Maria
Nuova, Istituto di Ricovero e Cura a Carattere
Scientifico-IRCCS, Reggio Emilia, Italy

MAŁGORZATA OLSZEWSKA, MD, PhD
Department of Dermatology, Medical
University of Warsaw, Warsaw, Poland

GIOVANNI PELLACANI, MD
Dermatology Unit, University of Modena and
Reggio Emilia, Modena, Italy

ALICE PHAN, MD, PhD
Department of Dermatology, Centre
Hospitalier Lyon Sud, Université Claude
Bernard Lyon 1, Piere Bénite Cedex, France

VINCENZO PICCOLO, MD
Department of Dermatology, Second
University of Naples, Naples, Italy

STEFANIA PIZZIGONI, MD
Skin Cancer Unit, First Medical Department,
Arcispedale Santa Maria Nuova, Istituto di
Ricovero e Cura a Carattere Scientifico-
IRCCS, Reggio Emilia, Italy

NICOLAS POULALHON, MD
Department of Dermatology, Centre
Hospitalier Lyon Sud, Université Claude
Bernard Lyon 1, Piere Bénite Cedex, France

PAULINE PRALONG, MD
Department of Dermatology, Centre
Hospitalier Lyon Sud, Université Claude
Bernard Lyon 1, Piere Bénite Cedex, France

SUSANA PUIG, PhD
Melanoma Unit, Dermatology Department,
Hospital Clinic of Barcelona, Institut
d'Investigacions Biomèdiques August Pi i
Sunyer and U726 Centros de Investigacion
Biomedica en Red de Enfermedades Raras,
Instituto de Salud Carlos III, Barcelona, Spain

HAROLD RABINOVITZ, MD
Department of Dermatology, Skin and Cancer
Associates, School of Medicine, University of
Miami, Miami, Florida

ADRIANA RAKOWSKA, MD, PhD
Department of Dermatology, CSK MSW,
Warsaw, Poland

CINZIA RICCI, MD
Dermatology and Skin Cancer Unit,
Arcispedale Santa Maria Nuova, Istituto di
Ricovero e Cura a Carattere Scientifico-
IRCCS, Reggio Emilia, Italy

LIDIA RUDNICKA, MD, PhD
Department of Dermatology, CSK MSW;
Department of Neuropeptides, Mossakowski
Medical Research Centre, Polish Academy of
Sciences; Faculty of Health Sciences, Medical
University of Warsaw, Warsaw, Poland

TOSHIAKI SAIDA, MD
Department of Dermatology, School of
Medicine, Shinshu University, Matsumoto,
Japan

TIZIANA SALVIATO, MD
Anatomic Pathology Unit, Department of
Laboratory Medicine, 'Santa Maria degli
Angeli' General Hospital, Pordenone, Italy

ALON SCOPE, MD
Department of Dermatology, Sheba Medical
Center, Sackler School of Medicine, Tel Aviv
University, Tel Aviv, Israel; Dermatology
Service, Memorial Sloan-Kettering Cancer
Center, New York, New York

STEFANIA SEIDENARI, MD
Department of Dermatology, University of
Modena and Reggio Emilia, Modena, Italy

H. PETER SOYER, MD, FACD
Dermatology Research Centre, Princess
Alexandra Hospital, The University of
Queensland School of Medicine, Brisbane,
Queensland, Australia

WILHELM STOLZ, MD
Clinic of Dermatology and Allergology, Hospital
Munich-Schwabing, Munich, Germany

LUC THOMAS, MD, PhD
Department of Dermatology, Centre
Hospitalier Lyon Sud, Université Claude
Bernard Lyon 1, Piere Bénite Cedex, France

DANICA TIODOROVIC-ZIVKOVIC, MD
Clinic of Dermatovenerology, Clinical Center of
Nis, Medical Faculty University of Nis, Nis,
Serbia

PHILIPP TSCHANDL, MD
Resident, Department of Dermatology,
Medical University of Vienna, Vienna, Austria

IRIS ZALAUDEK, MD
Department of Dermatology, Medical
University of Graz, Graz, Austria; Dermatology
and Skin Cancer Unit, Department of
Dermatology, Arcispedale Santa Maria Nuova,
IRCCS, Reggio Emilia, Italy

Contents

Dermoscopy has been shown in meta-analyses to improve the diagnostic accuracy of melanoma unequivocally compared with naked eye examination and to reduce excision rates of benign melanocytic lesions in clinical trials. Sequential digital dermoscopy imaging (SDDI) allows the detection of dermoscopic featureless melanoma. When used in high-risk individuals or on individual suspicious melanocytic lesions, it has a gross impact for detecting melanoma in clinical practice, with a range of 34% to 61% of melanomas detected exclusively using SDDI in these patients. Furthermore, SDDI has been shown to reduce the excision of benign lesions when used in combination with dermoscopy.

Dermoscopy is useful for skin cancer screening, but a detailed approach is required that integrates this tool into a rational clinical work flow. To investigate clinician perceptions and behavior in approaching patients with skin tumors, a survey was launched by electronic mail through the International Dermoscopy Society. After 4 months, the responses were analyzed and significant findings calculated. Considering the current approach of study participants in examining patients for skin cancer, an up-to-date system of triage is presented in this review, which aims to promote an improved diagnostic accuracy and more timely management of skin malignancy.

Melanoma in childhood is rare, and appears more commonly either in association with a preexisting (congenital) nevus, or with spitzoid features than de novo. Thus, problematic melanocytic lesions in children are essentially represented by congenital nevi and Spitz nevi that can be regarded as melanoma precursors and melanoma simulators, respectively. As a consequence, clinical and dermoscopic features of melanoma in children differ from those in an adult population. Herein we describe common clinical and dermoscopic features of problematic lesions in children, focusing on congenital and Spitz/Reed nevi, and including other problematic lesions, such as atypical, blue, acral, and scalp nevi.

As the population continues to age, clinicians and dermatologists are increasingly faced with geriatric patients presenting with a range of dermatologic manifestations, including benign and malignant skin tumors. Knowledge of epidemiologic and morphologic features, including dermoscopy of common and benign melanocytic and nonmelanocytic skin tumors, provides the basis for a better understanding and management of problematic skin tumors in this age group. This article provides an overview of common and problematic skin lesions in elderly patients and addresses epidemiologic, clinical, and dermoscopic clues that aid the differential diagnosis and management of challenging skin lesions.

Early recognition is the most effective intervention to improve melanoma mortality. Early diagnosis of melanoma in atypical mole syndrome patients, however, may be challenging. Skin self-examination and periodic physician-based total-body skin examinations are recommended in atypical mole patients but dermoscopy, total-body photography, and digital dermatoscopy have been proved to improve accuracy in early detection of melanoma in these high-risk patients. Digital follow-up in atypical mole syndrome patients allows detection of new lesions and changes in preexisting lesions.

The term "dysplastic nevus" is a misnomer and should be abandoned. Dysplastic nevus is not just a name, it is the root of the concept that histomorphology (or any morphologic examination including dermatoscopy) is able to predict the fate of a benign melanocytic proliferation. There is no evidence that this hypothesis is true but there are observations that falsify it. Preferably a specific diagnosis should be made based on dermatoscopic pattern and, if this is not possible, on clinical or dermatoscopic grounds alone the term "nevus, not otherwise specified" should be used.

Spitz nevus can clinically present either in the classical (reddish pink) or the pigmented (brownish black) variant. Dermoscopy demonstrates that the pigmented variant is much more common than the classical variant; however, none of these show dermoscopic patterns clearly distinguishable from melanoma. Even histopathologically, a clear-cut differentiation between benign and malignant spitzoid neoplasms is often difficult, so that intermediate diagnostic categories (atypical Spitz nevus and Spitz tumor) are admitted. Because of these difficulties in clinical and histopathologic evaluation, surgical excision is recommended for clinically atypical spitzoid lesions of childhood and for all spitzoid lesions of adulthood.

Differentiating dysplastic nevi from melanoma remains one of the main objectives of dermoscopy. Melanomas tend not to manifest any of the benign patterns described for nevi and instead usually display chaotic dermoscopic morphologies. Melanomas located on the face, chronically sun-damaged skin, volar surfaces, nails, and mucosal surfaces have additional features that can assist in their identification. However, some melanomas lack any defined dermoscopic structures. These so-called featureless melanomas can be identified via digital surveillance. This article reviews the melanoma-specific structures as a function of anatomic location (ie, melanomas on nonglabrous skin, face, volar surfaces, mucosae, and nails).

Although dermoscopy reflects the anatomy, skin anatomy is different on facial and acral skin as well as in the nail unit. Malignant patterns on acral sites include the parallel ridge pattern and irregular diffuse pigmentation, whose presence should lead to a biopsy. Malignant patterns on the face include features of follicular invasion (signet-ring images, annular granular images, and rhomboidal structures) and atypical vessels. Malignant patterns on the nail unit include the micro-Hutchinson sign and irregular longitudinal lines.

The anatomic region influences the dermoscopic features of different lesions. In this article, the particular characteristics of the scalp, mucosal membranes, and lesions located on the milk line are explained. In histopathology, the benign melanocytic lesions in these locations are also named nevi of special sites, considering the difficulty of the histopathologic diagnosis.

Blue color is found in a wide range of malignant and benign melanocytic and nonmelanocytic lesions and in lesions that result from penetration of exogenous materials, such as radiation or amalgam tattoo or traumatic penetration of particles. Discriminating between different diagnostic entities that display blue color relies on careful patient examination and lesion assessment. Dermoscopically, the extent, distribution, and patterns created by blue color can help diagnose lesions with specificity and differentiate between benign and malignant entities. This article provides an overview of the main diagnoses whereby blue color can be found, providing simple management rules for these lesions.

Dermoscopy (dermatoscopy or surface microscopy) is an ancillary dermatologic tool that in experienced hands can improve the accuracy of diagnosis of a variety of benign and malignant pigmented skin tumors. The early and more accurate diagnosis of nonpigmented, or pink, tumors can also be assisted by dermoscopy. This review focuses on the dermoscopic diagnosis of pink lesions, with emphasis on blood vessel morphology and pattern. A 3-step algorithm is presented, which facilitates the timely and more accurate diagnosis of pink tumors and subsequently guides the management for such lesions.

DERMATOLOGIC CLINICS

RELATED INTEREST

Pattern Classification of Dermoscopy Images: A Perceptually Uniform Model
Qaisar Abbas, M.E. Celebi, Carmen Serrano, Irene Fondón García, and Guangzhi Ma, *Editors*
Pattern Recognition, Volume 46, Issue 1, January 2013, Pages 86–97

NOW AVAILABLE FOR YOUR iPhone and iPad

Preface

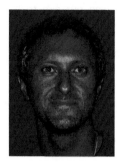

Giuseppe Argenziano, MD

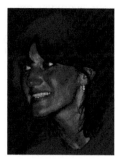

Iris Zalaudek, MD

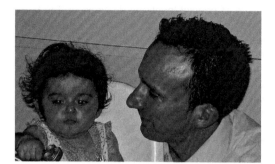

Jason Giacomel, MBBS

Editors

In this issue of *Dermatologic Clinics*, most of the hot topics relevant to the field of dermoscopy are reviewed by a panel of internationally renowned researchers. As mentioned in the introductory article by Scott Menzies, dermoscopy and sequential digital dermoscopy imaging have been shown to unequivocally improve the diagnostic accuracy of melanoma (compared with naked eye examination) and to reduce excision rates of benign melanocytic lesions.

Although dermoscopy has been proven to be useful for skin cancer screening, a detailed approach is still required that integrates this tool into a rational clinical workflow. In the second article, we report the results of a survey conducted by the International Dermoscopy Society to investigate clinician perceptions and behavior in approaching patients with skin tumors and to propose an updated system of triage.

In articles 3 to 5, specific guidelines are given with respect to patients of different age groups. Clinicians do not screen lesions but patients and, in this context, dermoscopy plays a key role only when used as part of the overall clinical examination of the patient. Lesions in children may have similar clinicodermoscopic features as those occurring in the elderly, but they often should be interpreted and managed very differently. Adult patients with multiple nevi should be managed differently as compared to patients consulting for solitary lesions. In sum, patients of different age groups present special challenges that are, therefore, specifically addressed in the previously mentioned articles.

In article 6, Harald Kittler reviews the never-ending story surrounding dysplastic nevi. The article is titled, "Dysplastic Nevus: Why This Term Should Be Abandoned in the Dermatoscopy Era." The reader may, therefore, easily understand from the outset the author's viewpoint, which can also be summarized by the two following statements: (1) "The terms 'dysplastic' and 'atypical' nevus are often used by clinicians and pathologists to express their diagnostic uncertainty but it has nothing to do with biologic uncertainty"; and (2) "There are parts of a melanoma that may look like a nevus clinically, dermatoscopically, and histopathologically, which led to the unjustified assumption that the inconspicuous part of the melanoma is a precursor nevus."

In article 7, Gerardo Ferrara provides an overview on Spitzoid lesions that, together with dysplastic nevi, are the most common simulators of melanoma both clinicodermoscopically and histopathologically. His core message can be summarized as follows: "No single clinicodermoscopic feature can allow reliable differentiation of Spitz nevus from melanoma. In patients up to 12 years of age, small (up to 1 cm) and dermoscopically 'typical' Spitzoid lesions can be submitted to follow-up with controls every 3 to 6 months; conversely, all Spitzoid lesions must be excised in patients older than 12 years."

In article 8, Natalia Jaimes and Ash Marghoob summarize the morphologic universe of melanoma by providing textual and visual descriptions of classic and new melanoma-specific dermoscopic criteria. In articles 9 and 10, Luc Thomas and

Dermatol Clin 31 (2013) xiii–xiv
http://dx.doi.org/10.1016/j.det.2013.07.002
0733-8635/13/$ – see front matter © 2013 Published by Elsevier Inc.

Rainer Hofmann-Wellenhof deal with the particular dermoscopic criteria that become apparent in lesions of special locations. Lesions on the face, palms/soles, nails, scalp, mucosae, and milk-line exhibit specific features related to the special anatomy of these areas.

In article 11, Giovanni Pellacani and Caterina Longo provide an overview of lesions with predominant blue color on dermoscopy, whereas pink tumors are reviewed in article 12. Both blue lesions and pink tumors can be difficult to diagnose accurately; both can often be nodular, thus both should be managed cautiously because of the possibility of misinterpreting a fast-growing melanoma. Special attention is thus deserved for these lesions by providing specific clues for diagnostic differentiation.

Finally, in articles 13 and 14, alternative uses of dermoscopy are reviewed by Aimilios Lallas, Zoe Apalla, and Lidia Rudnicka. Dermoscopy is not anymore only a tool for dermato-oncologists but a sort of dermatologic stethoscope in the pocket of every clinician dealing with inflammatory and infectious skin disorders, as well as hair and scalp diseases.

We hope that you enjoy reading this issue of *Dermatologic Clinics*, and that it proves useful in your everyday practice. It was our aim to help physicians provide the best level of care for their patients, assisted by the fascinating and ever-evolving technique of dermoscopy.

Giuseppe Argenziano, MD
Iris Zalaudek, MD
Dermatology and Skin Cancer Unit
Arcispedale Santa Maria Nuova, IRCCS
Viale Risorgimento 80
42100 Reggio Emilia, Italy

Jason Giacomel, MBBS
Skin Spectrum Medical Services
400 Canning Highway Como, Perth
Western Australia 6152, Australia

E-mail addresses:
g.argenziano@gmail.com (G. Argenziano)
iris.zalaudek@gmail.com (I. Zalaudek)
jasongiacomel@hotmail.com (J. Giacomel)

Evidence-Based Dermoscopy

Scott W. Menzies, MBBS, PhD[a,b,*]

KEYWORDS

- Dermoscopy • Evidence • Sequential digital dermoscopy imaging • Melanoma

KEY POINTS

- Dermoscopy improves the diagnostic accuracy for melanoma compared with naked eye examination.
- Dermoscopy results in a reduction of excisions in addition to an increased sensitivity for the diagnosis of melanoma.
- Sequential digital dermoscopy imaging (SDDI) allowed the detection of suspicious dermoscopic change in melanomas that lack dermoscopic evidence of melanoma at a particular time.
- When used in high-risk individuals or on individual suspicious melanocytic lesions, SDDI has a gross impact for detecting melanoma in clinical practice, with a range of 34% to 61% of melanomas detected exclusively using SDDI in these patients.
- SDDI has been shown to reduce the excision of benign lesions when used in combination with dermoscopy, in both dermatologists and primary care physicians.

Dermoscopy (dermatoscopy, oil epiluminescence microscopy, surface microscopy) is a technique that uses a hand-held magnification device following the application of a liquid at the skin-device interface or uses cross-polarized instruments. This technique allows the visualization of diagnostic submacroscopic, morphologic key structures of pigmented and nonpigmented skin lesions located in the epidermis down to the upper dermis not seen with the naked eye. In 2008 the evidence-based Clinical Practice Guidelines for the Management of Melanoma in Australia and New Zealand gave the recommendation that training and utilization of dermoscopy is recommended for clinicians routinely examining pigmented skin lesions.[1] This recommendation was given the highest grade (grade A: body of evidence can be trusted to guide practice). The following outlines the evidence leading to this recommendation and the subsequent published literature that further supports it.

Meta-analyses performed on studies in a variety of clinical and experimental settings have shown that dermoscopy improves the diagnostic accuracy for melanoma compared with naked eye examination.[2–4] The 2 earliest meta-analyses included studies in both prospective clinical and experimental settings, the latter using retrospectively collected photographs.[2,3] These studies, which were mainly conducted in a specialist setting, demonstrated a relative diagnostic odds ratio 4.7[2] and 3.7[3] times higher for dermoscopy compared to naked eye examination. The larger meta-analysis[2] of 13 studies published from 1987 to 2000 showed that diagnostic accuracy for melanoma, expressed as log odds ratio, was 4.0 for dermoscopy versus 2.7 for naked eye examination ($P = .001$). The other meta-analysis[3] of 8 studies involving only experienced users found similar results: log odds ratio 4.3 for dermoscopy versus 2.8 for naked eye examination ($P = .008$). These 2 meta-analyses showed that dermoscopy is significantly better (49%[2] and 56%[3]) at discriminating between melanoma and nonmelanoma than naked eye examination.

Financial Disclosures: None.

[a] Sydney Melanoma Diagnostic Centre, Royal Prince Alfred Hospital, Missenden Road, Camperdown, NSW 2050, Australia; [b] Discipline of Dermatology, Sydney Medical School, The University of Sydney, NSW 2006, Australia
* Sydney Melanoma Diagnostic Centre, Royal Prince Alfred Hospital, Missenden Road, Camperdown, NSW 2050, Australia.
E-mail address: scott.menzies@sswahs.nsw.gov.au

derm.theclinics.com

Following these 2 studies, a more recent meta-analysis was performed that restricted the analysis to include only prospective studies on consecutive patients in a clinical setting (published between 1987 and January 2008) (**Fig. 1**).[4] Nine studies were included in the analysis, which found the relative diagnostic odds ratio for melanoma compared with naked eye examination to be 15.6 (95% CI 2.9–83.7, $P = .016$). Summary estimates showed the sensitivity was 18% (95% CI 9–27; $P = .002$) higher than for naked eye examination, but there was no evidence of an effect on specificity.

Like other diagnostic techniques, some training in dermoscopy is needed to achieve improvement in diagnostic accuracy. It has been shown in an experimental setting that dermoscopy may decrease diagnostic performance on pigmented skin lesions for dermatologists without any formal training in the technique.[5,6] Most of the included studies in the latter described meta-analysis were performed by experienced dermoscopy users, but the participating primary care physicians in one clinical trial[7] had only received a 2-hour teaching session in a simple dermoscopic algorithm for distinguishing benign and malignant tumors.

Although these studies have shown a greater impact in detecting unrecognized melanomas by naked eye examination (ie, improved sensitivity) in comparison with detection of benign lesions, a dramatic effect of dermoscopy on specificity is best examined by its effect on excision rates. In a randomized trial in a specialist setting of naked eye versus naked eye and dermoscopy examination, there was a 42% reduction in patients referred to biopsy in the dermoscopy arm ($P = .01$),[8] which is consistent with the retrospective findings of a significant reduction of the benign/malignant ratio of excised melanocytic lesions in clinicians trained in the use of dermoscopy from 18:1 (predermoscopy era) to 4:1 (post-dermoscopy era) ($P = .04$).[9] In contrast, nonusers of dermoscopy continued their diagnostic performance without improvement (from 12:1 to 14:1). In a clinical trial looking at the impact of the combination of dermoscopy and sequential digital dermoscopy imaging compared with naked eye examination in primary care physicians, a reduction of 63.5% of benign pigmented lesions excised or referred was achieved ($P<.0005$).[10] Recently, in a study looking at the role of dermoscopy in a group of general dermatologists, a significant 9% reduction in excisions of recruited pigmented lesions occurred with the use of dermoscopy.[11]

Such studies showing a reduction of excisions in addition to an increased sensitivity for the diagnosis of melanoma with the use of dermoscopy were crystallized recently in a large 10-year international multicenter survey of the number-needed-to-excise (NNE) values for melanoma detection comparing specialized clinical versus nonspecialized settings.[12] The participating clinics contributed a total of greater than 300,000 cases, including 17, 000 melanomas and 283,000 melanocytic nevi. The overall NNE values achieved in specialized (clinics purely dedicated to skin cancer detection) and nonspecialized clinics in the 10-year period (1998–2007) were 8.7 and 29.4, respectively. The NNE improved over time in the specialized clinics (from 12.8 to 6.8), but seemed unchanged in the nonspecialized clinics. In particular, it was noted that there was a significantly greater number of excised melanomas in the specialized clinics. Although formal data on dermoscopy usage were not obtained, it is reasonable to conclude that dermoscopy had a highly significant impact on the results.

There is now widespread literature on the dermoscopic features of both pigmented and nonpigmented skin tumors. Nevertheless, most evidence-based studies on the effectiveness of the technique have assessed the impact of pigmented skin lesions, more often melanocytic

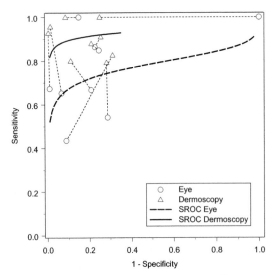

Fig. 1. The summary receiver operator curves following a meta-analysis of high-level diagnostic clinical studies comparing dermoscopy and naked eye examination for the diagnosis of melanoma. The 2 estimates for each study are joined by a line. (*Data from* Vestergaard M, Macaskill P, Holt P, et al. Dermoscopy compared to naked eye examination for the diagnosis of primary melanoma: a meta-analysis of studies performed in a clinical setting. Br J Dermatol 2008;159:669–76.)

lesions, and in particular, melanoma. It should be noted that in a recent study there was a greater impact on the improvement in the diagnosis of pigmented nonmelanocytic versus melanocytic lesions.[13]

Sequential digital dermoscopy imaging (SDDI) involves the capture and assessment of successive dermoscopic images, separated by an interval of time, of one or many melanocytic lesions to detect suspicious change. This imaging is performed in 2 settings: short-term digital monitoring (over a period of 3 months) for suspicious melanocytic lesions, and long-term surveillance (usually at intervals of 6–12 months).[14] In a recent meta-analysis[14] that grouped both short-term and long-term SDDI together, it was shown the number of lesions needed to monitor one detected melanoma ranged from 31 to 1008 depending on the clinical setting (lower number of lesions needed to monitor for short-term monitoring of suspicious lesions). For every additional month of monitoring, one additional melanoma was detected, with the chances to detect a melanoma during surveillance shown to increase as the length of follow-up extended. Furthermore, the proportion of in situ melanoma and thin melanomas detected by SDDI were higher than expected in the general population.

In 2008 the aforementioned Clinical Practice Guidelines for the Management of Melanoma in Australia and New Zealand gave the recommendation to consider the use of sequential digital dermoscopy imaging to detect melanomas that lack dermoscopic features of melanoma.[1] This recommendation was given a grade B: body of evidence can be trusted to guide practice in most situations. The basis of the recommendation was 4 high-level diagnostic studies that consistently showed that SDDI allowed detection of suspicious dermoscopic change in melanomas that lack dermoscopic evidence of melanoma at a particular time.[15–18] In these studies featureless melanomas were more frequently found with short-term versus long-term SDDI. Importantly, in one study that reviewed the lesion baseline images, there was no difference in the prevalence of specific dermoscopy melanoma features found in melanoma versus nevi, highlighting the importance of change to detect featureless melanomas.[16]

Since the Australian and New Zealand guidelines have been published, there have been many studies describing the impact of SDDI in clinical practice. In one cohort of moderate-risk to high-risk patients, 34% of melanomas were found exclusively using SDDI.[18] In a follow-up study, these researchers showed lower risk individuals (those with >50 nevi but <4 atypical nevi) had a high benign/melanoma ratio (79:1) of excised changed lesions using SDDI, compared with higher risk groups (atypical mole syndrome 15:1, and familial atypical mole and multiple melanoma syndrome 4:1).[19] The conclusion of these researchers was long-term SDDI of nevi is less efficacious in lower risk individuals; this has also been noted by others.[20]

In a prospective observational study of dermatologists comparing the use of dermoscopy versus dermoscopy with SDDI (short-term and long-term), there was a significant improvement in the excised benign/melanoma ratio in the group using SDDI (8.1 vs 2.4).[21] Furthermore, 55% of melanomas were detected exclusively by SDDI in the latter group. In this arm, melanomas detected with SDDI were significantly thinner than those detected without SDDI. The 10-year experience of following another cohort of high-risk melanoma patients using total body photography and SDDI (short-term and long-term) showed 61% of melanomas were detected with SDDI.[22] In contrast with the previous study, there was no difference in the thickness of melanomas detected with SDDI or without.

As mentioned previously, in a sequential intervention clinical trial in Australian primary care physicians, the combination of dermoscopy and short-term SDDI reduced excision/referrals of benign lesions by 64%, with the benign/melanoma ratio of excised/referred lesions decreasing from 9.5:1 to 3.5:1.[10] Furthermore, the sensitivity for the diagnosis of melanoma using the techniques nearly doubled compared with baseline naked eye examination (72% vs 38%). When isolating the effect of SDDI by analyzing only those lesions undergoing monitoring, there was a gross increase in sensitivity for the diagnosis of melanoma (73%) compared with only 18% achieved with naked eye examination. This increase in sensitivity occurred without any loss of specificity.[10]

In conclusion, dermoscopy unequivocally improves the diagnostic accuracy of melanoma compared with naked eye examination. It has also been shown to reduce excision rates of benign melanocytic lesions. SDDI allows the detection of dermoscopically featureless melanoma. When used in high-risk individuals or on individual suspicious melanocytic lesions, SDDI has a gross impact for detecting melanoma in clinical practice, with a range of 34% to 61% of melanomas detected exclusively using SDDI in these patients. Furthermore, SDDI has been shown to reduce the excision of benign lesions when used in combination with dermoscopy, in both dermatologists and primary care physicians.

REFERENCES

1. Australian Cancer Network Melanoma Guidelines Revision Working Party. Clinical Practice Guidelines for the Management of Melanoma in Australia and New Zealand. Wellington (New Zealand): Cancer Council Australia and Australian Cancer Network, Sydney and New Zealand Guidelines Group; 2008.
2. Kittler H, Pehamberger H, Wolff K, et al. Diagnostic accuracy of dermoscopy. Lancet Oncol 2002;3: 159–65.
3. Bafounta ML, Beauchet A, Aegerter P, et al. Is dermoscopy (epiluminescence microscopy) useful for the diagnosis of melanoma? Arch Dermatol 2001; 137:1343–50.
4. Vestergaard M, Macaskill P, Holt P, et al. Dermoscopy compared to naked eye examination for the diagnosis of primary melanoma: a meta-analysis of studies performed in a clinical setting. Br J Dermatol 2008;159:669–76.
5. Binder M, Puespoeck-Schwarz M, Steiner A, et al. Epiluminescence microscopy of small pigmented skin lesions: short-term formal training improves the diagnostic performance of dermatologists. J Am Acad Dermatol 1997;36:197–202.
6. Binder M, Schwarz M, Winkler A, et al. Epiluminescence microscopy. A useful tool for the diagnosis of pigmented skin lesions for formally trained dermatologists. Arch Dermatol 1995;131:286–91.
7. Argenziano G, Puig S, Zalaudek I, et al. Dermoscopy improves accuracy of primary care physicians to triage lesions suggestive of skin cancer. J Clin Oncol 2006;24:1877–82.
8. Carli P, de Giorgi V, Chiarugi A, et al. Addition of dermoscopy to conventional naked-eye examination in melanoma screening: a randomized study. J Am Acad Dermatol 2004;50:683–9.
9. Carli P, De Giorgi V, Crocetti E, et al. Improvement of malignant/benign ratio in excised melanocytic lesions in the "dermoscopy era": a retrospective study 1997-2001. Br J Dermatol 2004;150:687–92.
10. Menzies SW, Emery J, Staples M, et al. Impact of dermoscopy and short-term sequential digital dermoscopy imaging for the management of pigmented lesions in primary care: a sequential intervention trial. Br J Dermatol 2009;161:1270–7.
11. van der Rhee JI, Bergman W, Kukutsch NA. The impact of dermoscopy on the management of pigmented lesions in everyday clinical practice of general dermatologists: a prospective study. Br J Dermatol 2010;162:563–7.
12. Argenziano G, Cerroni L, Zalaudek I, et al. Accuracy in melanoma detection: a 10-year multicenter survey. J Am Acad Dermatol 2012;67:54–9.
13. Rosendahl C, Tschandl P, Cameron A, et al. Diagnostic accuracy of dermatoscopy for melanocytic and nonmelanocytic pigmented lesions. J Am Acad Dermatol 2011;64:1068–73.
14. Salerni G, Terán T, Puig S, et al. Meta-analysis of digital dermoscopy follow-up of melanocytic skin lesions: a study on behalf of the International Dermoscopy Society. J Eur Acad Dermatol Venereol 2013;27:805–14.
15. Menzies SW, Gutenev A, Avramidis M, et al. Short-term digital surface microscopic monitoring of atypical or changing melanocytic lesions. Arch Dermatol 2001;137:1583–9.
16. Kittler H, Guitera P, Riedl E, et al. Identification of clinically featureless incipient melanoma using sequential dermoscopy imaging. Arch Dermatol 2006;142:1113–9.
17. Robinson JK, Nickoloff BJ. Digital epiluminescence microscopy monitoring of high-risk patients. Arch Dermatol 2004;140:49–56.
18. Haenssle HA, Krueger U, Vente C, et al. Results from an observational trial: digital epiluminescence microscopy follow-up of atypical nevi increases the sensitivity and the chance of success of conventional dermoscopy in detecting melanoma. J Invest Dermatol 2006;126:980–5.
19. Haenssle HA, Korpas B, Hansen-Hagge C, et al. Selection of patients for long-term surveillance with digital dermoscopy by assessment of melanoma risk factors. Arch Dermatol 2010;146:257–64.
20. Schiffner R, Schiffner-Rohe J, Landthaler M, et al. Long-term dermoscopic follow-up of melanocytic naevi: clinical outcome and patient compliance. Br J Dermatol 2003;149:79–86.
21. Tromme I, Sacré L, Hammouch F, et al. Availability of digital dermoscopy in daily practice dramatically reduces the number of excised melanocytic lesions: results from an observational study. Br J Dermatol 2012;167:778–86.
22. Salerni G, Carrera C, Lovatto L, et al. Characterization of 1152 lesions excised over 10 years using total-body photography and digital dermatoscopy in the surveillance of patients at high risk for melanoma. J Am Acad Dermatol 2012;67:836–45.

A Clinico-Dermoscopic Approach for Skin Cancer Screening
Recommendations Involving a Survey of the International Dermoscopy Society

Giuseppe Argenziano, MD[a],*, Jason Giacomel, MBBS[b],
Iris Zalaudek, MD[a], Andreas Blum, MD[c], Ralph P. Braun, MD[d],
Horacio Cabo, MD[e], Allan Halpern, MD[f],
Rainer Hofmann-Wellenhof, MD[g], Josep Malvehy, PhD[h],
Ashfaq A. Marghoob, MD[f], Scott Menzies, MBBS, PhD[i],
Elvira Moscarella, MD[a], Giovanni Pellacani, MD[j],
Susana Puig, PhD[h], Harold Rabinovitz, MD[k], Toshiaki Saida, MD[l],
Stefania Seidenari, MD[j], H. Peter Soyer, MD[m], Wilhelm Stolz, MD[n],
Luc Thomas, MD, PhD[o], Harald Kittler, MD[p]

KEYWORDS

- Melanoma • Skin cancer • Clinical diagnosis • Dermoscopy • Dermatoscopy • Triage

KEY POINTS

- A survey consisting of 29 questions was given to members of the International Dermoscopy Society to investigate clinician perceptions and behavior in approaching patients with skin tumors and to propose an updated system of triage.
- Although 81.7% of the respondents reported using dermoscopy for patients presenting with skin tumors, only 37.4% screened all patients regardless of the presenting condition.

Continued

Financial Disclosure or Conflicts of Interest: None.
Study supported in part by the Italian Ministry of Health (RF-2010-2316524).
[a] Dermatology and Skin Cancer Unit, Arcispedale Santa Maria Nuova IRCCS, Viale Risorgimento 80, Reggio Emilia 42100, Italy; [b] Skin Spectrum Medical Services, Como, Perth, Western Australia 6152, Australia; [c] Public, Private and Teaching Practice of Dermatology, Konstanz, Germany; [d] Department of Dermatology, University Hospital Geneva, Geneva, Switzerland; [e] Department of Dermatology, Instituto de Investigaciones Médicas A. Lanari, University of Buenos Aires, Buenos Aires, Argentina; [f] Dermatology Service, Department of Dermatology, Memorial Sloan-Kettering Cancer Centre, 160 East 53rd street, New York, NY 10022, USA; [g] Department of Dermatology, Medical University of Graz, Auenbruggerplatz 8, Graz A-8038, Austria; [h] Melanoma Unit, Dermatology Department, Hospital Clinic, Institut d'Investigacions Biomèdiques August Pi i Sunyer and U726 Centros de Investigacion Biomedica en Red de Enfermedades Raras, Instituto de Salud Carlos III, Barcelona, Spain; [i] Sydney Medical School, Sydney Melanoma Diagnostic Centre, Royal Prince Alfred Hospital, The University of Sydney, Camperdown, Australia; [j] Dermatology Unit, University of Modena and Reggio Emilia, Modena 41121, Italy; [k] Department of Dermatology, Skin and Cancer Associates, School of Medicine, University of Miami, Miami, FL, USA; [l] Department of Dermatology, School of Medicine, Shinshu University, Matsumoto, Japan; [m] Dermatology Research Centre, Princess Alexandra Hospital, The University of Queensland School of Medicine, Brisbane, Queensland, Australia; [n] Clinic of Dermatology and Allergology, Hospital Munich-Schwabing, Munich, Germany; [o] Department of Dermatology, Centre Hospitalier Lyon Sud, Lyon 1 University, Pierre Bénite, France; [p] Department of Dermatology, Medical University of Vienna, Währinger Gürtel 18-20, Vienna 1090, Austria
* Corresponding author. Dermatology and Skin Cancer Unit, Arcispedale Santa Maria Nuova IRCCS, Viale Risorgimento 80, Reggio Emilia 42100, Italy.
E-mail address: g.argenziano@gmail.com

derm.theclinics.com

Continued

- The average waiting time for a regular patient consultation exceeded 1 month for 38.1% of the respondents (48.9% of those in public positions).
- More than half of the respondents (57%) performed monitoring in at least 30% of their patients.
- An up-to-date system of triage should be implemented to promote an improved diagnostic accuracy and more timely management of skin malignancy.

BACKGROUND

Skin malignancy is a major global health concern in white populations because of the significant incidence of melanoma and nonmelanoma skin cancer (NMSC) in fair-skinned individuals, coupled with its potential morbidity and mortality. Screening for melanoma in particular is considered challenging for 2 main reasons: the first is related to the potential mortality of melanoma if early recognition and removal is not carried out and the second concerns the high incidence of its benign counterpart, the melanocytic nevus. In some instances, nevi can mimic melanoma in clinical appearance and are present as multiple lesions in many individuals in the population. Consequently, even targeted screening for melanoma involves many patients.

Recently, with heightened emphasis on skin cancer prevention, there has been an increasing congestion of specialist dermatology clinics with patients referred from primary care, requiring assessment of possible skin malignancy. Waiting times for dermatology clinics have consequently usually increased, and dermatologists are faced with the task of assessing numerous referred benign lesions (including seborrheic keratoses, hemangiomas, and benign nevi) in lower-risk patients to detect but a few malignancies.[1,2] This circumstance places a strain on limited specialist resources and can create a paradoxic and counterproductive situation whereby an early diagnosis becomes increasingly difficult for those patients who actually do harbor a skin cancer.

Dermoscopy has become an important tool in the diagnostic armamentarium of clinicians dealing with skin cancer detection. In the current guidelines for the management of melanoma and NMSC, dermoscopy is mentioned as a useful technique for clinicians screening skin lesions because it can increase diagnostic accuracy and prompt earlier excision. Dermoscopy is also helpful for monitoring multiple pigmented lesions whereby recording digital dermoscopic images over time can provide evidence of significant (suspicious) morphologic change (level IA, grade A).[3,4] Despite these general recommendations, details

of a rational, stepwise approach integrating dermoscopy into a daily clinical work flow are largely absent. In this context, specific guidelines are needed to optimize the overall process of skin cancer screening.

The main objectives of the present study were twofold: (1) to investigate by questionnaire the attitudes and behaviors of International Dermoscopy Society (IDS) members in approaching patients with skin tumors and (2) to propose an updated, rational system of triage for skin cancer screening, based on current published evidence. The ultimate aim of the latter system of triage is to improve the accuracy of diagnosis of skin malignancy and promote a more timely and effective management of skin cancers by both general/family physicians (GFP) and dermatologists. Where the surveyed behavior of clinicians was found to depart from these evidence-based guidelines, the authors propose addressing these areas of concern through focused physician education campaigns.

METHODS

An e-mail of invitation for the questionnaire-type survey was sent on July 29, 2011 to all 5361 members of the IDS (http://www.dermoscopy-ids.org). The objective of the survey was to determine the attitudes and clinical behaviors of the survey participants in approaching patients with skin tumors, including the implementation of dermoscopy in their clinical work. The survey consisted of 29 questions (**Fig. 1**) that had previously been developed and ratified by the executive board members of the IDS. Questions included those inherent to (1) the participant's professional profile; (2) his or her attitudes on patient and lesion selection; (3) the method, waiting time, and outcome of triage; and (4) the methods used during the follow-up examination.

The survey was posted on the IDS Web site and took approximately 10 minutes to be completed. Participants were permitted to respond to the survey anonymously (without logging in) and were prevented from responding to the survey more

1. Your age
2. Sex
3. Country
4. **Qualification**: general/family physician; dermatologist; other medical specialist (specify); nurse practitioner or physician assistant; medical student; other non-medical qualification

5. **In what setting do you see most of your patients?** Private; hospital; academic; referral center (e.g., pigmented lesion clinic, melanoma clinic, etc)

6. **What percentage of your patients ask to be checked for skin tumors?** Less than 10%; 10-30%; 30-50%; more than 50%

7. **What proportion of patients presenting with skin tumors do you examine with dermoscopy?** Basically all of them; about half of them; less than half of them

8. **How long have you been using dermoscopy in your practice?** Less than 1 year; 1-2 years; 3-5 years; more than 5 years

9. **How many patients do you examine per week with dermoscopy?** Less than 10 patients; 10-30 patients; 30-50 patients; 50-100 patients; more than 100 patients

10. **How many new (previously un-biopsied) melanomas do you see per year?** Less than 10 melanomas; 10-30 melanomas; 30-50 melanomas; more than 50 melanomas

11. **Which patients do you examine for skin cancer?** Only patients referred/demanding for a skin check; referred/demanding patients plus those with risk factors for melanoma; basically all patients coming to the office for any medical conditions

12. **Which lesions do you examine with dermoscopy?** Only lesions highlighted by the patient or by another doctor; clinically

suspicious lesions selected by you during un-aided visual examination of the skin; almost all lesions (both clinically concerning and random benign-looking lesions)

13. **What instrument do you use mostly at the baseline examination of a new patient?** Hand-held polarized dermatoscope (Dermlite or similar); hand-held non-polarized dermatoscope (Heine or similar); both the previous (including Dermlite hybrid); digital video camera attached to a computer system (Molemax, Fotofinder or similar); digital photo camera attached to a hand-held dermatoscope

14. **Which instrument do you consider more reliable for the diagnosis at the baseline examination of a new patient?** Hand-held polarized dermatoscope (Dermlite or similar), hand-held non-polarized dermatoscope (Heine or similar); both the previous (including Dermlite hybrid); digital video camera attached to a computer system (Molemax, Fotofinder or similar); digital photo camera attached to a hand-held dermatoscope

15. **On average how long does it take you to perform a baseline exam on a new patient (excluding the time spent taking patient history, disrobing of the patient, acquiring any images, discussion of findings with patient, and paper work)?** Less than 5 minutes; 5-10 minutes; 10-15 minutes; 15-20 minutes; more than 20 minutes

16. **What is the main benefit of the instrument you use at the baseline visit of a new patient?** Diagnostic reliability; time effectiveness; cost effectiveness; patient satisfaction; reimbursement

17. **Do you have a fast track for seeing patients with concerning lesions who are referred by another doctor or are self-referred?** Yes; no

18. **What is the average wait time for a regular (not referred) patient to see you**

for the first time? Less than 1 month; 1-3 months; 3-6 months; more than 6 months

19. **When a patient's skin reveals only a few lesions at the baseline visit, but 1 or 2 of them are atypical (doubtful), what do you usually do?** Recommend excision of the atypical/doubtful lesions; recommend a short-term dermoscopic digital follow-up (2-4 months); recommend a long-term dermoscopic digital follow-up (6-12 months); recommend a non-digital follow-up (clinical follow-up with or without baseline clinical images)

20. **When a patient has many nevi on the skin, what do you recommend?** Recommend excision of all atypical/doubtful lesions (independent of the number of atypical lesions seen); perform a comparison of the lesion's morphology with the morphology of the patient's other nevi and, eventually, recommend excision of the ugly duckling, if present

21. **If you see an atypical/doubtful raised/palpable lesion, what do you recommend?** Recommend excision or follow-up depending on the patient risk factors and number of nevi; recommend excision irrespective of the other patient characteristics

22. **How many of your patients seen at the baseline consultation are scheduled for follow-up?** None; 1-10%; 10-20%; 30-40%; 40-50%; More than 50%

23. **Which patients do you schedule for follow-up?** Patients with multiple nevi or previous skin cancer and/or relevant risk factors; patients with single doubtful lesions (no previous skin cancer nor relevant risk factors); both the above; almost all patients, independent from their risk for developing skin cancer and independent from the number of nevi or their morphology

24. **In patients with multiple nevi (>50) what is the average number of lesions you monitor with digital dermoscopy?**

Less than 10 lesions; 10-30 lesions; most of them

25. **Which follow-up schedule do you recommend for patients with multiple nevi?** Short-term follow-up (2-4 months); long-term follow-up (6-12 months); a combination of short-term and long-term follow-up

26. **What instrument do you use mostly during the follow-up examination of the patient?** Hand-held polarized dermatoscope (Dermlite or similar); hand-held non-polarized dermatoscope (Heine or similar); both the previous (including Dermlite hybrid); digital video camera attached to a computer system (Molemax, Fotofinder or similar); digital photo camera attached to a hand-held dermatoscope; both hand-held and digital systems

27. **Which instrument do you consider more reliable for the diagnosis during the follow-up examination?** Hand-held polarized dermatoscope (Dermlite or similar); hand-held non-polarized dermatoscope (Heine or similar); both the previous (including Dermlite hybrid); digital video camera attached to a computer system (Molemax, Fotofinder or similar); digital photo camera attached to a hand-held dermatoscope; both hand-held and digital systems

28. **On average how long does it take you to perform a follow-up examination (excluding the time spent taking patient history, disrobing of the patient, acquiring any images, discussion of findings with patient, and paper work)?** Less than 5 minutes; 5-10 minutes; 10-15 minutes; 15-20 minutes; more than 20 minutes

29. **What is the main benefit of the instrument you use during follow-up examinations?** Diagnostic reliability; time effectiveness; cost effectiveness; patient satisfaction; reimbursement

Fig. 1. The IDS survey, consisting of 29 questions.

than once (by cookie). Participants were given 30 days to answer, edit, and complete the survey once connected for the first time. Three reminder e-mails were sent 1 month apart to invite additional members to join the survey.

On November 30, 2011 the survey was closed and responses collected on a data sheet. Continuous data are given as mean ± standard deviation unless otherwise specified. Chi-square tests were used for the comparisons of proportions. All given P values are 2-tailed, and a P value of less than .05 indicates statistical significance. Ethics committee approval was waived.

RESULTS
Participants General Data

Of the 5361 IDS members invited to join the survey, 1214 registered in 4 months and 1123 were considered eligible because they responded to more than 70% of the 29 questions. The mean age of eligible respondents was 46 years (SD, 11 years) and 563 (50.1%) were women. Participants were from 89 countries, with Australia, Italy, Spain, United Kingdom, United States, Romania, and Brazil being the most highly represented and

accounting for 577 (51.4%) responses. Most of the participants were dermatologists (849, 75.6%); 193 (17.2%) were GFP; and 69 (6.1%) were other medical specialists, nurses, or residents (12, not declared). A total of 562 (50%) participants were in private practice, and 553 participants (49.2%) held public positions (in a hospital, referral center, or academic institution).

Almost half of the participants (n = 559, 49.8%) reported that at least 30% of their patients asked to be checked for skin neoplasms, and 81.7% (n = 917) declared that they use dermoscopy for basically all patients presenting with a skin neoplasm. Most of the surveyed members (n = 591, 52.6%) had been using dermoscopy in their practice for more than 5 years, 54.8% (n = 616) used dermoscopy on more than 30 patients per week, and 46.7% (n = 525) saw more than 10 new (previously unbiopsied) melanomas per year.

Attitudes on Patient and Lesion Selection

When asked which patients they examine for skin cancer, only 37.4% (n = 420) of the respondents declared that they would carry out a formal skin cancer screening examination on all their patients, regardless of the presenting condition (39.1% of dermatologists and 29% of GFP [P = .009], 42.2% in private practice and 32.5% in public positions [P = .007]). Five hundred (44.5%) respondents performed a screening examination on patients either referred for or requesting a skin cancer check as well as those with risk factors for melanoma, and 17.4% (n = 195) would perform such an examination only for those patients referred for or specifically requesting a skin check.

Most of the participants (n = 619, 55.1%) declared using dermoscopy to examine almost all lesions (both clinically suspicious and random, clinically benign-looking lesions) of the given patient (no differences between dermatologists and GFP or between private and public practices), and 42.6% (n = 478) examined dermoscopically only clinically suspicious lesions selected during the unaided visual examination of the skin.

Triage Method and Waiting Time

Most of the respondents (n = 890, 79.3%) declared using hand-held dermatoscopes at the baseline examination of a new patient, mainly because of their diagnostic reliability. Although only 14.8% of the participants in public positions used digital systems, almost double (25.1%) the number of respondents who operated in private practice used digital dermoscopy (P = .004). More than half (n = 628, 55.9%) of all respondents declared performing a baseline examination on a new patient in less than 10 minutes, whereas only 6.9% (n = 78) required more than 20 minutes. When comparing participants from private versus public practices, 50.5% and 61.7%, respectively, performed an examination in less than 10 minutes, whereas 10.1% and 3.6%, respectively, required more than 20 minutes.

Although most respondents (n = 776, 69.1%) reported having a fast-track system for seeing patients with concerning lesions (who are referred by another doctor or are self-referred), the average waiting time for a regular (ie, routine, nonurgent) initial patient consultation was more than 1 month for 38.1% (n = 428) of the participants overall (48.9% in public positions and 27.6% in private practice; $P<.001$). Less than 1 month of waiting time was declared by 76.7% of GFP but only by 54.1% of dermatologists ($P<.001$).

Triage Outcome

When a patient's skin revealed only a few lesions at the baseline examination, and 1 or 2 lesions were doubtful (atypical), 90.5% (n = 1016) of surveyed members elected to perform excision (45%) or short-term follow-up (45.5%) for such

lesions. When a patient presented with multiple nevi, 91.3% (n = 1025) of participants first compared the (clinical-dermoscopic) morphology of these lesions with that of the patient's other nevi and recommended excision of any ugly duckling lesions (no differences between dermatologists and GFP were present or between private and public practices). Only 6% (n = 67) of the respondents recommended excision of all atypical/doubtful lesions (independent of the number of atypical lesions seen). If a raised or palpable atypical/doubtful lesion was encountered, 54.9% (n = 617) of the respondents recommended excision regardless of the other patient characteristics; but 41.9% (n = 470) recommended excision or follow-up depending on the patient risk factors and number of nevi.

More than half of the respondents (n = 640, 57%) reported that they would schedule a follow-up for at least 30% of their patients seen at the baseline consultation (62.6% of respondents in private practice and 51.5% in public positions, $P<.001$). When asked which patients they schedule for follow-up, 73.2% (n = 822) of the surveyed members declared that they would monitor patients with multiple nevi or previous skin cancer and/or relevant risk factors, patients with single doubtful lesions (no previous skin cancer nor relevant risk factors), or both. Of note, 22.2% (n = 249) of respondents would monitor almost all patients independent of their risk of developing skin cancer and independent of the number of nevi or their morphology (28.8% of respondents in private practice and 15.4% in public positions, $P<.001$).

Follow-up Examination

In patients with multiple nevi (>50 lesions), most of the participants (n = 922, 82.1%) recommended long-term (6–12 month) follow-up (39%) or a combination of short-term (2–4 month) and long-term follow-up (43.1%). A total of 452 (40.2%) respondents monitored less than 10 lesions per patient with digital dermoscopy, whereas 27.2% (n = 306) monitored 10 to 30 lesions, and 25.3% (n = 284) monitored most of the patient's lesions. At the follow-up examination of the patient, 47.1% (n = 528) declared using hand-held dermatoscopes, 24.7% (n = 277) a digital system, and 23.0% (n = 258) both hand-held and digital dermoscopy (no differences were noted between dermatologists and GFP or between private and public practices). Performing a follow-up examination took less than 10 minutes, 10 to 20 minutes, and more than 20 minutes for 45.7% (n = 513),

39.5% (n = 443), and 10.0% (n = 112) of the respondents, respectively.

DISCUSSION

Skin cancer is a significant worldwide health problem because of its high incidence in white populations, combined with its potential morbidity and mortality. Recently, with increasing emphasis on skin cancer prevention, there has been a progressive inundation of specialist dermatology clinics with patients referred from primary care, requiring assessment of possible skin malignancy. Limited specialist resources have subsequently become overtaxed with many benign lesions in lower-risk patients. This scenario can create a counterproductive situation wherein an early appointment and diagnosis becomes increasingly difficult for other (higher-risk) patients who actually do harbor a skin cancer.

In the United Kingdom, patients referred from primary care with suspected skin cancer (ie, melanoma or invasive squamous cell carcinoma) should be, as a rule, seen at a public hospital dermatology clinic within 2 weeks (and treatment commenced within 62 days).[1,5] However, the feasibility of this program is challenged by the problems mentioned earlier; in many countries, the waiting time is longer than 1 month. In the United States, for example, patients with a changing pigmented lesion (a possible indicator of malignancy) face waiting times just as long as those for patients with routine complaints (more than 38 days).[6] In the authors' survey involving 1123 clinicians from 89 countries, the average waiting time for a regular (nonurgent) initial patient consultation was more than 1 month for 38.1% of respondents overall and for about half (48.9%) of the clinicians working in public hospitals.

In the authors' estimation, this difficult situation is not only caused by the increasing demand for skin cancer screening but also stems from several factors currently hampering efficiency in the general clinical approach to patients with skin tumors. By investigating the screening behavior of clinicians particularly devoted to skin cancer detection and after evaluating current published evidence in this field, the authors propose an updated, rational system of triage. The latter primarily aims to improve the accuracy of diagnosis and lead to a more efficient management of skin cancers (particularly melanoma) by both GFP and dermatologists. If it can achieve these objectives, this triage system has the potential to reduce the number of unnecessary referrals of benign skin lesions to specialist dermatology clinics, to decrease the number of unnecessary removals of benign skin lesions in primary and secondary care, and to reduce waiting times for dermatologic and surgical clinics.

Over the last decade, dermoscopy has been shown to improve the accuracy of diagnosis of a variety of skin lesions over clinical inspection alone.[7–13] Although largely expected, 81.7% of the surveyed members declared examining all patients with dermoscopy who presented with skin tumors. This finding demonstrates that dermoscopy has become a well-used method in the diagnostic armamentarium of clinicians dealing with skin cancer detection. Current guidelines for the management of melanoma and NMSC cite dermoscopy as a useful tool for clinicians screening skin lesions.[3,4] Despite this, details of a methodology that integrates dermoscopy into a rational clinical work flow for skin cancer screening are essentially absent, and a proposal for such an integrated clinico-dermoscopic approach is, therefore, presented.

Choice of Dermoscopy Device

To optimize screening, clinicians should be equipped with a manual (hand-held) dermatoscope. These devices are relatively inexpensive optical instruments that are capable of producing high-quality images while also allowing a relatively quick examination for most patients. Regarding the latter, a recent study estimated that the time required to complete a total body skin examination with manual dermatoscopy was in the order of only 2 to 3 minutes.[14] These benefits of hand-held dermoscopy seem to be reflected in the survey results whereby most of the respondents (79.3%) reported using a hand-held dermatoscope at the baseline examination of a new patient, and more than half of all respondents (55.9%) performed a baseline examination on a new patient in less than 10 minutes.

The characteristic ease and rapidity of examination when using a hand-held dermatoscope enables an examination of all lesions by dermoscopy, which is particularly important for diagnosing early melanoma and NMSC. Early melanoma often does not present as an ugly duckling lesion by clinical inspection. These clinically featureless melanomas may be pigmented or non-pigmented and may be small, regular in shape, and/or fairly uniform in color, in effect escaping clinical diagnosis based on the classic ABCD (asymmetry, border, color, diameter) criteria. However, these melanomas frequently have suspicious features on dermoscopy, which permits an early diagnosis.[15] This point should be underlined because only 55.1% of the surveyed members used dermoscopy to examine almost all lesions of a given patient (both clinically concerning and random, benign-looking lesions), and 42.6% examine dermoscopically only clinically suspicious lesions selected during the unaided visual examination of the skin. The latter method of applying dermoscopy may be effective in reducing the excision of benign (false positive) lesions, thus improving specificity for melanoma detection, but may result in missing early, clinically inconspicuous melanoma (ie, potentially reducing sensitivity for melanoma diagnosis).

In contrast to hand-held dermatoscopes, video dermatoscopes are digital tools that do not generally provide the high image quality required for precision in dermoscopic diagnosis but are very useful for performing digital monitoring of patients with multiple nevi.[16,17] In effect, they aid in the detection of melanocytic lesions that develop dermoscopic change over time. Of note, video dermatoscopes are usually incorporated into more expensive computerized instrumentation, and nevus monitoring increases the time required for patient assessment.[18] This general concept seems to be reflected in the authors' survey responses. Although only 14.8% of participants in public positions used digital systems, almost double (25.1%) that number of respondents in private practice used digital dermoscopy. When analyzing the time needed to perform a baseline patient examination using any instrument, participants from private practice required a significantly greater amount of time compared with clinicians in public positions.

Improving Patient Selection

In line with previous reports,[19] in the authors' survey, only 37.4% of the respondents performed a general skin cancer examination on all patients presenting to their office for any medical condition. Of the remaining respondents, 44.5% examined patients who were referred for (or who requested) a skin cancer check plus those with risk factors for melanoma, and 17.4% examined only those patients who were referred for (or who requested) a skin cancer check.

As discussed previously, a significant problem of screening for melanoma in the general population is the extremely high prevalence of individuals with melanocytic nevi. Unselected screening of vast numbers of patients in the population is possible but rather difficult with respect to the available resources and cost.[20] Targeted screening of higher-risk individuals has, therefore, become advocated.[21] Opportunistic full skin examinations of higher-risk patients by GFP and dermatologists may assist in the detection of skin cancer, including melanoma. For example, a US study estimated that more than 60% of patients with melanoma had visited their GFP in the year before diagnosis for problems not related to the skin. Therefore, opportunistic screening of high-risk GFP patients could potentially lead to an earlier diagnosis of such melanoma, with improved prognosis.[22] A second point concerns dermatologists: a recent clinical study has calculated that the risk of missing a skin cancer in patients who are seen by a dermatologist for a localized problem (which does not involve examination of the whole cutaneous surface) is in the order of 1 in 50 patients, whereas the risk of missing a melanoma is about 1 in 400 patients.[23]

These sobering figures lead us to consider, at least for the specialist, the possibility of offering a total body skin examination to all patients; but if that is not feasible, then it should be offered to patients in the following higher-risk groups:

1. Patients with a personal history of any skin malignancy or a family history of melanoma (in first-degree relatives)
2. Patients younger than 50 years who present with more than 50 nevi in total or more than 20 nevi on the arms
3. Patients older than 50 years who present with evidence of chronic solar damage

This scheme, a modification of a recent French study, may allow a quick and effective selection of patient groups who are at increased risk of melanoma and NMSC.[24]

Improving Triage Outcome

Once examined clinically and by hand-held (manual) dermoscopy, patients will follow 2 distinct management paths, depending on their risk profile: (1) patients who have a single lesion or few lesions and (2) patients with multiple nevi.

Patients with a single lesion or few lesions

Simply put, if a lesion seems benign it may be left; but if it is suspicious, it should be removed. This approach, although apparently straightforward and obvious, is not so easily applied in daily practice because of the high prevalence of lesions appearing slightly irregular by clinical or dermoscopic examination. Clinicians may choose to monitor such mildly atypical melanocytic lesions in low-risk patients over time; but in the authors' view, monitoring is a specific procedure that helps reduce the number of unnecessary excisions in higher-risk patients, particularly those with multiple nevi (see later discussion). In contrast, for low-risk patients with a single or a few slightly atypical melanocytic lesions, a simple dichotomous approach (ie, no further examination versus excision) can be adopted. The latter approach has the advantage of prompting the excision of an eventual melanoma as early as possible and to acquire more appointment space for new, higher-risk patients to be screened.

An alternate method to manage indeterminate or equivocal melanocytic lesions is short-term clinical and dermoscopic follow-up.[17,25] Short-term follow-up is useful in ensuring that the lesion being monitored follows a benign evolutionary course, thus helping to avoid unnecessary biopsy of benign lesions. Conversely, if there is any morphologic change in the lesion after short-term follow-up (generally 2–4 months), then the lesion is removed for histopathologic testing. In this way, short-term monitoring aims to detect early melanoma that may otherwise have been missed. This overall approach seems to be well reflected in the authors' survey, in which 90.5% of respondents reported that they would perform excision or short-term follow-up for single atypical lesions.

Patients with multiple nevi

A patient with multiple nevi is identified by the presence of more than 50 common nevi in total (excluding lentigines or freckles and common nevi less than 2 mm in diameter) and/or the presence of multiple clinically atypical moles. The latter are characterized by their relatively large diameter (>6 mm) and irregularity in shape and color. With or without an additional family history of melanoma, these patients are at a higher risk of developing melanoma and benefit from long-term monitoring of their lesions.

During the initial visit, the patients' nevi are each analyzed with the manual dermatoscope for any suspicious features. This approach is the traditional *analytic* or *morphologic* approach for the dermoscopic diagnosis of melanoma. Next, the predominant dermoscopic nevus pattern of the patients are determined (ie, reticular, globular, or homogeneous dermoscopic pattern or a combination thereof). By recognizing the predominant dermoscopic morphology of the patients' nevi (also called the *signature* nevus pattern), the dermatologist can then identify any possible dermoscopic ugly duckling lesion that differs from the others and, therefore, should be targeted for excision.[26,27] This approach is the *comparative* dermoscopic approach for diagnosing melanoma. By adding the comparative to the analytic dermoscopic approach for recognizing melanoma, dermoscopists in a recent study were able to reduce the number of unnecessary removals of benign lesions by approximately 75%.[28] In other words, specificity for the diagnosis of melanoma was improved, which the authors found occurred without missing a case of melanoma.

Employment of this comparative approach is confirmed in the authors' survey results, in which 91.3% of the respondents reported performing a comparison of the lesion's morphology with the morphology of the patient's other nevi and subsequently recommended excision of any ugly duckling lesions.

Once the aforementioned process is completed at the first visit, patients with multiple nevi should be included in a long-term clinical and dermoscopic monitoring program for the detection of subsequent melanoma.[29–33] This procedure is a time consuming but is justified for 2 main reasons: (1) A dermoscopically featureless melanoma, such as an amelanotic/hypomelanotic melanoma or very early pigmented melanoma, may already be present. Such melanomas can be very difficult to diagnose at the initial visit and typically lie covertly among other benign-looking lesions. (2) Patients with numerous nevi have a significant risk of developing a cutaneous melanoma at some subsequent time in their life, and diagnosis at the earliest possible stage (when prognosis is most favorable) is vital. Formal clinico-dermoscopic monitoring of such high-risk patients in specialist care has been shown to result in the diagnosis of thinner melanomas than if patients are left in the community without specific surveillance.[34]

For patients with more than 50 common nevi and several atypical nevi (but without a family history of melanoma), the risk of developing a primary melanoma is approximately 3%,[35] whereas for patients with multiple nevi and a positive family history of melanoma (or previous melanoma), the risk is at least 10%.[29,33,36] Conversely, the probability of developing melanoma is exceedingly low for monitored patients who exhibit less than 50 nevi and have no other risk factors for melanoma.[37]

The latter point should be emphasized because most respondents (57%) declared scheduling for follow-up at least 30% of their patients seen at the baseline consultation, and 22.2% scheduled for follow-up almost all patients independent of their risk for developing skin cancer and independent of the number of nevi or their morphology. These high rates of dermoscopic monitoring or follow-up may represent a significant problem inherent to current skin cancer screening practices, which could limit access of other higher-risk patients to screening facilities. In addition, digital follow-up of a few lesions in a given patient with multiple nevi must never replace total body examination with dermoscopy. As previously reported, up to 30% of melanomas in high-risk patients may develop in unmonitored lesions.[35]

Before embarking on long-term monitoring, the specialist should first ensure that patients are able to adhere to a strict follow-up regimen. If agreement between the physician and the patient is reached, the long-term monitoring protocol requires an initial (baseline) inspection of all nevi. In addition to this, video dermoscopic recording of a collection of lesions is carried out, usually consisting of those lesions having the most atypical appearance, but small and dermoscopically unremarkable lesions can also be monitored. No data are available concerning the optimal number of lesions to be monitored per patient; but in the authors' survey, 40.2% of the respondents declared performing digital dermoscopic monitoring of 1 to 10 lesions per patient, and 52.5% monitored more than 10 lesions.

This procedure is repeated after a 3-month interval. This first follow-up review facilitates the detection of any changes in the selected existing lesions on short-term video dermoscopic examination. Such changing lesions should be excised for histopathologic examination to exclude melanoma. Of note, patient compliance is typically significantly higher for short-term (2–4 month) as compared with longer-term (6–12 month) reviews.[35]

Following the 3-month review, if no suspicious lesions are identified, patients should be followed on a 6- to 12-month basis. This approach is reflected in the authors' survey results, in which 82.1% of the respondents recommended long-term follow-up or a combination of short-term and long-term follow-up for patients with multiple nevi. It should be noted that only clinically flat (nonpalpable) melanocytic lesions with a predominantly reticular pattern on dermoscopy are suitable for monitoring. Clinically elevated (palpable) equivocal lesions or those with significant regression (>50% of the area of the lesion), and a predominant globular, starburst, or multicomponent pattern on dermoscopy should not be monitored, as a general rule. The latter is advocated as a safeguard against the possibility of delaying the diagnosis of potentially invasive melanoma, particularly an elevated nodular melanoma with aggressive biologic behavior, or an invasive melanoma undergoing regression. In other words, elevated indeterminate lesions and those demonstrating significant regression should be excised at the outset rather than monitored. Elevated lesions that are clearly benign (eg long-standing, soft dermal nevi or clear-cut seborrheic keratoses) do not require monitoring.

The overall schema detailed earlier (**Fig. 2**) should be strongly emphasized because in the authors' survey, a relatively high percentage of clinicians (41.9%) declared that they would not necessarily excise a doubtful palpable lesion at the outset but that their decision would depend on patient risk factors for skin malignancy and the total nevus count. This practice is a point of concern because it may potentially result in the nonexcision of an aggressive invasive malignancy, such as a rapidly growing nodular melanoma.[38]

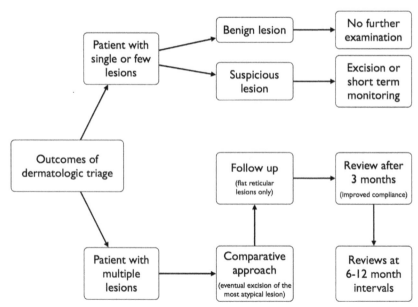

Fig. 2. Work flow summarizing the 2 outcomes of the clinician triage using dermoscopy.

Physician education campaigns could address this issue by focusing on the clinico-dermoscopic recognition and early removal of aggressive skin cancers, particularly nodular melanoma. Regarding the clinical recognition of the nodular melanoma, the EFG mnemonic is a helpful aid and signifies an elevated, firm, and growing lesions present for more than a month.[39,40] Furthermore, dermoscopic features may be a useful aid to the recognition of nonpigmented and pigmented nodular melanoma; the former often harbors an atypical vascular pattern and remnants of pigmentation,[41] and the latter frequently shows areas of blue and black coloration (which can be coupled with other melanoma-specific dermoscopic criteria).[42]

In conclusion, despite general limitations of the survey study technique, including a relatively brief questionnaire formulated to encourage a high response rate, the questions and choice of answers being fixed or closed ended, and respondents being unable to explain their responses, and the specific limitation of the preselected profile of the interviewed clinicians (all members of the IDS), this study confirms that dermoscopy is acknowledged and used as a standard skin cancer screening tool. Based on available evidence, up-to-date recommendations for the screening and management (ie, triage) of patients with skin cancer are presented. These recommendations aim to improve the accuracy of diagnosis and promote a more timely and effective management of melanoma and other skin cancers. Areas are highlighted where current (surveyed) clinical behavior departs from these recommendations, and these potential areas of concern could be addressed through focused physician education programs.

REFERENCES

1. Cox NH. Evaluation of the U.K. 2-week referral rule for skin cancer. Br J Dermatol 2004;150:291–8.
2. Baughan P, Keatings J, O'Neill B. Urgent suspected cancer referrals from general practice: audit of compliance with guidelines and referral outcomes. Br J Gen Pract 2011;61:700–6.
3. Marsden JR, Newton-Bishop JA, Burrows L, et al. Revised U.K. guidelines for the management of cutaneous melanoma 2010. Br J Dermatol 2010; 163:238–56.
4. Australian Cancer Network Melanoma Guidelines Revision Working Party. Clinical practice guidelines for the management of melanoma in Australia and New Zealand. Wellington (New Zeland): Cancer Council Australia and Australian Cancer Network, Sydney and New Zealand Guidelines Group; 2008.
5. May C, Giles L, Gupta G. Prospective observational comparative study assessing the role of store and forward teledermatology triage in skin cancer. Clin Exp Dermatol 2008;33:736–9.
6. Tsang MW, Resneck JS. Even patients with changing moles face long dermatology appointment wait-times: a study of simulated patient calls to dermatologists. J Am Acad Dermatol 2006;55:54–8.
7. Bafounta ML, Beauchet A, Aegerter P, et al. Is dermoscopy (epiluminescence microscopy) useful for the diagnosis of melanoma? Results of a meta-analysis using techniques adapted to the evaluation of diagnostic tests. Arch Dermatol 2001; 137:1343–50.
8. Kittler H, Pehamberger H, Wolff K, et al. Diagnostic accuracy of dermoscopy. Lancet Oncol 2002;3: 159–65.
9. Argenziano G, Soyer HP, Chimenti S, et al. Dermoscopy of pigmented skin lesions: results of a consensus meeting via the Internet. J Am Acad Dermatol 2003;48:679–93.
10. Carli P, De Giorgi V, Chiarugi A, et al. Addition of dermoscopy to conventional naked-eye examination in melanoma screening: a randomized study. J Am Acad Dermatol 2004;50:683–9.
11. Carli P, De Giorgi V, Crocetti E, et al. Improvement of malignant/benign ratio in excised melanocytic lesions in the "dermoscopy era": a retrospective study 1997-2001. Br J Dermatol 2004;150:687–92.
12. Vestergaard ME, Macaskill P, Holt PE, et al. Dermoscopy compared with naked eye examination for the diagnosis of primary melanoma: a meta-analysis of studies performed in a clinical setting. Br J Dermatol 2008;159:669–76.
13. Argenziano G, Cerroni L, Zalaudek I, et al. Accuracy in melanoma detection: a 10-year multicenter survey. J Am Acad Dermatol 2011;67(1):54–9.
14. Zalaudek I, Kittler H, Marghoob AA, et al. Time required for a complete skin examination with and without dermoscopy: a prospective, randomized multicenter study. Arch Dermatol 2008;144:509–13.
15. Argenziano G, Ferrara G, Francione S, et al. Dermoscopy–the ultimate tool for melanoma diagnosis. Semin Cutan Med Surg 2009;28:142–8.
16. Kittler H, Seltenheim M, Dawid M, et al. Morphologic changes of pigmented skin lesions: a useful extension of the ABCD rule for dermatoscopy. J Am Acad Dermatol 1999;40:558–62.
17. Menzies SW, Emery J, Staples M, et al. Impact of dermoscopy and short-term sequential digital dermoscopy imaging for the management of pigmented lesions in primary care: a sequential intervention trial. Br J Dermatol 2009;161:1270–7.
18. Malvehy J, Puig S. Follow-up of melanocytic skin lesions with digital total-body photography and digital dermoscopy: a two-step method. Clin Dermatol 2002;20:297–304.

19. Federman DG, Kravetz JD, Kirsner RS. Skin cancer screening by dermatologists: prevalence and barriers. J Am Acad Dermatol 2002;46:710–4.

20. Breitbart EW, Waldmann A, Nolte S, et al. Systematic skin cancer screening in Northern Germany. J Am Acad Dermatol 2012;66:201–11.

21. Geller AC, O'Riordan DL, Oliveria SA, et al. Overcoming obstacles to skin cancer examinations and prevention counseling for high-risk patients: results of a national survey of primary care physicians. J Am Board Fam Pract 2004;17:416–23.

22. Geller AC, Koh HK, Miller DR, et al. Use of health services before the diagnosis of melanoma: implications for early detection and screening. J Gen Intern Med 1992;7:154–7.

23. Argenziano G, Zalaudek I, Hofmann-Wellenhof R, et al. Total body skin examination for skin cancer screening in patients with focused symptoms. J Am Acad Dermatol 2012;66:212–9.

24. Quéreux G, Moyse D, Lequeux Y, et al. Development of an individual score for melanoma risk. Eur J Cancer Prev 2011;20:217–24.

25. Altamura D, Avramidis M, Menzies SW. Assessment of the optimal interval for and sensitivity of short-term sequential digital dermoscopy monitoring for the diagnosis of melanoma. Arch Dermatol 2008;144:502–6.

26. Suh KY, Bolognia JL. Signature nevi. J Am Acad Dermatol 2009;60:508–14.

27. Scope A, Dusza SW, Halpern AC, et al. The "ugly duckling" sign: agreement between observers. Arch Dermatol 2008;144:58–64.

28. Argenziano G, Catricalà C, Ardigo M, et al. Dermoscopy of patients with multiple nevi: improved management recommendations using a comparative diagnostic approach. Arch Dermatol 2011;147:46–9.

29. Haenssle HA, Korpas B, Hansen-Hagge C, et al. Selection of patients for long-term surveillance with digital dermoscopy by assessment of melanoma risk factors. Arch Dermatol 2010;146:257–64.

30. Haenssle HA, Krueger U, Vente C, et al. Results from an observational trial: digital epiluminescence microscopy follow-up of atypical nevi increases the sensitivity and the chance of success of conventional dermoscopy in detecting melanoma. J Invest Dermatol 2006;126:980–5.

31. Kittler H, Guitera P, Riedl E, et al. Identification of clinically featureless incipient melanoma using sequential dermoscopy imaging. Arch Dermatol 2006;142:1113–9.

32. Kittler H, Binder M. Risks and benefits of sequential imaging of melanocytic skin lesions in patients with multiple atypical nevi. Arch Dermatol 2001;137:1590–5.

33. Marghoob AA, Kopf AW, Rigel DS, et al. Risk of cutaneous malignant melanoma in patients with "classic" atypical-mole syndrome. A case-control study. Arch Dermatol 1994;130:993–8.

34. Salerni G, Lovatto L, Carrera C, et al. Melanomas detected in a follow-up program compared with melanomas referred to a melanoma unit. Arch Dermatol 2011;147:549–55.

35. Argenziano G, Mordente I, Ferrara G, et al. Dermoscopic monitoring of melanocytic skin lesions: clinical outcome and patient compliance vary according to follow-up protocols. Br J Dermatol 2008;159:331–6.

36. Salerni G, Carrera C, Lovatto L, et al. Benefits of total body photography and digital dermatoscopy ("two-step method of digital follow-up") in the early diagnosis of melanoma in patients at high risk for melanoma. J Am Acad Dermatol 2011;67(1):e17–27.

37. Schiffner R, Schiffner-Rohe J, Landthaler M, et al. Long-term dermoscopic follow-up of melanocytic naevi: clinical outcome and patient compliance. Br J Dermatol 2003;149:79–86.

38. Liu W, Dowling JP, Murray WK, et al. Rate of growth in melanomas: characteristics and associations of rapidly growing melanomas. Arch Dermatol 2006;142:1551–8.

39. Kelly JW, Chamberlain AJ, Staples MP, et al. Nodular melanoma. No longer as simple as ABC. Aust Fam Physician 2003;32:706–9.

40. Chamberlain AJ, Fritschi L, Kelly JW. Nodular melanoma: patients' perceptions of presenting features and implications for earlier detection. J Am Acad Dermatol 2003;48:694–701.

41. Menzies SW, Kreusch J, Byth K, et al. Dermoscopic evaluation of amelanotic and hypomelanotic melanoma. Arch Dermatol 2008;144:1120–7.

42. Argenziano G, Longo C, Cameron A, et al. Blue-black rule: a simple dermoscopic clue to recognize pigmented nodular melanoma. Br J Dermatol 2011;165:1251–5.

Problematic Lesions in Children

Elvira Moscarella, MD[a,*], Vincenzo Piccolo, MD[b],
Giuseppe Argenziano, MD[a], Aimilios Lallas, MD[a],
Caterina Longo, MD, PhD[a], Fabio Castagnetti, MD[a],
Stefania Pizzigoni, MD[a], Iris Zalaudek, MD[a,c]

KEYWORDS

- Childhood • Melanoma • Melanocytic nevi • Congenital nevi • Spitz nevi • Atypical spitz tumor

KEY POINTS

- Problematic melanocytic lesions in the pediatric setting are represented by congenital nevi and Spitz nevi.
- Congenital melanocytic nevi carry a higher risk of melanoma development as compared with common nevi. The risk of melanoma is proportional to the nevus size; thus, particular attention should be paid to large congenital nevi.
- Childhood melanoma often lacks the classical features of pigmented melanoma, and it is more often an amelanotic and nodular lesion resembling pyogenic granuloma or nonpigmented Spitz nevus.
- A classical or pigmented Spitz nevus appearing up to puberty, clinically and dermoscopically readily diagnosed, can be managed conservatively. Large (>1 cm), nodular, ulcerated, rapidly changing, and atypical Spitz tumors of childhood must be excised.

INTRODUCTION

Pediatric melanoma is extremely rare, especially before puberty.[1–3] During the last congress of the American Academy of Dermatology, a famous pediatric dermatologist compared childhood melanoma to the legend of "Bigfoot," a figure everybody is concerned about, but that only a few actually declare to have seen in their life. Of course she was not questioning the existence of childhood melanoma, but wanted to point the accent on the extreme rarity of this event and on the fact that, because of its rarity, no clear-cut clinical features and patterns of presentation are actually known.[4] Most physicians will probably never be confronted with this malignancy, but even if they do encounter it, they might not readily recognize it. Recent findings in fact[5] corroborated previous studies indicating that childhood melanoma does not present with conventional ABCDE criteria for melanoma.[6–8] Most frequently it may mimic clinically nonmelanocytic lesions, such as angioma, pyogenic granuloma, viral wart, and molluscum. The same lesions are in the differential diagnosis of amelanotic/hypomelanotic Spitz nevi, which actually represent the main clinically and histopathologically challenging lesions to be differentiated from melanoma in this age group.[9–11] In this scenario, it is not surprising that accuracy in melanoma detection in children still remains low. A recent study tested the accuracy in melanoma

The authors have no conflict of interest to declare.

Funding Sources: Study supported in part by the Italian Ministry of Health (RF-2010-2316524).

[a] Skin Cancer Unit, First Medical Department, Arcispedale Santa Maria Nuova, IRCCS, Viale Risorgimento, 80, Reggio Emilia 42100, Italy; [b] Department of Dermatology, Second University of Naples, Via Pansini 5, 80131 Naples, Italy; [c] Department of Dermatology, Medical University of Graz, Auenbruggerplatz 2, 8036 Graz, Austria

* Corresponding author. Skin Cancer Unit, Arcispedale S. Maria Nuova, IRCCS, Viale Risorgimento, 80, Reggio Emilia 42100, Italy.

E-mail address: elvira.moscarella@gmail.com

detection in children and adolescents over a 10-year period, using the NNE value (number needed to excise; obtained dividing the total number of excised lesions by the number of melanomas).[12] The NNE value for this pediatric population (0–18 years) was 20 times higher than the rates usually found in adult patients, meaning that a very high number of benign nevi (ie, approximately 594) were excised to detect one melanoma.[12] An effective strategy to reduce the number of unnecessary excisions would be to focus on problematic lesions. Epidemiologic data indicate that, apart from immune suppression and genetic conditions (such as xeroderma pigmentosum), the main risk factor for developing melanoma in a pediatric population is represented by the presence of a large congenital nevus.[13,14] Thus, spitzoid lesions and congenital nevi have to be considered the true problematic lesions in children, representing melanoma simulator and melanoma precursor, respectively. In this article, we describe the main clinical and dermoscopic characteristics and the management options for problematic lesions in children.

SPITZ/REED NEVI

Since the first description by Sophie Spitz in 1948,[15] much work has been conducted in elucidating the clinico/pathologic variability of spitzoid lesions. Currently, common Spitz and Reed nevi are considered benign melanocytic proliferations that frequently occur in children and are histopathologically classified as benign without difficulty.[16–20] At the other end of the spectrum of spitzoid lesions, we place "Spitzoid melanomas," a morphologic type of melanoma with Spitzoid features, which are promptly identified as malignant on histopathologic examination. Between these 2 extremes are a series of Spitzoid lesions that present varying features of clinical and histopathologic atypia and unknown malignant potential that have been referred to with a variety of terms such as "Spitz nevus with atypia," "atypical Spitz nevus," "atypical Spitz tumors (AST)" and melanocytic tumors of uncertain malignant potential (MELTUMP).[21,22] Some investigators have suggested the term of AST as the more widely accepted; however, no adequate histologic criteria exist to clearly classify these lesions as benign or malignant, and even experienced pathologists are unable to predict, in most cases, the outcome of this group of atypical Spitz lesions based on morphologic criteria. These uncertainties are the major reason why evidence-based management guidelines for Spitz tumors have not yet been established.[18,23–26]

From a clinical point of view, a "classical" Spitz nevus presents as a pink or flesh-colored papule or nodule, rapidly growing, and appearing most frequently on the lower extremities or the head/neck region in childhood or adolescence. The histopathologic hallmark of Spitz nevi is the presence of large spindle and/or epithelioid cells, usually in the paucity or absence of melanin.[27]

"Reed nevus" is the eponymic designation for a benign melanocytic lesion described by Reed and colleagues[28] in 1975 as "pigmented spindle cell nevus." It is mostly found in young adults on the lower extremities as a rapidly growing brownish-black macule or papule. On histopathology, it is described as made up of interconnecting junctional fascicles of heavily pigmented spindle cells. The autonomy of Reed nevus from Spitz nevus has been questioned because of the occurrence of cases of spindle and/or epithelioid cell nevi with heavy pigmentation,[16] thus ascribing Reed nevus to the morphologic spectrum of Spitz nevus. At present, some investigators still maintain that Reed nevus is an entity that can be readily differentiated from pigmented spindle cell Spitz nevus.[29,30] However, a clinicopathologic evaluation of a large case series showed that the histopathologic distinction between these 2 diagnostic categories is often a matter of great debate.[27]

Dermoscopy

On dermoscopy, Spitz/Reed nevi can display 6 main dermoscopic patterns: vascular, globular, starburst, reticular, homogeneous, and atypical.[27,31]

The vascular pattern is mainly composed of dotted vessels,[32,33] which are monomorphic, regularly distributed throughout the lesion, and surrounded by regularly intersecting white lines, the so-called "reticular depigmentation."[34] A slight pigmentation can be present as a diffuse brownish to grayish hue with regular gray-brown, small to medium-sized globules.

In frankly pigmented lesions, globules are brown to black, large, and regularly distributed at the periphery, or surrounded by reticular depigmentation. In most cases of pigmented Spitz nevi, peripheral globules are fused with the central body of the lesion; these regular radial projections, the so-called streaks, give rise to a "starburst" appearance. In a minority of cases, a heavy pigmentation also determines the presence of a regular superficial black network.[35] The homogeneous pattern is characterized by a diffuse dark brown to black-bluish color, which lacks the evidence of clear-cut streaks at the periphery.

Several of these features can be simultaneously present or irregularly distributed within a given lesion, thus giving an atypical pattern. Dermoscopic atypia also can be increased by the presence of a blue-whitish veil. As a general rule, Spitz nevus can be considered as potentially showing all the dermoscopic features of melanoma. The occurrence of an atypical dermoscopic pattern in Spitz nevus is well recognized and is an important mimic of melanoma.[27] Moreover, melanoma may at times show very few or no dermoscopic features suggestive of malignancy, but may mimic Spitz nevus in exhibiting either the globular or the starburst pattern. The latter patterns have been described in such melanomas occurring in adulthood (**Fig. 1**).[36]

Management

Based on the inverse age distribution of Spitz nevi versus melanoma,[20,37] with the number of Spitz nevi being highest in the first decade of life, some investigators have proposed conservative management for a classical or pigmented Spitz nevus appearing up to puberty. Relatively small (up to 1 cm) Spitz/Reed nevi, showing no atypical clinical and dermoscopic features,[38] can be managed conservatively, with clinical and dermoscopic controls every 3 to 6 months. In the absence of sudden and marked changes in color, shape, or size, such a follow-up protocol can be continued until the appearance of a homogeneous pattern; thereafter, annual follow-up can be performed. During monitoring, the observed changes in dermoscopic patterns appear to represent different phases of the natural evolution of the nevus: the globular and starburst pattern are typical of the growth phase and the homogeneous or reticular pattern appears when the lesion becomes stable (**Figs. 2** and **3**).[39,40] During the growth phase, a marked increase in the diameter of the lesion, and substantial changes in the dermoscopic features, can be observed. These changes can sometimes produce a somewhat worrisome clinical and dermoscopic appearance, even after a very short follow-up period. In a recent study by Argenziano and colleagues,[40] the investigators followed a series of 64 lesions in pediatric patients (mean age: 10.4 years) for a mean follow-up period of 25 months. In this study, 79.7% (n = 51) of the lesions showed an involution pattern and 20.3% (n = 13) showed a growing (n = 4) or stable pattern (n = 9). The great majority of growing lesions were pigmented or partially pigmented (92.3%), whereas 47.1% of lesions in involution were amelanotic (P = .005).[40] One

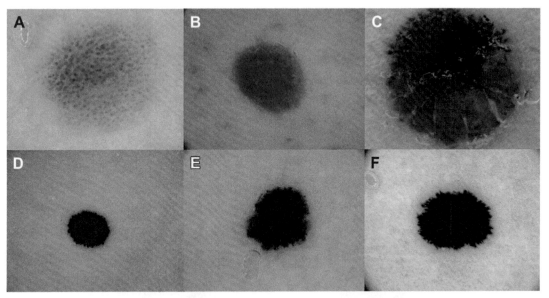

Fig. 1. The many dermoscopic faces of Spitz/Reed nevi. (*A*) Hypomelanotic Spitz nevus showing a vascular pattern composed of dotted vessels regularly distributed throughout the lesion, and intersected by a white network. A few, regular, light brown globules are visible at the periphery. (*B*) Amelanotic Spitz nevus showing fairly regularly arranged dotted vessels on a "milky pink" background. (*C*) Atypical dermoscopic pattern of a Spitz nevus, showing linear irregular vessels, and an atypical pigment network on the upper right side of the lesion. (*D*) Typical starburst pattern in a small ("baby") Reed nevus. (*E*) Dark brown and black globules irregularly distributed in a pigmented Spitz nevus. Blue-white blotches are also present centrally. (*F*) Heavily pigmented lesion (Reed nevus), with streaks at the periphery and a very evident superficial black network.

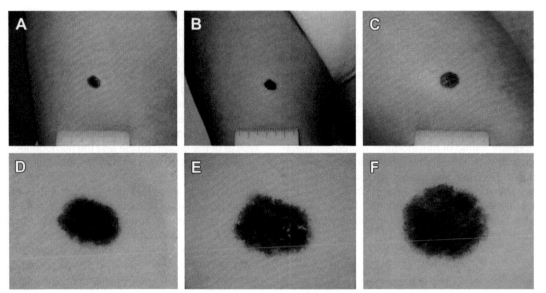

Fig. 2. Different phases in the evolution of a pigmented Spitz nevus arising on the leg of a 2-year-old girl. (*A–C*) Clinical view at baseline, and after 4-month, and 12-month follow-up, respectively. (*D–F*) Corresponding dermoscopic images, showing a marked increase in the size of the nevus and increase in the number of peripheral globules and streaks around the lesion.

pigmented growing lesion was excised by the investigators, and 6 were excised per patient request. All were histopathologically classified as Spitz nevi.

AST

A clear-cut description of the clinico-dermoscopic features of ASTs has not yet been formally defined.

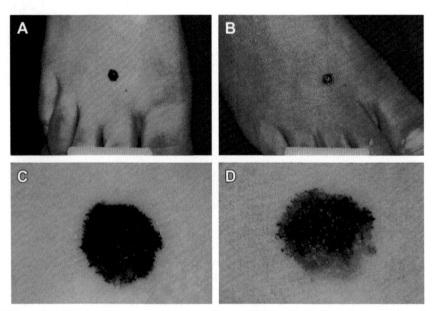

Fig. 3. Involuting pigmented Spitz nevus arising in a 9-year-old boy. (*A, B*) Clinical view at baseline and after 8 months follow-up, respectively. (*C*) Heavily pigmented, reticular pattern under dermoscopy. (*D*) Partial involution of the network pattern, a blue-gray area of peppering is now visible in approximately half of the lesion surface.

However, according to retrospective histopathology studies,[21,22,41] AST could be broadly outlined as a medium to large, nodular, sometimes ulcerated, hypopigmented or amelanotic spitzoid lesion. Thus, large (>1 cm), nodular, ulcerated, rapidly changing, or otherwise atypical Spitz nevi of childhood must be excised. Surgical excision is also recommended when Spitz nevi appear after puberty and during adulthood, regardless the presence of atypical clinical/dermoscopic features. Because of the absence of criteria that allow an accurate differentiation of nonpigmented Spitz nevi from pyogenic granuloma (lobular hemangioma), histopathologic examination is also recommended for those lesions showing features of pyogenic granuloma, independently of age (**Fig. 4**). Of note, Requena and colleagues,[9] in a recent clinico-pathologic study on 349 histologically proven Spitz nevi, found that only 18% of lesions were correctly diagnosed clinically. Clinical diagnoses included, among others, hemangioma, viral wart, xanthogranuloma, and molluscum contagiosum.[9]

When a diagnosis of AST is given by histopathologic examination, the clinician is faced with the challenging responsibility of choosing the best management option for their young patients (**Fig. 5**). The management of AST is matter of great debate. In 2000, Kelley and Cockerell[42] proposed that, in addition to wide excision, sentinel lymph node biopsy (SLN biopsy) should be considered for these patients. The presence of metastatic tumor deposits in the lymph node would support the malignant nature of the primary tumor. Against this theory is the evidence that none of the patients with primary ambiguous Spitz tumor and positive lymph nodes in the 7 published series died of metastatic melanoma to date.[43–49] These findings may support the hypothesis that not all atypical Spitz tumors represent misdiagnosed conventional melanomas, but are perhaps a distinct category of "less aggressive" melanocytic tumors with locoregional malignant behavior.[50] Thus, SLN biopsy cannot be considered a diagnostic procedure, and moreover it has not been proven to represent a valuable prognostic tool in children. In addition to the known controversies around its survival benefit in adults, these considerations support the conclusion that, currently, the best treatment option for children diagnosed with AST is represented by complete excision of the primary lesion (ie, with sufficiently wide margin) and careful follow-up.

A recent survey among 175 pediatric dermatologists in the United States and around the world revealed that the previously mentioned management for Spitz nevi and atypical spitzoid lesions

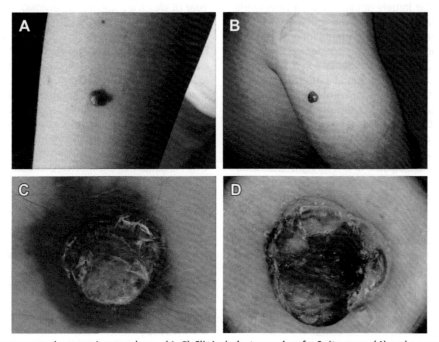

Fig. 4. Spitz nevus and pyogenic granuloma. (*A, B*) Clinical photographs of a Spitz nevus (*A*) and a pyogenic granuloma (*B*) arising on the upper arm of an 11-year-old and 4-year-old boy, respectively. (*C, D*) Corresponding dermoscopy shows 2 amelanotic nodules surrounded by a collarette. The presence of a brownish background pigmentation and a few brown globules in the first lesion (*C*) could suggest the diagnosis of a melanocytic tumor; however, the exclusion of nonpigmented melanoma in both cases is extremely difficult and histopathologic examination is warranted.

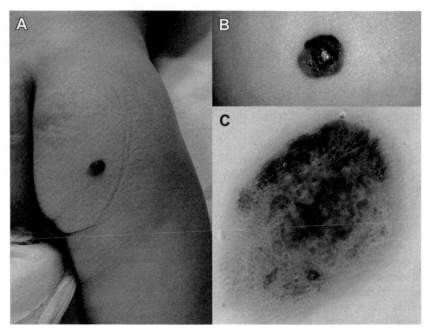

Fig. 5. Atypical Spitz tumor. (*A*) A 2-cm plaque arising on the gluteal region of a 2-year-old girl. (*B*) Close-up view showing the presence of a central nodular area and variegated pigmentation. (*C*) Under dermoscopy, the lesion is spitzoid, showing reticular depigmentation, dot vessels, and peripheral streaks, but also displays centrally located milky red areas. Complete excision with narrow margins was performed and the histopathologic diagnosis of AST was confirmed by 2 experienced pathologists.

appears to be largely applied among physicians. Interestingly, in this survey, clinical follow-up was chosen by 49.3% of respondents for small, stable, and nonpigmented clinically suspected Spitz nevi, and by 29.7% of respondents for a pigmented lesion with a typical starburst pattern on dermoscopy. Furthermore, approximately 80% of the dermatologists surveyed reported using dermoscopy for their lesion assessments. These data show that conservative management for typical Spitz nevi is a clinical option chosen by many pediatric dermatologists, and highlight the widespread use of dermoscopy for the diagnosis of melanocytic lesions in the pediatric population.[51] Importantly, the respondents to the survey had cared for only 2 patients who were thought to have died because of a lesion initially diagnosed as a Spitz nevus or atypical spitzoid neoplasm, an extremely small fraction of the approximately 20,000 Spitz nevi diagnosed by these dermatologists. Moreover, no deaths had resulted from the approximately 10,000 Spitz nevi and atypical spitzoid neoplasms seen by the 91 respondents with academic or hospital-based practices.[51]

CONGENITAL NEVI

Congenital melanocytic nevi (CMN) are defined as nevi present at birth or appearing within the first year of life. They can be subdivided into 3 groups based on their size: small (<1.5 cm), medium (1.5–20 cm), and large or giant (>20 cm in their projected adult size) (**Fig. 6**).[52] Giant CMN may be further classified as G1 (21–30 cm), G2 (31–40 cm), and G3 (>40 cm). They are genetically determined and persist throughout all life. The estimated prevalence of CMN ranges from 0.5% to 31.7%, depending on the study cited.[52] Giant CMN have an estimated incidence of 1 in 20,000 to 500,000 live births.[52] The clinical diagnosis of CMN is usually straightforward because of the history of a pigmented lesion being present since (or shortly following) birth. Clinically, CMNs are usually larger than common nevi, may present color variegation, and tend to become palpable and covered with terminal hair. Giant CMNs involve a large area of the skin surface and are often associated with scattered "satellite nevi,"[53] defined as smaller CMNs that are present at birth or arise months to years later.

Dermoscopy

By dermoscopy, the main pattern seen in CMN is the so called "cobblestone pattern," constituted of large, angulated globules, resembling cobblestones. Additional dermoscopic criteria include perifollicular hypopigmentation, milialike cysts,

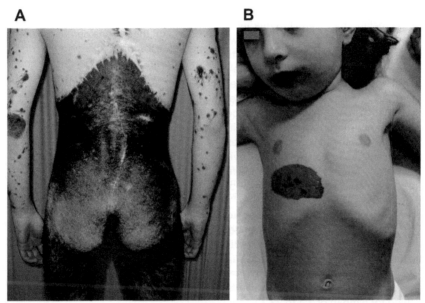

Fig. 6. (*A*) A giant congenital ("bathing trunk") nevus with multiple satellite nevi, occurring in a 15-year-old boy. Note the presence of multiple scars due to serial, partial excisions of the giant nevus during childhood. (*B*) Medium-sized congenital nevus on the chest of a 3-year-old girl. Clinical and dermoscopic follow-up was preferred by the parents rather than surgical excision.

and the presence of coarse hairs (hypertrichosis). Dotted and comma vessels may also be apparent in some CMNs (**Fig. 7**).[11,54] CMNs on the head, neck, and trunk of children frequently exhibit a globular pattern, whereas those arising on the extremities (particularly the lower limb) often display a reticular pattern.[11]

Two main areas of concern associated with CMN are, first, the risk of melanoma development and, second, cosmetic and psychological issues.

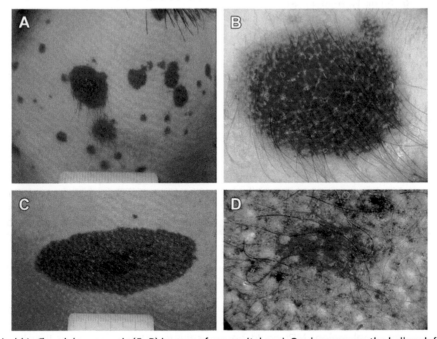

Fig. 7. Clinical (*A, C*) and dermoscopic (*B, D*) images of congenital nevi. On dermoscopy, the hallmark features are the presence of a cobblestone pattern, with large, angulated globules (*B*) and a reticular pattern with numerous small globules (*D*). Hairs also cover the lesion surfaces. In addition, perifollicular hypopigmentation is present (*D*).

There is a substantial lack of consensus on the risk of developing melanoma in small to medium-sized CMN; however, this risk seems to be low. It has been estimated that up to 1% of patients with small and medium CMNs will develop a melanoma over a lifetime.[55] Other physicians consider the risk of melanoma development related to age; children younger than 10 years have an incidence of approximately 0.7 per million, whereas for children aged 15 to 19 years, the incidence increases up to 13.2 per million.[56] Moreover, there is evidence that melanomas tend to arise earlier in life in giant CMNs than in small ones. In a review of melanoma in children younger than 12 years,[57] one-third of cases were found to be related to the presence of giant CMN. Similarly, Krengel and colleagues[58] reported the frequency of melanoma in patients with CMN, ranging between 0.05% and 10.7%, and being significantly higher in smaller studies. On a total of 6571 patients with CMN followed for a mean of 3.4 to 23.7 years, only 0.7% developed melanoma. The median age at diagnosis of melanoma was 7 years and the melanoma risk was strongly dependent on the nevus size, being highest for giant CMN, with a maximum risk during childhood.[58]

Concerning the depth of origin of melanomas arising from CMN, some investigators believe that melanoma arising within a giant CMN originates from a greater depth, being nodular from the beginning.[53] Conversely, melanomas arising in the context of small to medium-sized CMNs tend to develop from the dermoepidermal junction, being of the superficial spreading type on histology. However, data on this hypothesis appear limited at this time.

Large CMNs can be associated with systemic diseases, and in particular with neurocutaneous melanocytosis (NCM). This is a melanocytic proliferation involving the central nervous system, associated with giant CMN, especially those with multiple satellitosis.[59] The presence of NCM could alter the prognosis of the affected patients because of increased intracranial pressure. A fatal outcome has been reported in more than half of the patients affected by symptomatic NCM; death occurred within about 3 years after the appearance of symptoms, mostly in individuals younger than 10 years of age.[60] Brain magnetic resonance imaging (MRI) is indicated for patients at risk for NCM, namely children with giant CMN; satellite nevi or multiple CMN; and head, neck, or posterior midline location. Moreover, in children with large or medium-sized nevi affecting the lumbosacral region, MRI could be used to detect spinal abnormalities, such as tethered cord syndrome.

Management

Based on these considerations, treatment of CMN has to be individualized and address malignant melanoma risk, and aesthetic and psychosocial matters. Given the low risk of melanoma development within small and medium-sized congenital nevi, early excision or, alternatively, regular clinical and dermoscopic follow-up can be both considered as valuable management options. If no atypical clinical and dermoscopic features are detected, these nevi can be managed on an individual basis depending on patient compliance to follow-up and also depending on cosmetic concerns of parents and patients. Clinical follow-up should be performed annually for these lesions, and digital clinical dermoscopic imaging can be useful to detect early changes in an otherwise clinically banal CMNs, before the development of any nodular component. It is also important to explain to parents that the lesion can gradually increase in size over time, but it should be always proportional to the growth of the child. In large CMNs, early excision has often been justified as prophylaxis against malignant transformation; however, this prophylactic role is difficult to quantify.[61] Moreover, because melanoma can develop outside of the nevus, surgery seems unable to negate all giant CMN-associated melanoma risk. Thus, management of giant CMN should be individualized with respect not only to melanoma risk, but also to aesthetic and psychosocial aspects.

OTHER PROBLEMATIC LESIONS

The total number of melanocytic nevi varies with age, following a dynamic evolution. Nevus counts and nevus density increase from youth to midlife and thereafter decrease.[11] Thus, usually children present with very few nevi, especially if considering children before puberty. Nevi with atypical features generally arise after puberty, representing a marker of increased risk for melanoma development. Therefore, regular follow-up is recommended after puberty, especially in children presenting additional risk factors, such as positive family history of melanoma, fair skin phototype, and history of sunburns. The main objective in managing patients with multiple nevi consists of the identification of early melanoma and its differentiation from atypical nevi. However, given the peculiar clinical and dermoscopic characteristics of melanoma in children, the rules used to avoid missing melanoma that clinicians usually apply for adults, are only partially useful in children.[62] A higher threshold for malignancy should probably be applied when dealing with pediatric patients, to avoid unnecessary excisions of benign lesions.[12] A peculiar clinical and dermoscopic confounding feature is the presence of focal eccentric hyperpigmentation (also called Bolognia sign).[4] This is a rather common finding in childhood nevi, but it can be mistaken as a sign of melanoma by clinicians. However, in contrast to melanoma, nevi with eccentric hyperpigmentation exhibit dermoscopically brown to gray-black homogeneous pigmentation, in the absence of any melanoma-specific feature. In addition, this hyperpigmentation may often disappear during follow-up. Scalp nevi in children and teenagers are known indicators for a higher total nevus count in adulthood, being considered as a marker of the so-called "moley child." Common scalp nevi in children and teenagers may reveal a uniform globular pattern under dermoscopy or alternatively a pigmented network with perifollicular hypopigmentation that may give rise to border irregularity. In children with fair skin types, scalp nevi may present with central hypopigmentation, and are also called eclipse nevi. Despite the high level of concern among clinicians in the past regarding these melanocytic proliferations, nowadays these lesions are widely considered as benign and can usually be managed conservatively.[4] Similarly, acral nevi, which are often a matter of concern for parents, can be managed conservatively when displaying a typically benign clinical and dermoscopic pattern.[63] Under dermoscopy, these lesions display a parallel pattern of pigmentation distributed along the skin furrows. Less frequently, a latticelike and a fibrillar pattern can also be detected.[63] Conversely, a parallel ridge pattern is highly suggestive of melanoma on acral sites.

Blue nevi (BN) are benign neoplasms characterized histologically by a dermal proliferation of melanin-laden dendritic melanocytes. There are a number of variants of BN, the 2 main types being common BN and cellular BN. Common BN usually appear as bluish, smooth-surfaced papules, nodules, and plaques. Dermoscopic examination of common BN shows a typical steel-blue homogeneous coloration generated by the presence of heavily pigmented melanocytes in the dermis. This dermoscopic finding occurs in the absence of any other dermoscopic feature, in particular a pigment network, dots, globules, and vessels. The main clinical difference between common and cellular BN is the diameter, with the latter being larger (up to 30 mm) than the former (<10 mm). Cellular BN may also have a polychromatic appearance (ie, mixed blue, brown, and white in color). Other types of BN may show color variations (eg, "white" or hypochromic BN), but nonetheless still show a fairly homogeneous color (or combination of colors) in the absence of the local dermoscopic structures, as mentioned previously (ie, network, dots/globules, and vessels) (**Fig. 8**).[11] BNs with peripheral satellitosis mimicking malignant melanoma (MM)[64] have also been described. Finally, combined BNs are defined as BNs in which the dermal component arises in combination with a more superficial junctional or compound proliferation, and the overall appearance of the lesions may give rise to a worrisome presentation. In these cases, excision may be necessary to confirm the benign nature of the melanocytic proliferation (**Fig. 9**).

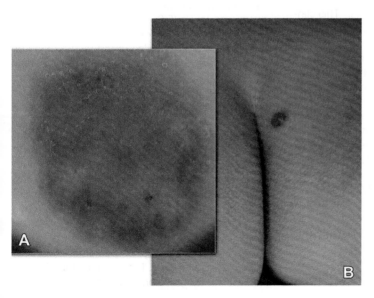

Fig. 8. Blue nevus in a 2-year-old boy, (*A*) showing a structureless blue-gray color under dermoscopy, in the absence of any other local dermoscopic structure (*B*).

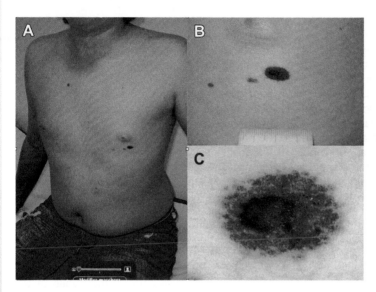

Fig. 9. Combined nevus (congenital nevus and blue nevus) on the chest of a 12-year-old boy. (*A*) Close-up photograph (*B*) of the 1-cm-diameter lesion, showing color variegation. On dermoscopy, there is an overall cobblestone pattern, with a central homogeneous bluish area (*C*). The lesion was excised to rule out melanoma, and histopathology showed a combined lesion, constituted by a combination of congenital and blue nevus.

MELANOMA

Childhood melanoma is extremely rare, accounting for approximately 2% of childhood malignancy. In the United States, 1% to 4% of all melanomas arise in patients younger than 20 years[4]; however, only 0.3% occur before puberty. In addition to its rarity, childhood melanoma seems to be characterized by different patterns of presentation, risk factors, and survival rates as compared with melanoma of adults. A large retrospective study of children given the diagnosis of melanoma, or ambiguous melanocytic tumors treated as melanoma, before the age of 20 years, revealed that melanoma in most cases did not present with conventional ABCDE criteria.[5] Rather, amelanosis, bleeding, "bumps," uniform color, variable diameter, and de novo development were the most common clinical findings.[5] This clinical description is in line with previous reports, describing childhood melanoma presenting more often as an amelanotic and nodular lesion resembling pyogenic granuloma or nonpigmented Spitz nevus.[6–8] Moreover, melanoma seems to behave differently in children compared with adults, with higher Breslow thickness at presentation, a higher incidence of lymph node involvement, but an overall better prognosis.[6,65] A marked difference seems also to exist among pediatric patients in relation to age, in terms of incidence and survival rates, with a clear cutoff represented by puberty. Concerning risk factors, the importance of a family history of melanoma has been recently confirmed in children of all ages.[5] However, the contribution of numerous acquired melanocytic nevi and personal history of more than 3 sunburns was found to be a significant risk factor for melanoma in older children, whereas the presence of darker-skinned, non-white subjects in younger pediatric cohorts (0–9 years of age) suggests the impact of genetic predisposition in younger children and the larger influence of environmental exposures for melanoma development in older children.[5] Concerning histopathologic subtypes, Paradela and colleagues[66] have recently compared the biologic behavior between spitzoid (SM) and nonspitzoid (N-SM) childhood melanoma. The authors reported children with SM to be significantly younger than those with N-SM, to have more frequently a nodular melanoma subtype with vertical growth phase, high Breslow thickness and mitotic rate, positive sentinel lymph node biopsy, and a more advanced stage. Conversely, N-SM was more often associated with a nevus (**Fig. 10**). Interestingly, the mortality rate in the SM group was lower (5.9%) than in the N-SM group (12.0%).[66] The difference in melanoma prognosis in relation to age was also reported in a study on melanoma deaths among children younger than 20 years. A total of 643 deaths were registered between 1968 and 2004 in the United States, an average of 18 per year. The overall age-adjusted mortality rate for melanoma in children was 2.25 deaths per year.[67] Interestingly, mortality rates were strongly associated with age, being 8- to 18-times higher after puberty.[67] The less aggressive behavior of childhood melanoma could be due to a lower potential for widespread distant metastases than conventional melanomas in children of a younger age who have SM. The question is open as to whether an alternative explanation for the more favorable biology of pediatric melanoma could be misdiagnosis. In several histopathologic studies, in fact, lesions initially diagnosed as

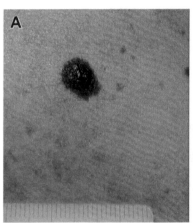
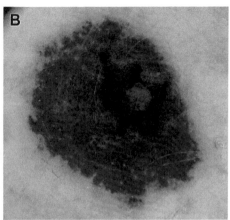

Fig. 10. (A) Melanoma in situ arising within a congenital nevus in a 17-year-old girl. The patient had a fair skin phototype and multiple nevi. (B) Dermoscopy shows a diffuse cobblestone pattern with a focal area of blue-white structures (the latter corresponding to in situ melanoma).

melanoma were reclassified as Spitz nevi/tumors when reviewed retrospectively.[68]

In this scenario, given the higher rate of sentinel lymph node involvement and overall less aggressive behavior of pediatric melanoma, the role of sentinel node biopsy as a prognostic factor in children with melanoma is highly debated. Because definitive data are currently lacking, the management of childhood melanoma should not differ from management in adults. Early detection remains the mainstay in treatment to ensure a favorable prognosis. When a suspect lesion is detected, narrow margin excision is recommended. Histopathologic evaluation should be performed by an expert dermatopathologist. In the case that a diagnosis of melanoma is confirmed, surgical excision with sufficient wide margins should be performed. The role of sentinel node biopsy and adjuvant therapies requires future clarification and needs to be considered critically, discussing the pros and cons with the parents. After surgical removal, regular clinical and dermoscopic follow-up should be scheduled according to established protocols.

SUMMARY

In the great majority of cases, children present with few, banal, nonproblematic melanocytic lesions. Thus, melanoma screening in pediatric patients is not routinely recommended before puberty. After puberty, clinical and dermoscopic follow-up is indicated for those adolescents presenting a higher total nevus count and additional risk factors, such as a family history of melanoma, fair skin phototype, and history of sunburns. In the presence of medium-sized to large or giant congenital nevi, annual clinical and dermoscopic follow-up is recommended to detect potential melanoma development at an early stage. Small, typical, pigmented or nonpigmented Spitz nevi of childhood can be managed conservatively up to puberty. Large, ulcerated, rapidly growing, nodular lesions, at any age, should be excised to rule out melanoma, keeping in mind that paradoxically the main differential diagnosis of melanoma in children is not an atypical nevus but banal nonmelanocytic lesions, such as angioma or pyogenic granuloma. The most challenging situation for clinicians dealing with pediatric patients is the excision of a spitzoid lesion that has an equivocal interpretation on histopathology. Until more definite conclusions about the benign or malignant nature of atypical Spitz tumors are available, the best management option remains wide local excision and careful follow-up. A better understanding of the biology of spitzoid lesions is mandatory to improve the clinical management of these neoplasms.

REFERENCES

1. Pappo AS. Melanoma in children and adolescents. Eur J Cancer 2003;39:2651–61.
2. Lange JR, Balch CM. Melanoma in children: heightened awareness of an uncommon but often curable malignancy. Pediatrics 2005;115:802–3.
3. Strouse JJ. Pediatric melanoma: risk factor and survival analysis of the surveillance, epidemiology and end results database. J Clin Oncol 2005;23:4735–41.
4. Schaffer JV. Pigmented lesions in children: when to worry. Curr Opin Pediatr 2007;19:430–40.
5. Cordoro KM, Gupta D, Frieden IJ, et al. Pediatric melanoma: results of a large cohort study and proposal for modified ABCD detection criteria for children. J Am Acad Dermatol 2013. http://dx.doi.org/10.1016/j.jaad.2012.12.953.

6. Ferrari A, Bono A, Baldi M, et al. Does melanoma behave differently in younger children than in adults? A retrospective study of 33 cases of childhood melanoma from a single institution. Pediatrics 2005;115:649–54.

7. Mones JM, Ackerman AB. Melanomas in prepubescent children: review comprehensively, critique historically, criteria diagnostically, and course biologically. Am J Dermatopathol 2003;25:223–38.

8. Lange JR, Palis BE, Chang DC, et al. Melanoma in children and teenagers: an analysis of patients from the National Cancer Data Base. J Clin Oncol 2007;25:1363–8.

9. Requena C, Requena L, Kutzner H, et al. Spitz nevus: a clinicopathological study of 349 cases. Am J Dermatopathol 2009;31:107–16.

10. Luo S, Sepehr A, Tsao H. Spitz nevi and other spitzoid lesions part I. Background and diagnoses. J Am Acad Dermatol 2011;65:1073–84.

11. Haliasos EC, Kerner M, Jaimes N, et al. Dermoscopy for the pediatric dermatologist part III: Dermoscopy of melanocytic lesions. Pediatr Dermatol 2012. http://dx.doi.org/10.1111/pde.12041.

12. Moscarella E, Zalaudek I, Cerroni L, et al. Excised melanocytic lesions in children and adolescents—a 10-year survey. Br J Dermatol 2012;167:368–73.

13. Tannous ZS, Mihm MC, Sober AJ, et al. Congenital melanocytic nevi: clinical and histopathologic features, risk of melanoma, and clinical management. J Am Acad Dermatol 2005;52:197–203.

14. Richardson SK, Tannous ZS, Mihm MC. Congenital and infantile melanoma: review of the literature and report of an uncommon variant, pigment-synthesizing melanoma. J Am Acad Dermatol 2002;47:77–90.

15. Spitz S. Melanomas of childhood. Am J Pathol 1948;24:591–609.

16. Paniago-Pereira C, Maize JC, Ackerman AB. Nevus of large spindle and/or epithelioid cells (Spitz's nevus). Arch Dermatol 1978;114:1811–23.

17. Spatz A, Barnhill RL. The Spitz tumor 50 years later: revisiting a landmark contribution and unresolved controversy. J Am Acad Dermatol 1999;40:223–8.

18. Barnhill RL, Argenyi ZB, From L, et al. Atypical Spitz nevi/tumors: lack of consensus for diagnosis, discrimination from melanoma, and prediction of outcome. Hum Pathol 1999;30:513–20.

19. LeBoit PE. 'Safe' spitz and its alternatives. Pediatr Dermatol 2002;19:163–5.

20. Dal Pozzo V, Benelli C, Restano L, et al. Clinical review of 247 case records of spitz nevus (epithelioid cell and/or spindle cell nevus). Dermatology 1997;194:20–5.

21. Ferrara G, Zalaudek I, Argenziano G. Spitz nevus: an evolving clinicopathologic concept. Am J Dermatopathol 2010;32:410–4.

22. Ferrara G, Errico ME, Donofrio V, et al. Melanocytic tumors of uncertain malignant potential in childhood: do we really need sentinel node biopsy? J Cutan Pathol 2012;39:1049–51.

23. Smith KJ, Barrett TL, Skelton HG, et al. Spindle cell and epithelioid cell nevi with atypia and metastasis (malignant spitz nevus). Am J Surg Pathol 1989;13:931–9.

24. Cerroni L. A new perspective for spitz tumors? Am J Dermatopathol 2005;27:366–7.

25. Urso C. A new perspective for spitz tumors? Am J Dermatopathol 2005;27:364–6.

26. Luo S, Sepehr A, Tsao H. Spitz nevi and other spitzoid lesions part II. Natural history and management. J Am Acad Dermatol 2011;65:1087–92.

27. Ferrara G, Argenziano G, Soyer HP, et al. The spectrum of Spitz nevi: a clinicopathologic study of 83 cases. Arch Dermatol 2005;141:1381–7.

28. Reed RJ, Ichinose H, Clark WH, et al. Common and uncommon melanocytic nevi and borderline melanomas. Semin Oncol 1975;2:119–47.

29. Barnhill RL, Mihm MC. Pigmented spindle cell naevus and its variants: distinction from melanoma. Br J Dermatol 1989;121:717–25.

30. Smith NP. The pigmented spindle cell tumor of Reed: an underdiagnosed lesion. Semin Diagn Pathol 1987;4:75–87.

31. Peris K, Ferrari A, Argenziano G, et al. Dermoscopic classification of Spitz/Reed nevi. Clin Dermatol 2002;20:259–62.

32. Argenziano G, Zalaudek I, Corona R, et al. Vascular structures in skin tumors: a dermoscopy study. Arch Dermatol 2004;140:1485–9.

33. Zalaudek I, Kreusch J, Giacomel J, et al. How to diagnose nonpigmented skin tumors: a review of vascular structures seen with dermoscopy: part I. Melanocytic skin tumors. J Am Acad Dermatol 2010;63:361–74 [quiz: 375–6].

34. Zalaudek I, Kittler H, Hofmann-Wellenhof R, et al. 'White' network in Spitz nevi and early melanomas lacking significant pigmentation. J Am Acad Dermatol 2013. http://dx.doi.org/10.1016/j.jaad.2012.12.974.

35. Argenziano G, Soyer HP, Ferrara G, et al. Superficial black network: an additional dermoscopic clue for the diagnosis of pigmented spindle and/or epithelioid cell nevus. Dermatology 2001;203:333–5.

36. Argenziano G, Scalvenzi M, Staibano S, et al. Dermatoscopic pitfalls in differentiating pigmented Spitz naevi from cutaneous melanomas. Br J Dermatol 1999;141:788–93.

37. Herreid PA, Shapiro PE. Age distribution of Spitz nevus vs malignant melanoma. Arch Dermatol 1996;132:352–3.

38. Brunetti B, Nino M, Sammarco E, et al. Spitz naevus: a proposal for management. J Eur Acad Dermatol Venereol 2005;19:391–3.

39. Argenziano G, Zalaudek I, Ferrara G, et al. Involution: the natural evolution of pigmented Spitz and Reed nevi? Arch Dermatol 2007;143: 549–51.

40. Argenziano G, Agozzino M, Bonifazi E, et al. Natural evolution of Spitz nevi. Dermatology 2011;222: 256–60.

41. Urso C, Borgognoni L, Saieva C, et al. Sentinel lymph node biopsy in patients with 'atypical Spitz tumors.' A report on 12 cases. Hum Pathol 2006; 37:816–23.

42. Kelley SW, Cockerell CJ. Sentinel lymph node biopsy as an adjunct to management of histologically difficult to diagnose melanocytic lesions: a proposal. J Am Acad Dermatol 2000; 42:527–30.

43. Lohmann CM, Coit DG, Brady MS, et al. Sentinel lymph node biopsy in patients with diagnostically controversial spitzoid melanocytic tumors. Am J Surg Pathol 2002;26:47–55.

44. Su LD, Fullen DR, Sondak VK, et al. Sentinel lymph node biopsy for patients with problematic spitzoid melanocytic lesions: a report on 18 patients. Cancer 2003;97:499–507.

45. Urso C, Gelli R, Borgognoni L, et al. Positive sentinel node biopsy in a 30-month-old boy with atypical Spitz tumour (Spitzoid melanoma). Histopathology 2006;48:884–6.

46. Gamblin TC, Edington H, Kirkwood JM, et al. Sentinel lymph node biopsy for atypical melanocytic lesions with spitzoid features. Ann Surg Oncol 2006;13:1664–70.

47. Murali R, Sharma RN, Thompson JF, et al. Sentinel lymph node biopsy in histologically ambiguous melanocytic tumors with spitzoid features (so-called atypical spitzoid tumors). Ann Surg Oncol 2008;15:302–9.

48. Ludgate MW, Fullen DR, Lee J, et al. The atypical Spitz tumor of uncertain biologic potential: a series of 67 patients from a single institution. Cancer 2009;115:631–41.

49. Hung T, Piris A, Lobo A, et al. Sentinel lymph node metastasis is not predictive of poor outcome in patients with problematic spitzoid melanocytic tumors. Hum Pathol 2013;44:87–94.

50. Busam KJ, Pulitzer M. Sentinel lymph node biopsy for patients with diagnostically controversial Spitzoid melanocytic tumors? Adv Anat Pathol 2008; 15:253–62.

51. Tlougan BE, Orlow SJ, Schaffer JV. Spitz nevi: beliefs, behaviors, and experiences of pediatric dermatologists. JAMA Dermatol 2013;149:283–91.

52. Alikhan A, Ibrahimi OA, Eisen DB. Congenital melanocytic nevi: where are we now? Part I. Clinical presentation, epidemiology, pathogenesis, histology, malignant transformation, and neurocutaneous melanosis. J Am Acad Dermatol 2012;67: 495.e1–17 [quiz: 512–4].

53. Marghoob AA. Congenital melanocytic nevi. Evaluation and management. Dermatol Clin 2002;20: 607–16, viii.

54. Seidenari S, Pellacani G. Surface microscopy features of congenital nevi. Clin Dermatol 2002;20: 263–7.

55. Alikhan A, Ibrahimi OA, Eisen DB. Congenital melanocytic nevi: Where are we now? Part II. Treatment options and approach to treatment. J Am Acad Dermatol 2012;67:515.e1–13 [quiz: 528–30].

56. Rhodes AR, Melski JW. Small congenital nevocellular nevi and the risk of cutaneous melanoma. J Pediatr 1982;100:219–24.

57. Bonifazi E, Bilancia M, Berloco A, et al. Malignant melanoma in children aged 0-12. Review of 289 cases of the literature. Eur J Pediatr Dermatol 2001;11:157–75.

58. Krengel S, Hauschild A, Schafer T. Melanoma risk in congenital melanocytic naevi: a systematic review. Br J Dermatol 2006;155:1–8.

59. Bett BJ. Large or multiple congenital melanocytic nevi: occurrence of neurocutaneous melanocytosis in 1008 persons. J Am Acad Dermatol 2006;54: 767–77.

60. Kadonaga JN, Frieden IJ. Neurocutaneous melanosis: definition and review of the literature. J Am Acad Dermatol 1991;24:747–55.

61. Vourc'h-Jourdain M, Martin L, Barbarot S, et al. Large congenital melanocytic nevi: therapeutic management and melanoma risk. J Am Acad Dermatol 2013;68:493–498.e1–14.

62. Lallas A, Zalaudek I, Apalla Z, et al. Management rules to detect melanoma. Dermatology 2013. http://dx.doi.org/10.1159/000346645.

63. Saida T, Oguchi S, Miyazaki A. Dermoscopy for acral pigmented skin lesions. Clin Dermatol 2002;20: 279–85.

64. Piana S, Grenzi L, Albertini G. Cellular blue nevus with satellitosis: a possible diagnostic pitfall. Am J Dermatopathol 2009;31:401–2.

65. Moore-Olufemi S, Herzog C, Warneke C, et al. Outcomes in pediatric melanoma. Ann Surg 2011;253: 1211–5.

66. Paradela S, Fonseca E, Pita-Fernández S, et al. Spitzoid and non-spitzoid melanoma in children. A prognostic comparative study. J Eur Acad Dermatol Venereol 2012. http://dx.doi.org/10.1111/j.1468-3083.2012.04686.x.

67. Lewis KG. Trends in pediatric melanoma mortality in the United States, 1968 through 2004. Dermatol Surg 2007;34:152–9.

68. Leman JA, Evans A, Mooi W, et al. Outcomes and pathological review of a cohort of children with melanoma. Br J Dermatol 2005;152:1321–3.

Problematic Lesions in the Elderly

Iris Zalaudek, MD[a,b],*, Aimilios Lallas, MD[a],
Caterina Longo, MD, PhD[a], Elvira Moscarella, MD[a],
Danica Tiodorovic-Zivkovic, MD[c], Cinzia Ricci, MD[a],
Giuseppe Albertini, MD[a], Giuseppe Argenziano, MD[a]

KEYWORDS

- Melanoma • Non-melanoma skin cancer • Dermoscopy • Geriatric • Elderly

KEY POINTS

- The age shift in the population has resulted in an overall increase in total number of melanoma and nonmelanoma skin cancers.
- Compared with younger individuals, older persons participate less frequently in skin cancer screening programs, and therefore opportunistic skin cancer screening should be promoted in this age group.
- Signs of actinic damage or the presence of suspicious skin lesions at visible body sites, such as the face or forearms, should be considered important risk factors for additional melanoma or nonmelanoma skin cancer located on generally uncovered body sites, such as the torso.
- Nevus count decreases after the fourth decade of life, and therefore elderly patients usually present with few, mainly banal intradermal nevi.
- Any newly developing, growing, or large melanocytic skin lesion in elderly patients should raise the suspicion of melanoma or nonmelanoma skin cancer.
- Awareness of the clinical and dermoscopic features of histopathologically challenging melanocytic skin lesions helps avoid misclassification of melanoma and inadequate treatment.
- Knowledge of the clinical and dermoscopic features of the most common benign skin lesions in the elderly aids the recognition of potentially suspicious skin lesions.

INTRODUCTION
Defining the Elderly

The boundary between middle and old age cannot be defined exactly, because it does not have the same meaning in all races and societies. Accordingly, the definition of an "elderly" or "old" person is somewhat arbitrary. However, most developed world countries have accepted the chronologic age of 60 years and older as a definition of "elderly."[1]

The Process of Skin Aging

Human skin undergoes chronologic changes, which affect the structure and function of the skin. The process of aging is influenced by intrinsic (physiologic aging) and extrinsic (photoaging) factors.[2,3]

Age-related changes include progressive thinning of the epidermis with loss of undulating rete pattern, decreased cell replacement of the epidermis, increased blood vessel fragility, dryness,

Study supported in part by the Italian Ministry of Health (RF-2010-2316524).
[a] Dermatology and Skin Cancer Unit, Arcispedale Santa Maria Nuova, Istituto di Ricovero e Cura a Carattere Scientifico-IRCCS, Viale Risorgimento 80, Reggio Emilia 42100, Italy; [b] Department of Dermatology, Medical University of Graz, Auenbruggerplatz 8, Graz 8036, Austria; [c] Clinic of Dermatovenerology, Clinical Center of Nis, Medical Faculty University of Nis, Bul. Dr Zorana Djindjica 81, Nis 18000, Serbia
* Corresponding author. Dermatology and Skin Cancer Unit, Arcispedale Santa Maria Nuova, IRCCS, Viale Risorgimento 80, Reggio Emilia 42100, Italy.
E-mail address: iris.zalaudek@gmail.com

derm.theclinics.com

and reduced wound healing. The number of melanocytes, fibroblasts, and Langerhans cells is decreased, causing changes in skin pigmentation, elasticity, and barrier function.

All of these changes contribute to certain dermatologic conditions, which are more commonly ascribed to the elderly. These disorders encompass a diverse array of etiologically unrelated degenerative, autoimmune, idiopathic, and neoplastic conditions that may impact quality of life and produce significant morbidity and mortality.[4–6]

As the population ages, a more complete understanding of clinical and histopathologic features unique to the geriatric dermatologic patient becomes essential.

The Magnitude of the Problem

More than 36 million people older than 65 years were alive in the United States in 2004, representing approximately 12% of the population. By 2030, this number will increase to 71 million, accounting for approximately 20% of the population.[7]

Skin diseases of the elderly will therefore represent a significant part of general dermatology in the near future.[4] Studies evaluating the prevalence of skin diseases in geriatric dermatology identified benign and malignant skin tumors among common reasons for consultation.[5]

This article reviews the epidemiologic, clinical, and dermoscopic features of common and problematic skin tumors in the elderly, and provides clues and rules for their diagnosis, management, and treatment.

COMMON MELANOCYTIC SKIN LESIONS
Age-Related Nevus Pattern

The nevus count and prevailing nevus patterns are well documented as being influenced by age and body site.[8] Nevus count increases from childhood to midlife, and decreases thereafter.[9] This dynamic is reflected by the phrase "we are born and we will die without nevi" (**Fig. 1**).

Histopathologic and dermoscopic studies report on a high prevalence of intradermal and compound nevi in both children and the elderly, dermoscopically characterized by a globular and structureless pattern, respectively.[10–20] Moreover, a small subset of compound nevi in adolescents will exhibit a peripheral rim of small brown globules; this dermoscopic pattern is a sign of growth as these nevi enlarge symmetrically with time, accompanied by a progressive development of reticular pattern, until the disappearance of peripheral globules indicates their growth stabilization.[21–24] Finally, most adults are prone to junctional or superficial compound nevi (eg, Clark nevi) with a dermoscopic reticular pattern.[11,14,25–28]

The age-related differences between nevus subtypes have led to the hypothesis that nevogenesis occurs through at least 2 distinct pathways.[29–32] One, the congenital or constitutional pathway, gives rise to globular or structureless nevi, with onset during childhood. These nevi are thought to derive from predominantly dermal melanoblasts (ie, not fully mature melanocytes), which represent persisting small congenital nevus-like proliferations that acquire the typical

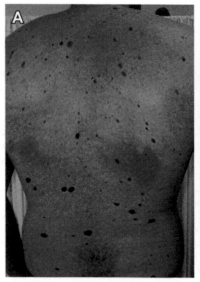
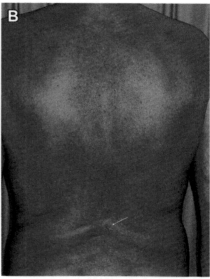

Fig. 1. In contrast to adolescents or adults, elderly people usually harbor only few, mostly intradermal nevi. (*A*) Clinical overview of the back of a 31-year-old man showing multiple, heavily pigmented nevi. (*B*) Clinical overview of the back of a 73-year-old man. Only one intradermal nevus is seen on the lower back (*arrow*).

appearance of an intradermal nevus of the Miescher or Unna type with time.

In contrast, the acquired or exogenous pathway is responsible for the formation of reticular nevi (ie, flat, Clark nevi), which initially exhibit a peripheral rim of small brown globules. These nevi are hypothesized to derive from predominantly intraepidermal melanocytes (ie, mature melanocytes), which proliferate in response to factors such as intermittent ultraviolet light exposure. These nevi seem to progressively disappear after the fourth decade of life because of involution, regression, or apoptosis.[33–35]

The dynamic of reticular nevi is further supported by 2 recent studies. The first study investigated the frequency of dermoscopic nevus subtypes by age and body site in a study cohort aged between 2 to 101 years, and showed that the number of evolving nevi, dermoscopically characterized by a peripheral rim of brown globules, increases from childhood until the second decade of life, and thereafter decreases rapidly.[22] Notably, no evolving nevus was detected in subjects older than 60 years.

The second study investigated the frequency of nevus subtypes by body site and age in a cohort aged between 60 and 89 years, and reported that nevus counts in persons older than 60 years continue to decrease, noting that this reduction was largely attributable to a reduction of flat, reticular (Clark) nevi.[34] In contrast, structureless intradermal nevi (Unna and Miescher type) persisted even into the oldest age (ie, >89 years).

Body Site–Related Patterns of Melanocytic Nevi

In addition to the age-related patterns, studies suggest that the prevailing nevus type and pattern are also influenced by the anatomic body site.

Several clinical and dermoscopic studies report a high frequency of nodular nevi (ie, intradermal nevi) on the head and neck area and upper trunk (shoulders), compared with flat and reticular nevi (ie, mostly superficial compound or junctional nevi), which can be seen in any area of the trunk but are particularly common on the extremities.[13,14,18,22,27,28]

These epidemiologic and morphologic data show that most elderly present with few, mostly intradermal, common nevi, whereas evolving nevi showing peripheral globules or large, flat, junctional (ie, reticular) melanocytic proliferations can be regarded as uncommon. This knowledge has practical implications for the diagnosis and management of some, potentially conflicting, melanocytic skin lesions in the elderly.

PROBLEMATIC MELANOCYTIC SKIN LESIONS IN THE ELDERLY
Growing Melanocytic Lesions

Although evolving nevi in adolescence are an expected finding, and therefore do not require further interventions, a melanocytic skin lesion showing signs of growth (ie, with peripheral rim of brown globules) after 50 years of age should be viewed with great caution.[21,22] The presence of peripheral globules in these older individuals can be the clue to the diagnosis of an otherwise elusive melanoma; management options include excision or close observation (Fig. 2).

Regarding the choice of monitoring (ie, short-term monitoring after 3 months or long-term monitoring after 12 months), a recent study investigating the growth patterns of melanomas detected during digital dermoscopic monitoring revealed that melanomas exhibiting globules may grow faster than melanomas characterized by a reticular pattern (ie, slow-growing melanoma).[36] As a consequence, an equivocal melanocytic skin lesion showing globules or streaks dermoscopically (both are important signs of growth) should be scheduled for short-term monitoring (ie, follow up after 2–3 months), because long-term monitoring (ie, follow up after 12 months) in the case of fast-growing melanoma could result in significant increase of tumor thickness and its related consequences.

Another interesting aspect regarding changing melanocytic nevi is provided by a recent study, which assessed the age-related frequency of changing nevi during short-term monitoring.[37] As expected, changing nevi were significantly associated with young age (0–18 years), and most nevi were reported to be banal on histopathology. Surprisingly, changing nevi were also significantly more frequent in the oldest age group (>65 years) than in middle-aged patients (36–65 years); however, in contrast to the younger age group, excised changing nevi in the elderly were more often histopathologically referred to as "dysplastic." Whether this may be related to a histopathologic underestimation of early melanomas in this age group remains to be further clarified. However, signs associated with involution (ie, any loss of structure or pigmentation) were seen in approximately 38% of changing nevi, whereas 27.6% of nevi showed an increase in size (of which 62.5% showed an asymmetric size increase). Further studies are needed to better understand the biologic significance of changing lesions in the elderly.

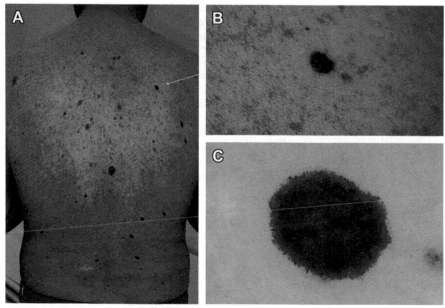

Fig. 2. Clinical overview (*A*) and close up (*B*) of a clinically symmetric and inconspicuous-appearing melanoma (thickness, 0.5 mm) located on the right shoulder of a 58-year-old man. Although the clinical appearance is unremarkable, dermoscopy displays a clear growth pattern consisting of a peripheral rim of brown globules and brown, white, red, and gray colors (*C*). (*Arrow* in [*A*] indicates the lesion shown in [*B*] and [*C*])

Atypical Lentiginous Junctional Melanocytic Nevus

In 1991, Steven Kossard described a peculiar histopathologic type of melanocytic proliferation commonly located on chronically sun-damaged skin of elderly patients, which he named *atypical lentiginous junctional nevus of the elderly*.[38,39]

Ongoing debate exists regarding whether atypical lentiginous junctional melanocytic proliferations of the elderly should be regarded as nevi with a potential risk of progression toward melanoma, or instead represent a very initial form of slow-growing melanoma in situ on sun-damaged skin. The latter view is further supported by studies reporting on associated melanomas in 38% to 75% of these junctional lesions, and the often-large size of the lesions, suggesting continuous growth.[39–41]

From a clinical standpoint, these discussions are practically irrelevant, because these lesions should be managed as if they would be melanoma in situ; in other words, complete excision with clear margins is recommended.

Clinically, these atypical lentiginous junctional melanocytic proliferations of the elderly are commonly located on the upper back, shoulders, or extremities, and present as solitary, often large (>8 mm), ill-defined macules with nuances of black, brown, gray, or white. Dermoscopically,

these lesions are typified by a more or less atypical pigmented network, diffuse structureless brown pigmentation, and areas of regression (**Fig. 3**). Digital dermoscopic follow-up studies suggest that these lentiginous atypical melanocytic proliferations may belong to a group of slow-growing melanomas, which show only subtle time-related changes and occasionally require several years to be finally recognized by digital monitoring.[41–45]

Nested Melanoma of the Elderly

Nested melanoma of the elderly was only recently described, and represents a distinct morphologic variant of superficial spreading melanoma. Given its recent identification, epidemiologic and prognostic data are scarce. Histopathologically, nested melanoma is characterized by large intraepidermal nests of melanocytes, which correspond dermoscopically to variable, large, brown to black globules over a structureless brown background that do not follow any specific arrangement.[46,47]

PROBLEMATIC LESIONS RELATED TO SPECIAL ANATOMIC BODY AREAS
Flat Pigmented Facial Lesions

The clinical recognition of lentigo maligna in the mottled chronic sun-damaged skin can be challenging, because it shares many clinical features

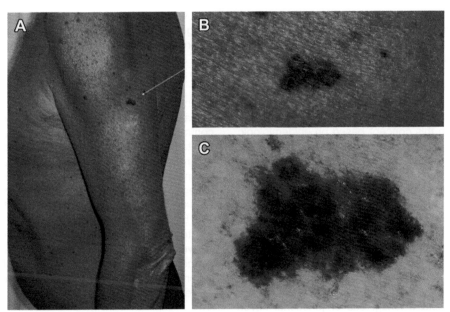

Fig. 3. Clinical overview (*A*) (*arrow* indicates the lesion shown in *B* and *C*), close up (*B*), and dermoscopy of a melanocytic lesion compatible with the diagnosis atypical junctional lentiginous melanocytic nevus versus early lentiginous melanoma. Clinically, the lesion is clearly noticeable because of its size and clinical asymmetry. In contrast to the striking clinical asymmetry, dermoscopy reveals a relatively regular network and some irregular dots and blotches (*C*).

with other pigmented macules that commonly arise on sun-damaged skin. These macules include particularly nonmelanocytic skin lesions, such as solar lentigo, flat seborrheic keratosis, regressing seborrheic keratosis (lichen planus–like keratosis), and pigmented actinic keratosis (AK).[48–52]

Notably, the list of differentials never includes "melanocytic nevus"; this can be explained by the fact that nevi on the head/neck area of elderly are usually dome-shaped, well-defined, often hypopigmented nodules (ie, intradermal nevus of the Miescher type), whereas lentigo maligna is flat and pigmented (**Fig. 4**).[11,12,18–20]

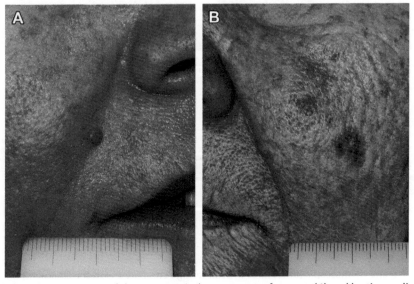

Fig. 4. The side-by-side comparison of the stereotypical appearance of a nevus (*A*) and lentigo maligna (*B*) on the face of an elderly patient explains why nevus is not included in the differential diagnosis of melanoma at this body site.

Accordingly, the clinical appearance of a nevus on the head and neck differs from that of lentigo maligna, and therefore a nevus is not considered in the differential diagnosis of flat, facial pigmented macules. This omission is further supported by a study in which no single, flat, dermoscopically reticular nevus was found on the face of subjects older than 60 years.[34]

Although this concept based on epidemiologic and clinical data sounds simple and logic, it is often only unconsciously applied in clinical practice and, accordingly, the histopathologic diagnosis of a "junctional or lentiginous nevus" of a flat, often large (>6 mm) pigmented macule on the head and neck region in an elderly patient is accepted without sufficient criticism of its clinico-pathologic validity.

In fact, on histopathologic analysis, early lentigo maligna may lack significant cytologic atypia or architectural disarrangement, making its differentiation from a lentiginous or junctional nevus challenging[51,52]; however, knowledge about the stereotypical clinical appearance of facial nevi in the elderly provides an important criterion and clue to avoid misdiagnosing an early facial melanoma as a junctional nevus.

Nevertheless, the differential diagnosis between lentigo maligna, solar lentigo, pigmented AK, and lichen planus–like keratosis remains challenging and requires consideration of important criteria, such as number of lesions, lesions surface, and color.

In the authors' experience, lentigo maligna commonly presents as a solitary, brown, poorly demarcated macule with a smooth surface; in contrast, solar lentigines and pigmented actinic keratoses are commonly numerous and reveal a rough-to-scaly surface. On dermoscopy, the single most important criterion for differentiating between benign and potentially malignant macules is related to the color; solar lentigo usually exhibits only brown color, whereas lentigo maligna or pigmented AK commonly reveal a combination of brown and gray (**Fig. 5**).[50,53,54] One exception is pigmented AK and lichen planus–like keratosis, which also show gray color on dermoscopy.[55] In these cases, a biopsy is required.[56]

Differential Diagnosis of Nodular Facial Lesions

Similar to nevi, the morphologic patterns of basal cell carcinoma (BCC) are influenced by age and

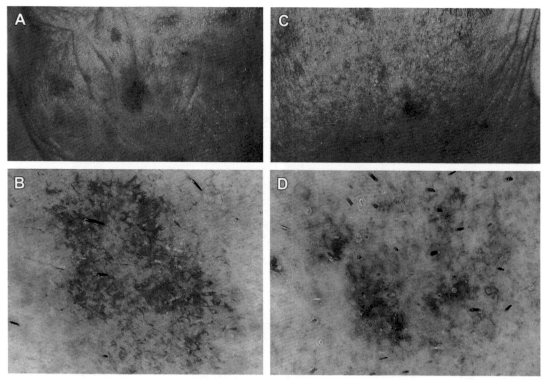

Fig. 5. Clinical (*A*) and dermoscopic (*B*) features of solar lentigo compared with the clinical (*C*) and dermoscopic (*D*) features of lentigo maligna. Although both lesions represent as flat pigmented and ill-defined macules, dermoscopy in the case of solar lentigo reveals only brown color. In contrast, lentigo maligna reveals a combination of brown and gray colors.

body site.[57–59] Most BCCs on the head and neck area are nodular, whereas flat, superficial BCCs are most commonly located on the trunk and lower extremities. Accordingly, the leading differential diagnosis of facial dermal nevus is nodular BCC.

Dermoscopy is helpful to differentiate between both entities through disclosing different vascular and/or pigmented patterns.[60,61] Vessels in intradermal nevi are usually blurred, curved, and show few ramifications. If pigment is present, it will often appear as structureless brown-gray. Instead, vessels in nodular BCC are usually dull red and sharply focused, and reveal ramifications into the finest capillaries (**Fig. 6**). In the case of pigmentation, often blue-gray roundish structures of variable size are seen.

Benign Nonmelanocytic Skin Lesions in the Elderly

In contrast to generally few nevi, skin tags, hemangiomas, and seborrheic keratosis are benign nonmelanocytic skin lesions that are frequently encountered in the elderly.[62,63] In most cases,

their clinical diagnosis does not prompt significant difficulties; however, it is has become a rule to examine all lesions using dermoscopy, irrespective of whether they look clinically benign or suspicious. This rule is based on the fact that a certain proportion of melanomas or other malignancies may masquerade clinically as benign skin lesion, which are not routinely excised.[64–68] In these cases, dermoscopy helps demask these challenging melanomas through disclosing conflicting dermoscopic patterns that do not fit with the clinical diagnosis (**Fig. 7**).[68] However, benign lesions occasionally appear clinically highly suspicious. In these cases, dermoscopy can reduce the level of suspicion through allowing the observation of patterns associated with benign skin tumors (**Fig. 8**).

NONMELANOMA SKIN CANCER

The term *nonmelanoma skin cancer* (NMSC) encompasses all cutaneous malignancies that are not melanoma, but is mainly used to define BCC and squamous cell carcinoma (SCC). Both

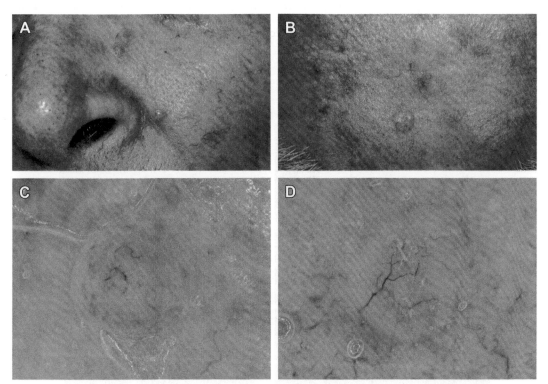

Fig. 6. The most important differential diagnosis of intradermal facial nevus (*A*) is nodular BCC (*B*). Although clinical criteria are often insufficient to differentiate between these entities, dermoscopy allows an accurate differentiation through exhibiting blurred vessels (similar to the surrounding normal dermal plexus), with few ramifications in dermal nevi (*C*), and focused bright red branching vessels in BCC (*D*). Comparing tumoral vessels with the vessels of the dermal plexus of the surrounding thinned skin is also helpful to assess the visibility of vessels.

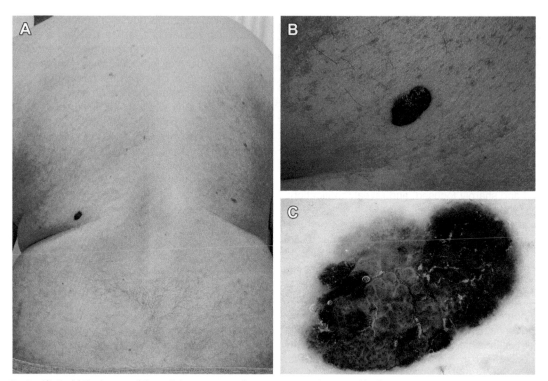

Fig. 7. Clinical (*A*), close up (*B*), and dermoscopy of a verrucous melanoma (thickness, 2.0 mm) mimicking clinically seborrheic keratosis. No criteria suggestive of seborrheic keratosis are present dermoscopically, but melanoma-associated patterns are seen, such as irregular black, brown and gray dots, blue-white structures, and irregular black blotches (*C*).

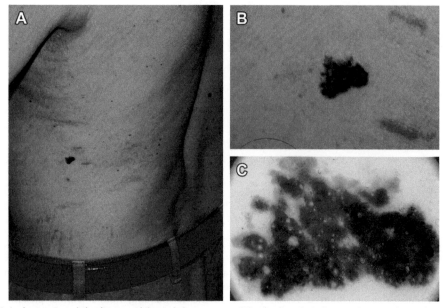

Fig. 8. Clinical overview (*A*), close up (*B*), and dermoscopy (*C*) of seborrheic keratosis mimicking clinically melanoma. Dermoscopy allows the diagnosis of seborrheic keratosis based on the presence of multiple come openings and milia cysts.

subtypes represent a common form of skin cancer in the elderly. With some exceptions, most BCCs and SCCs will not spread to other body sites. However, at advanced stages, they may cause significant morbidity, including functional and cosmetic disfigurement. Therefore, early diagnosis and adequate treatment represent key strategies for reducing BCC- and SCC-related morbidity and costs.[69,70]

FACTORS INFLUENCING THE PATTERNS OF BCC

The clinical and dermoscopic aspects of BCC are influenced by several factors, including histopathologic subtype, location, gender, age, and pigmentary trait.[57–59,71]

Most nodular BCCs occur on the head neck of elderly people (mean age, 65.5 years), whereas superficial BCCs are more common on the legs of younger individuals (mean age, 57.5 years), especially women.[57] Furthermore, nodular BCC prevails on the ears in men and the eyelids, lips, and neck in women. If BCC develops in persons of color, pigmentation is present in more than 50% of the tumors; in striking contrast, only approximately 5% of BCCs in fair-skinned individuals are pigmented (**Fig. 9**).[71] Most recently, the concept

of the signature pattern of BCC has been introduced.[72]

This concept refers to the observation that multiple BCC in an individual patient often harbor repetitive clinicodermoscopic patterns (**Fig. 10**). The fact that most BCCs in a patient reveal a similar appearance may help reduce the number of biopsies performed. This finding gains practical relevance in the presence of increasing availability of noninvasive, topical treatments of skin cancer (ie, topical chemotherapy).

PROGRESSION MODEL OF KERATINOCYTE SKIN CANCER

The term *SCC* refers to different stages in the progression of keratinocyte skin cancer, and includes AK, Bowen disease (intraepidermal carcinoma), and invasive SCC.

AKs are the most common neoplasms within the continuum of keratinocyte skin cancer. The actual risk of an individual AK progressing to fully developed is estimated to vary from as low as 0.1% to as high as 20%.[73,74]

Based on clinical characteristics, AK can be subdivided into 3 grades: grade 1 AKs are slightly palpable (better felt than seen), grade 2 are moderately thick (easily felt and seen), and grade 3 are very thick, hyperkeratotic, and/or obvious. The

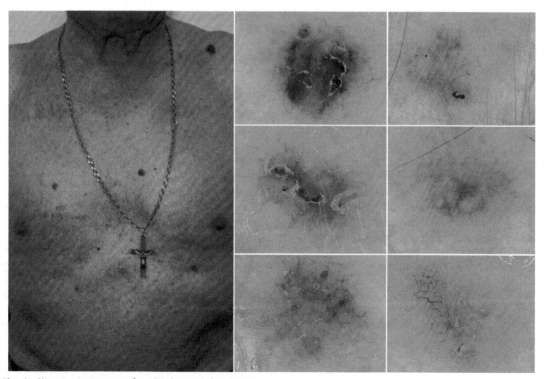

Fig. 9. Signature pattern of multiple superficial BCCs.

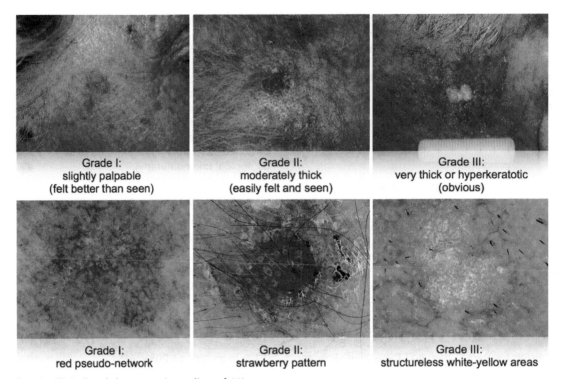

Fig. 10. Clinical and dermoscopic grading of AK.

clinical grading should aid to assess the SCC risk, whereby a high number of grade 3 AKs indicates the highest risk for developing invasive SCC. The 3 different clinical grades of AK correspond dermoscopically to 3 different patterns, namely a red pseudo-network pattern, a strawberry pattern, and a structureless yellow pattern, respectively (see **Fig. 10**).[75]

Instead, dotted vessels, diffuse yellow opaque scales, and microerosions are prevalent among SCC in situ. Hairpin vessels, linear-irregular vessels, targetoid hair follicles, white structureless areas, a central mass of keratin, and ulceration have been shown to be significantly associated with invasive SCC (**Fig. 11**).[75]

Based on the clinical and dermoscopic differences between these different types of keratinocyte skin cancer, a progression model of facial AK developing into intraepidermal carcinoma and invasive SCC has been proposed.

AKs that are at risk to progress tend to display initially a red pseudo-network (ie, expression of a dynamic horizontal growth), whereas tumoral neovascularization seen as clustered dotted and glomerular vessels are indicative of fully developed in situ SCC. With further progression of in situ to invasive SCC, the lesion thickens clinically, whereas dermoscopically, hairpin and/or linear-irregular vessels will appear. Along with these

vascular changes, dynamic changes of dyskeratinization will appear, characterized initially by fine scales in grade 1 and 2 AK, yellow opaque scales in grade 3 AK and SCC in situ, enlarged keratotic hair follicles over white background (white circles) in early invasive SCC, and lastly, the development of unordered masses of keratin.

PROBLEMS REGARDING MELANOMA AND NMSC SCREENING IN THE ELDERLY

The age shift in the population has resulted in an overall increase in the total number of skin cancers, because the incidence of both melanoma and NMSC increases with age. Indeed, 80% of NMSCs occur in people aged 60 years and older. The number of cases presenting to dermatologists is estimated to increase by 50% in 2030.[69,76]

Moreover, the incidence of melanoma in patients older than 65 years is up to 10 times higher than in patients younger than 40 years, reaching 100 cases per 100,000 in high-incidence regions of Australia.[70,77] As the geriatric age increases, especially in the United States and in Europe, melanoma will be an important public health issue during the new century.[70–74,77–81]

Although elderly patients encompass an important group among those with melanoma, studies report on a lower survival rate among elderly versus

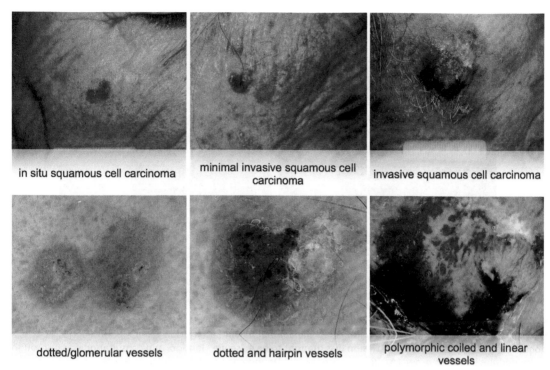

| in situ squamous cell carcinoma | minimal invasive squamous cell carcinoma | invasive squamous cell carcinoma |
| dotted/glomerular vessels | dotted and hairpin vessels | polymorphic coiled and linear vessels |

Fig. 11. Different vascular patterns at different stages of SCC progression.

younger persons.[70,77] Three main reasons seem to influence the poor outcome of melanoma in the elderly: patient awareness, tumor biology, and opportunistic skin cancer screening in the elderly.

Patient Awareness

Compared with younger individuals, older people are less attentive to skin changes, less frequently perform self-examination or partner examination (also because of loss of partner), and participate less frequently in skin cancer screening programs. Furthermore, the general low nevus density may contribute to a lower consciousness about melanoma risk (ie, undeveloped melanoma culture).[71–84] Expansion of current preventive strategies to include older age groups is therefore warranted (Fig. 12).

Tumor Biology

Studies suggest a higher frequency of biologically aggressive melanoma subtypes (ie, fast-growing nodular melanoma) in this age group.[78–83,85–91] Nodular melanoma develops de novo, grows rapidly, and lacks clinical parameters, such as asymmetry, border irregularity, color variegations, and large diameter (ABCD). By contrast, rapid growth (ie, evolution) is noted by approximately 80% of patients with nodular melanomas. This

finding has lead to the introduction of the EFG rule (elevation, firm on palpation, growth >1 month) to improve and enhance early recognition by clinicians and laypersons.[79,86] Promotion of these features to the population and primary care practitioners would be valuable in the secondary prevention of melanoma in older age groups (Fig. 13).

Opportunistic Skin Cancer Screening in the Elderly

Evidence shows that many physicians, including dermatologists, do not endorse the concept of opportunistic screening of their patients for skin cancer because of a lack of evidence for its efficacy, lack of reimbursement, and lack of time, among other factors.[84–87,91–94] However, a recent study showed that performing a total body skin examination (TBSE) for patients presenting with localized dermatologic problems allows detection of skin malignancies that would otherwise be missed.[88,95] In a population of patients who are not scheduled to undergo a complete skin examination, 47 patients need to be examined by TBSE to find 1 skin malignancy (including melanoma and NMSC), and 400 patients to find 1 melanoma. Factors that significantly increased the likelihood of finding a skin cancer by TBSE

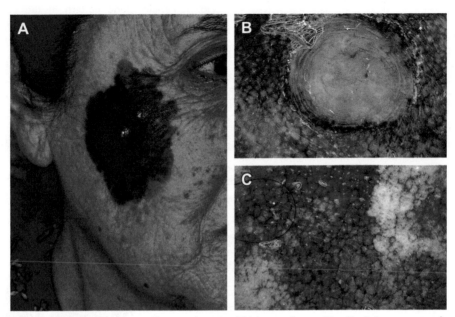

Fig. 12. This case of invasive lentigo maligna melanoma (thickness, 6 mm; 11 mitosis in correspondence to the nodular areas) suggests that poor awareness of melanoma may be one reason for the poor diagnosis of melanoma in the elderly. In this case, the lesion was thought to be a "senile" lentigo, and consultation was just sought when nodules began to grow. (*A*) Clinical overview. (*B*) Dermoscopy of the nodular area showing blue and black colors. (*C*) Dermoscopy of the flat part showing gray lines (rhomboidal structures).

were patient age (>60 years), male sex, previous NMSC, a fair skin type, and a skin tumor as the main reason of consultation. Translating these data into a simple clinical message indicates that approximately 1 of 10 patients older than 60 years and with a skin cancer on an uncovered body site will have additional suspicious lesions on covered body areas. Accordingly,

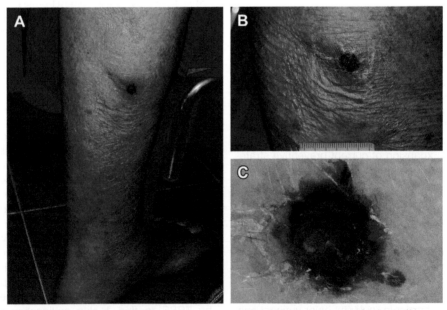

Fig. 13. Clinical overview (*A*), close up (*B*), and dermoscopy (*C*) of fast-growing and biologically aggressive melanoma (thickness, 1.7 mm) located on lower leg of an 88-year-old woman. A rapidly growing spot was noticed only 5 months before. At presentation, satellite metastases (*red* small nodules and macules in *A* and *B*) were already present.

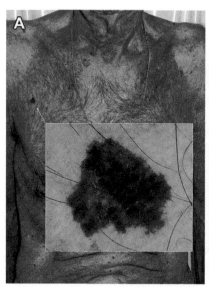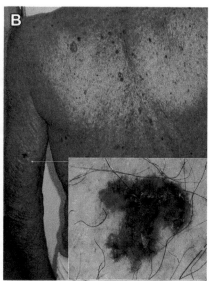

Fig. 14. Increased opportunistic screening in the elderly is likely to improve the detection of melanoma and NMSC. This patient is a 91-year-old man who was sent for the diagnosis and management of a nodular BCC on his front. On total body skin examination, 2 minimally invasive melanomas were detected on the chest and upper arm (thickness, 0.3 and 0.2 mm, respectively) (*A,B*). Dermoscopically, both melanomas showed similar patterns of a relatively regular network and diffuse areas of regression (*inserts*).

opportunistic screening, especially in older persons, has a significant chance to impact on early skin cancer detection (**Fig. 14**).[89,96]

REFERENCES

1. World Health Organization. Available at: http://www.who.int/healthinfo/survey/ageingdefnolder/en/index.html. Accessed July 19, 2013.
2. Yaar M, Gilchrest BA. Skin aging: postulated mechanisms and consequent changes in structure and function. Clin Geriatr Med 2001;17:617.
3. Debacq-Chainiaux F, Leduc C, Verbeke A, et al. UV, stress and aging. Dermatoendocrinol 2012; 4(3):236–40.
4. Makrantonaki E, Liakou AI, Eckardt R, et al. Skin diseases in geriatric patients. Epidemiologic data. Hautarzt 2012;63(12):938–46 [in German].
5. Rubegni P, Poggiali S, Nami N, et al. Skin diseases in geriatric patients: our experience from a public skin outpatient clinic in Siena. G Ital Dermatol Venereol 2012;147(6):631–6.
6. Kleinsmith DM, Perricone NV. Common skin problems in the elderly. Clin Geriatr Med 1989;5(1):189–211.
7. Administration on Aging Administration for Community Living U.S. Department of Health and Human Services. Available at: http://www.aoa.gov/Aging_Statistics/Profile/2012/3.aspx. Accessed July 19, 2013.
8. Zalaudek I, Docimo G, Argenziano G. Using dermoscopic criteria and patient-related factors for the management of pigmented melanocytic nevi. Arch Dermatol 2009;145(7):816–26.
9. Kincannon J, Boutzale C. The physiology of pigmented nevi. Pediatrics 1999;104:1042–5.
10. Worret WI, Burgdorf WH. Which direction do nevus cells move? Abtropfung reexamined. Am J Dermatopathol 1998;20(2):135–9.
11. Martinka M, Bruecks AK, Trotter MJ. Histologic spectrum of melanocytic nevi removed from patients >60 years of age. J Cutan Med Surg 2007; 11(5):168–73.
12. Yus ES, del Cerro M, Simón RS, et al. Unna's and Miescher's nevi: two different types of intradermal nevus: hypothesis concerning their histogenesis. Am J Dermatopathol 2007;29(2):141–51.
13. Scope A, Marghoob AA, Dusza SW, et al. Dermoscopic patterns of naevi in fifth grade children of the Framingham school system. Br J Dermatol 2008;158:1041–9.
14. Zalaudek I, Grinschgl S, Argenziano G, et al. Age-related prevalence of dermoscopy patterns in acquired melanocytic naevi. Br J Dermatol 2006;154:299–304.
15. Seidenari S, Pellacani G, Martella A, et al. Instrument-, age- and site-dependent variations of dermoscopic patterns of congenital melanocytic naevi: a multicentre study. Br J Dermatol 2006;155:56–61.
16. Changchien L, Dusza SW, Agero AL, et al. Age- and site-specific variation in the dermoscopic patterns

of congenital melanocytic nevi: an aid to accurate classification and assessment of melanocytic nevi. Arch Dermatol 2007;143:1007–14.

17. Niederkorn A, Ahlgrimm-Siess V, Fink-Puches R, et al. Frequency, clinical and dermoscopic features of benign papillomatous melanocytic naevi (Unna type). Br J Dermatol 2009;161(3):510–4.

18. Witt C, Krengel S. Clinical and epidemiological aspects of subtypes of melanocytic nevi (Flat nevi, Miescher nevi, Unna nevi). Dermatol Online J 2010;16(1):1.

19. Ackerman AB, Milde P. Naming acquired melanocytic nevi. Common and dysplastic, normal and atypical, or Unna, Miescher, Spitz, and Clark? Am J Dermatopathol 1992;14(5):447–53.

20. Sowa J, Kobayashi H, Ishii M, et al. Histopathologic findings in Unna's nevus suggest it is a tardive congenital nevus. Am J Dermatopathol 2008; 30(6):561–6.

21. Kittler H, Seltenheim M, Dawid M, et al. Frequency and characteristics of enlarging common melanocytic nevi. Arch Dermatol 2000;136:316–20.

22. Zalaudek I, Schmid K, Marghoob AA, et al. Frequency of dermoscopic nevus subtypes by age and body site: a cross-sectional study. Arch Dermatol 2011;147(6):663–70.

23. Zalaudek I, Guelly C, Pellacani G, et al. The dermoscopical and histopathological patterns of nevi correlate with the frequency of BRAF mutations. J Invest Dermatol 2011;131(2):542–5.

24. Pellacani G, Scope A, Ferrari B, et al. New insights into nevogenesis: in vivo characterization and follow-up of melanocytic nevi by reflectance confocal microscopy. J Am Acad Dermatol 2009; 61(6):1001–13.

25. Cohen LM, Bennion SD, Johnson TW, et al. Hypermelanotic nevus: clinical, histopathologic, and ultrastructural features in 316 cases. Am J Dermatopathol 1997;19(1):23–30.

26. Westhafer J, Gildea J, Klepeiss S, et al. Age distribution of biopsied junctional nevi. J Am Acad Dermatol 2007;56(5):825–7.

27. Douglas NC, Borgovan T, Carroll MJ, et al. Dermoscopic naevus patterns in people at high versus moderate/low melanoma risk in Queensland. Australas J Dermatol 2011;52(4):248–53.

28. Gamo R, Malvehy J, Puig S, et al. Dermoscopic features of melanocytic nevi in seven different anatomical locations in patients with atypical nevi syndrome. Dermatol Surg 2013;39(6):864–71.

29. Zalaudek I, Hofmann-Wellenhof R, Kittler H, et al. A dual concept of nevogenesis: theoretical considerations based on dermoscopic features of melanocytic nevi. J Dtsch Dermatol Ges 2007;5(11):985–92.

30. Zalaudek I, Catricalà C, Moscarella E, et al. What dermoscopy tells us about nevogenesis. J Dermatol 2011;38(1):16–24.

31. Zalaudek I, Leinweber B, Hofmann-Wellenhof R, et al. The epidermal and dermal origin of melanocytic tumors: theoretical considerations based on epidemiologic, clinical, and histopathologic findings. Am J Dermatopathol 2008;30(4):403–6.

32. Zalaudek I, Marghoob AA, Scope A, et al. Age distribution of biopsied junctional nevi–Unna's concept versus a dual concept of nevogenesis. J Am Acad Dermatol 2007;57(6):1096–7.

33. Terushkin V, Scope A, Halpern AC, et al. Pathways to involution of nevi: insights from dermoscopic follow-up. Arch Dermatol 2010;146:459–60.

34. Piliouras P, Gilmore S, Wurm EM, et al. New insights in naevogenesis: number, distribution and dermoscopic patterns of naevi in the elderly. Australas J Dermatol 2011;52(4):254–8.

35. Zalaudek I, Donati P, Catricalà C, et al. "Dying nevus" or regressing melanoma. Hautarzt 2011; 62(4):293–6 [in Italian].

36. Beer J, Xu L, Tschandl P, et al. Growth arte of melanoma in vivo and correlation with dermatoscopic and dermatopathologic findings. Dermatol Pract Concept 2011;1(1):13.

37. Menzies SW, Stevenson ML, Altamura D, et al. Variables predicting change in benign melanocytic nevi undergoing short-term dermoscopic imaging. Arch Dermatol 2011;147(6):655–9.

38. Kossard S, Commens C, Symons M, et al. Lentiginous dysplastic naevi in the elderly: a potential precursor for malignant melanoma. Australas J Dermatol 1991;32(1):27–37.

39. Kossard S. Atypical lentiginous junctional naevi of the elderly and melanoma. Australas J Dermatol 2002;43(2):93–101.

40. King R, Page RN, Googe PB, et al. Lentiginous melanoma: a histologic pattern of melanoma to be distinguished from lentiginous nevus. Mod Pathol 2005;18(10):1397–401.

41. Ferrara G, Zalaudek I, Argenziano G. Lentiginous melanoma: a distinctive clinicopathological entity. Histopathology 2008;52(4):523–5.

42. Terushkin V, Dusza SW, Scope A, et al. Changes observed in slow-growing melanomas during long-term dermoscopic monitoring. Br J Dermatol 2012;166(6):1213–20.

43. Argenziano G, Kittler H, Ferrara G, et al. Slow-growing melanoma: a dermoscopy follow-up study. Br J Dermatol 2010;162(2):267–73.

44. Roma P, Savarese I, Martino A, et al. Slow-growing melanoma: report of five cases. J Dermatol Case Rep 2007;1(1):1–3.

45. Argenziano G, Zalaudek I, Ferrara G. Fast-growing and slow-growing melanomas. Arch Dermatol 2007;143(6):802–3 [author reply: 803–4].

46. Kutzner H, Metzler G, Argenyi Z, et al. Histological and genetic evidence for a variant of superficial

spreading melanoma composed predominantly of large nests. Mod Pathol 2012;25(8):1178.

47. Pennacchia I, Garcovich S, Gasbarra R, et al. Morphological and molecular characteristics of nested melanoma of the elderly (evolved lentiginous melanoma). Virchows Arch 2012;461(4):433–9.

48. Tanaka M, Sawada M, Kobayashi K. Key points in dermoscopic differentiation between lentigo maligna and solar lentigo. J Dermatol 2011;38(1):53–8.

49. Sahin MT, Oztürkcan S, Ermertcan AT, et al. A comparison of dermoscopic features among lentigo senilis/initial seborrheic keratosis, seborrheic keratosis, lentigo maligna and lentigo maligna melanoma on the face. J Dermatol 2004;31(11):884–9.

50. Pralong P, Bathelier E, Dalle S, et al. Dermoscopy of lentigo maligna melanoma: report of 125 cases. Br J Dermatol 2012;167(2):280–7.

51. Situm M, Buljan M. Surgical and histologic pitfalls in the management of lentigo maligna melanoma. G Ital Dermatol Venereol 2012;147(1):21–7.

52. McGuire LK, Disa JJ, Lee EH, et al. Melanoma of the lentigo maligna subtype: diagnostic challenges and current treatment paradigms. Plast Reconstr Surg 2012;129(2):288e–99e.

53. Schiffner R, Schiffner-Rohe J, Vogt T, et al. Improvement of early recognition of lentigo maligna using dermatoscopy. J Am Acad Dermatol 2000; 42(1 Pt 1):25–32.

54. Stolz W, Schiffner R, Burgdorf WH. Dermatoscopy for facial pigmented skin lesions. Clin Dermatol 2002;20(3):276–8.

55. Bugatti L, Filosa G. Dermoscopy of lichen planus-like keratosis: a model of inflammatory regression. J Eur Acad Dermatol Venereol 2007; 21(10):1392–7.

56. Moscarella E, Zalaudek I, Pellacani G, et al. Lichenoid keratosis-like melanomas. J Am Acad Dermatol 2011;65(3):e85–7.

57. Bastiaens MT, Hoefnagel JJ, Bruijn JA, et al. Differences in age, site distribution, and sex between nodular and superficial basal cell carcinoma indicate different types of tumors. J Invest Dermatol 1998;110:880–4.

58. Betti R, Radaelli G, Mussino F, et al. Anatomic location and histopathologic subtype of basal cell carcinomas in adults younger than 40 or 90 and older: any difference? Dermatol Surg 2009;35(2): 201–6.

59. Scrivener Y, Grosshans E, Cribier B. Variations of basal cell carcinomas according to gender, age, location and histopathological subtype. Br J Dermatol 2002;147(1):41–7.

60. Zalaudek I, Kreusch J, Giacomel J, et al. How to diagnose nonpigmented skin tumors: a review of vascular structures seen with dermoscopy: part I. Melanocytic skin tumors. J Am Acad Dermatol 2010;63(3):361–74 [quiz: 375–6].

61. Zalaudek I, Kreusch J, Giacomel J, et al. How to diagnose nonpigmented skin tumors: a review of vascular structures seen with dermoscopy: part II. Nonmelanocytic skin tumors. J Am Acad Dermatol 2010;63(3):377–86 [quiz: 387–8].

62. Yeatman JM, Kilkenny M, Marks R. The prevalence of seborrhoeic keratoses in an Australian population: does exposure to sunlight play a part in their frequency? Br J Dermatol 1997;137(3):411–4.

63. Hafner C, Vogt T. Seborrheic keratosis. J Dtsch Dermatol Ges 2008;6(8):664–77.

64. Izikson L, Sober AJ, Mihm MC Jr, et al. Prevalence of melanoma clinically resembling seborrheic keratosis: analysis of 9204 cases. Arch Dermatol 2002; 138(12):1562–6.

65. Argenziano G, Rossiello L, Scalvenzi M, et al. Melanoma simulating seborrheic keratosis: a major dermoscopy pitfall. Arch Dermatol 2003;139(3): 389–91.

66. Chamberlain A, Ng J. Cutaneous melanoma—atypical variants and presentations. Aust Fam Physician 2009;38(7):476–82.

67. Zalaudek I, Ferrara G, Di Stefani A, et al. Dermoscopy for challenging melanoma: how to raise the 'red flag' when melanoma clinically looks benign. Br J Dermatol 2005;153(1):200–2.

68. Puig S, Argenziano G, Zalaudek I, et al. Melanomas that failed dermoscopic detection: a combined clinicodermoscopic approach for not missing melanoma. Dermatol Surg 2007;33(10): 1262–73.

69. Rubin AI, Chen EH, Ratner D. Basal cell carcinoma. N Engl J Med 2005;353(21):2262–9.

70. Alam M, Ratner D. Cutaneous squamous cell carcinoma. N Engl J Med 2001;344(13):975–83.

71. Bradford PT. Skin cancer in skin of color. Dermatol Nurs 2009;21(4):170–8.

72. Zalaudek I, Moscarella E, Longo C, et al. The "signature" pattern of multiple basal cell carcinomas. Arch Dermatol 2012;148(9):1106.

73. Glogau RG. The risk of progression to invasive disease. J Am Acad Dermatol 2000;42:23–4.

74. Marks R, Rennie G, Selwood TS. Malignant transformation of solar keratoses to squamous cell carcinoma. Lancet 1988;8589:795–7.

75. Zalaudek I, Giacomel J, Schmid K, et al. Dermatoscopy of facial actinic keratosis, intraepidermal carcinoma, and invasive squamous cell carcinoma: a progression model. J Am Acad Dermatol 2012; 66(4):589–97.

76. Madan V, Lear JT, Szeimies RM. Non-melanoma skin cancer. Lancet 2010;375(9715):673–85.

77. Lasithiotakis KG, Petrakis IE, Garbe C. Cutaneous melanoma in the elderly: epidemiology, prognosis and treatment. Melanoma Res 2010;20(3):163–70.

78. Pollack SV. Skin cancer in the elderly. Clin Geriatr Med 1987;3(4):715–28.

79. Austin PF, Cruse CW, Lyman G, et al. Age as a prognostic factor in the malignant melanoma population. Ann Surg Oncol 1994;1(6):487–94.

80. Keller KL, Fenske NA, Glass LF. Cancer of the skin in the older patient. Clin Geriatr Med 1997;13(2):339–61.

81. Janda M, Youl PH, Lowe JB, et al. What motivates men age > or =50 years to participate in a screening program for melanoma? Cancer 2006;107(4):815–23.

82. Aitken JF, Janda M, Lowe JB, et al. Prevalence of whole-body skin self-examination in a population at high risk for skin cancer (Australia). Cancer Causes Control 2004;15:453–63.

83. Geller AC, Sober AJ, Zhang Z, et al. Strategies for improving melanoma education and screening for men age Z 50 years: findings from the American academy of dermatological national skin cancer screening program. Cancer 2002;95:1554–61.

84. Oliveria SA, Christos PJ, Halpern AC, et al. Evaluation of factors associated with skin self-examination. Cancer Epidemiol Biomarkers Prev 1999;8:971–8.

85. Chamberlain AJ, Fritschi L, Kelly JW. Nodular melanoma: patients' perceptions of presenting features and implications for earlier detection. J Am Acad Dermatol 2003;48:694–701.

86. Chamberlain AJ, Kelly JW. Nodular melanomas and older men: a major challenge for community surveillance programs. Med J Aust 2004;180:432.

87. Lipsker D, Engel F, Cribier B, et al. Trends in melanoma epidemiology suggest three different types of melanoma. Br J Dermatol 2007;157(2):338–43.

88. Mar V, Roberts H, Wolfe R, et al. Nodular melanoma: a distinct clinical entity and the largest contributor to melanoma deaths in Victoria, Australia. J Am Acad Dermatol 2012;68(4):568–75.

89. Demierre MF, Chung C, Miller DR, et al. Early detection of thick melanomas in the United States: beware of the nodular subtype. Arch Dermatol 2005;141(6):745–50.

90. Hersey P, Sillar RW, Howe CG, et al. Factors related to the presentation of patients with thick primary melanomas. Med J Aust 1991;154(9):583–7.

91. Geller AC, O'Riordan DL, Oliveria SA, et al. Overcoming obstacles to skin cancer examinations and prevention counseling for high-risk patients: results of a national survey of primary care physicians. J Am Board Fam Pract 2004;17(6):416–23.

92. Oliveria SA, Christos PJ, Marghoob AA, et al. Skin cancer screening and prevention in the primary care setting: national ambulatory medical care survey 1997. J Gen Intern Med 2001;16(5):297–301.

93. Geller AC, Koh HK, Miller DR, et al. Use of health services before the diagnosis of melanoma: implications for early detection and screening. J Gen Intern Med 1992;7(2):154–7.

94. Altman JF, Oliveria SA, Christos PJ, et al. A survey of skin cancer screening in the primary care setting: a comparison with other cancer screenings. Arch Fam Med 2000;9(10):1022–7.

95. Argenziano G, Zalaudek I, Hofmann-Wellenhof R, et al. Total body skin examination for skin cancer screening in patients with focused symptoms. J Am Acad Dermatol 2012;66(2):212–9.

96. Fontaine J, Mielczarek S, Meaume S, et al. Incidence of undiagnosed skin cancers in a geriatric hospital. Ann Dermatol Venereol 2008;135(10):651–5.

Monitoring Patients with Multiple Nevi

Susana Puig, PhD, Josep Malvehy, PhD*

KEYWORDS

- Melanocytic nevi • Melanoma • Atypical mole syndrome • Dermoscopy • Follow-up

KEY POINTS

- Early recognition is the most effective intervention to improve melanoma prognosis.
- Early diagnosis of melanoma in atypical mole patients, with a reduced number of unnecessary biopsies of benign lesions, may be challenging.
- Stratification of risk in patients with multiple nevi is useful to guide the strategy for early diagnosis of melanoma. Clinical factors, such as age, number of nevi, atypical mole syndrome, history of melanoma, and/or genetic background, are of major importance. Dermoscopic information of the lesions (features of melanoma, complex pattern, and comparative analyses) should also be used in the evaluation of patients with multiple nevi.
- Patient-based skin self-examination (SSE) with the support of pictures (print books or digital images) and periodic physician-based total-body skin examination are recommended in patients with multiple nevi.
- Dermoscopy, total-body photography (TBD), and digital dermatoscopy (DD) have been proved to improve accuracy in the early detection of melanoma in high-risk patients with atypical mole syndrome.
- Digital follow-up (DFU) in atypical mole syndrome patients allows the detection of new lesions and changes in preexisting lesions.
- Some changes in dermoscopy have been associated with malignancy in the context of atypical mole syndrome patients.
- Risk factors to take into account when detecting malignant melanoma during follow-up are patient age and clinical background (previous melanoma, familial melanoma, and number of atypical lesions).

In patients with multiple nevi, management goals are early diagnosis of melanoma and avoidance of unnecessary biopsies of benign lesions.

Stratification of the risk of developing melanoma in cases of multiple nevi is of great importance to establish the best strategies and follow-up methods.

Atypical nevi count is confirmed to increase the risk factor for melanoma 10-fold in different studies. If a patient has a history of melanoma (personal or family) or genetic mutations in high penetrance genes, the risk increases significantly.

Strategies for early detection of melanoma in patients with multiple nevi include body self-examination, total-body examination, dermoscopy, digital monitoring with TBP and DD, and computer-assisted diagnosis.

Melanoma Unit, Dermatology Department, Hospital Clinic of Barcelona, IDIBAPS, Villarroel 170, Barcelona 08036, Spain
* Correspondence author.
E-mail address: jmalvehy@gmail.com

Dermatol Clin 31 (2013) 565–577
http://dx.doi.org/10.1016/j.det.2013.06.004
0733-8635/13/$ – see front matter © 2013 Published by Elsevier Inc.

INTRODUCTION

Early recognition is the most effective intervention to improve melanoma prognosis.[1] It has been demonstrated that dermoscopy improves the diagnostic accuracy of cutaneous neoplasms, and, to date, 3 meta-analyses concluded that dermoscopy is more accurate than naked eye examination for the diagnosis of cutaneous melanoma.[2–4]

Nevertheless, melanoma may be not only clinically but also dermoscopically indistinguishable from melanocytic nevi, especially in incipient lesions in which specific criteria for malignancy may not be present[5]; thus, in patients with many atypical moles, sometimes hundreds, a great number of excisions is not practical and does not avoid the misdiagnosis of an early melanoma.

On the basis of benign lesions remaining stable versus melanoma tending to change over time, various strategies have been proposed for melanoma detection in high-risk patients, such as SSE total cutaneous examination,[6,7] TBP,[8–10] dermoscopy,[11–14] and a combination of TBP and digital dermoscopy.[14–17]

Management goals

- Early diagnosis of multiple melanoma (MM)

Early recognition is the most effective intervention to improve melanoma prognosis.[18] A large body of evidence suggests that the number of melanocytic nevi represents a good predictor for cutaneous malignant melanoma and that atypical nevi may play an independent role.[19–23] Risk of melanoma changes with the type of nevi and number of lesions.[24]

- Avoidance of unnecessary biopsies

Early recognition of melanoma is challenging in patients with multiple nevi. The limitation of the identification of melanoma at early stages is even more evident in cases of atypical mole syndrome with multiple melanocytic lesions exhibiting clinical melanoma features. In this context, different methods are recommended to detect malignant lesions and reduce the number of excisions of benign equivocal melanocytic lesions.

- Optimize costs

The ideal strategies for early detection of melanoma in patients with multiple nevi have to consider the efficacy and cost of their implementation. The identification of risk factors in patients can optimize the impact of a surveillance program. From educational strategies to sophisticated digital imaging to detect changes or new lesions in high-risk patients, different strategies have to be considered.

Strategies

- Identification of risk factors for melanoma in patients with multiple nevi
  - Atypical mole syndrome
  - Total number of nevi
  - Personal and family history of melanoma
  - Genetic susceptibility: high penetrance genes
- Strategies for early detection of melanoma in patients with multiple nevi
  - Patient-based SSE
  - Physician-based total-body skin examination
  - Clinical comparative approach: ugly duckling sign
  - Dermoscopic examination
  - Dermoscopic comparative approach
  - The 4 × 4 × 6 rule
  - Digital Follow-up (DFU): Total-body photography (TBP) + Digital Dermoscopy (DD)
    - Methods of digital monitoring
    - Short-term versus medium/long-term follow-up
    - Patients to be included in digital monitoring
    - Interval and length of follow-up
    - Number of monitored lesions and melanomas
    - Length of follow-up and diagnosis of melanoma
    - Criteria for lesions to be monitored or excised
    - Characteristics of melanomas detected during DFU
    - Compliance of patients
  - Computer-assisted diagnosis and other strategies

IDENTIFICATION OF RISK FACTORS FOR MELANOMA IN PATIENTS WITH MULTIPLE NEVI

Stratification of the risk of developing melanoma in cases of multiple nevi is of great value. The identification of some or several such factors is mandatory to establish the best strategies and methods to follow-up patients. The main known risk factors may be classified as atypical mole syndrome and number of nevi, personal/familial history of melanoma, and genetic background. The efficacy of periodic surveillance is appropriate in high-risk subjects and the strategies of follow-up should be adapted to the risk assessment.[25,26]

Atypical Mole Syndrome

The first report on increased incidence of melanomas in families with multiple melanocytic nevi was published by Clark in 1978.[27] He introduced a pathogenetic model for the stepwise development of MM from dysplastic melanocytic nevi, originally using the term, B-K mole syndrome (B and K were the initials of the last names of the first individuals reported).

The atypical or dysplastic nevus syndrome (Clark nevus syndrome) is characterized by multiple atypical moles that continue to appear in adulthood. It was reported worldwide that persons with atypical mole (dysplastic nevus) syndrome are at much higher risk. Greene and colleagues[28] estimated that a person with dysplastic nevi and at least 2 family members with melanoma had a 500-fold increased melanoma risk. In unselected series, however, this syndrome accounts for less than 5% of the total melanoma incidence. Furthermore, in many of these families, dysplastic nevi and environmental factors are involved.

Statistically significant associations were found between nevi (common and atypical) count and melanoma in meta-analyses of the studies on the risk of developing melanoma.[24] Atypical nevi count is confirmed to be a highly significant risk factor for melanoma in several studies. Presence of any atypical nevus increases the risk 10-fold compared with the absence of atypical nevi (relative risk [RR] 10.12; 95% CI, 5.04, 20.32).

Total Number of Nevi

Individuals with a high nevus count (more than 100 nevi) have an almost 7-times (pooled RR 6.89; 95% CI, 4.63, 10.25) higher risk of developing melanoma than people with few nevi. The number of common nevi indicates a significant risk for melanoma even in individuals with a medium to low nevus count (<40 nevi count) compared with those with few nevi (<15 nevi) (pooled RR 1.47; 95% CI, 1.36, 1.59).[24]

It has been suggested that a high number of nevi on the arms may be considered an indicator for an increased total nevus count. It has been shown that the risk for melanoma in people with 11 to 15 common nevi on their arms is almost 5 times greater than risk for people with no nevi on arms (pooled RR 4.82; 95% CI, 3.05, 7.62).

Prophylactic excision of melanocytic nevi was proposed in the past with the assumption that this strategy reduces the risk of melanoma. The hypothesis that melanocytes in nevi are prone to

undergo malignant transformation is based on the observation that approximately two-thirds to three-quarters of patients with melanomas report a preexisting lesion at the site of melanoma. Moreover, nevus-associated melanomas comprise approximately 25% of all melanomas in histopathological series.[29] It should be kept in mind, however, that histopathologic studies are biased by considering only excised lesions. In light of the high number of nevi that are never excised, the effective risk of an individual nevus of developing melanoma during a lifetime is low and has been estimated at approximately 1 of 33,000 nevi. Therefore, the strategy of prophylactic excision of melanocytic nevi in patients with multiple lesions is not recommended, because it neither reduces the risk of melanoma (approximately 75% develop de novo) nor the need for regular surveillance in these patients.

Personal or Family History of Melanoma

Subjects with family history of melanoma, having 1 or more affected first-degree relatives, harbor a higher risk of melanoma. Moreover, families with multiple cases of melanoma often exhibit the atypical or dysplastic nevus syndrome (Clark nevus syndrome). The association of melanoma with a family history of the disease seems independent of the total nevus count. When the 2 factors are present in an individual, the risk is superior than the presence of either 1 of the 2 factors or their absence.

Genetic Susceptibility: High Penetrance Genes

Approximately 10% of cutaneous melanomas occur in a familial setting. Two main genes involved in melanoma susceptibility have been described: CDKN2A, located on chromosome 9p21, encoding 2 distinct proteins, p16INK4A and p14ARF, and CDK4, an oncogene located in 12q13.[30-33]

Germline CDKN2A mutations have been described in 10% to 50% of melanoma-prone families from several countries[33-38] and in patients with more than 1 primary cutaneous melanoma without a familial history.[36] These patients have an increased risk of carrying mutations in CDKN2A, which are detected in 8.3% to 15% of multiple primary melanoma patients irrespective of the family history,[14-16] in 9% to 12% of sporadic cases, and in 47.8% of familial cases.[38]

In patients with multiple primary melanomas it was demonstrated that atypical mole syndrome was a major risk factor with a genotype/phenotype correlation in patients and their families.[36] Atypical mole syndrome has been observed in approximately 80% of patients with multiple primary melanomas. This is more frequent than expected in sporadic melanoma, suggesting that the atypical mole phenotype may be a cofactor that contributes to the development of MMs.[23] Recently, different genetic loci have been shown involved in nevogenicity.[39–41]

Numerous moles might indicate a greater genetic tendency to develop melanoma. Although no major gene conferring an increasing risk has been identified, except for CDKN2A and CDK4 in melanoma-prone families, the possibility that some of the genes associated with nevi may play a direct role in melanoma progression cannot be excluded.

STRATEGIES FOR EARLY DETECTION OF MELANOMA IN PATIENTS WITH MULTIPLE NEVI

In patients with atypical moles, different strategies have been introduced to allow the early detection of melanoma, minimizing the number of unnecessary excisions. These strategies are SEE, total-body examination, dermoscopy, digital monitoring, TBP + DD, and computer-assisted diagnosis.

Patient-Based Skin Self-Examination

Approximately 75% of melanomas are detected by patients themselves or by spouses, friends, or other laypersons. SSE has been shown to result in significantly lower melanoma-related mortality because of earlier diagnosis.[42] Dermatologic and cancer societies recommend monthly, whole-body SSE for high-risk populations, such as melanoma survivors or patients with atypical mole syndrome. Despite this evidence and recommendation, the prevalence of systematic and regular SSE is low among patients.[43,44] This can be improved through patient education. Dermatologic education is effective, however, only in approximately 50% of the cases and little is known about the characteristics of those who do not respond to questionnaires in published studies. In the current literature, psychosocial variables, like distress, coping with cancer, and partner and physician support, have been shown essential for other health behaviors and for adherence to medical advice. The prevalence of thorough SSE diminishes during the months after standardized dermatologic education on SSE. Female gender in different studies predicts better SSE in terms of frequency and completeness. Psychosocial variables, including partner and physician support, psychological distress, and coping strategies, have a significant impact on SSE performance.

Physician and partner support of SSE play an important role for SSE. Strategies based on nurse-delivered intervention have been effective at increasing patient adherence to SSE. Using digital photographs as an adjunct to screening seems to increase patient adherence to performing SSE.[42,45] A recent proliferation of melanoma detection e-health tools—digital resources that facilitate screening in patients often outside the clinical setting—may offer new strategies to promote adherence and expand the proportion and range of individuals performing SSE.

SSE, with the aid of photo-print books or digital images, has been advocated in pigmented skin lesion clinics.[46] Patients are advised to check their moles to detect changes or new moles. In France, a method consisting of SSE with full-resolution posters of the body is used in patients with multiple nevi (Narcissus method). Patients use the poster at home to compare their moles and detect changes. The recent proliferation of e-health tools for melanoma detection—digital resources that facilitate screening in patients often outside the clinical setting—may be useful to promote adherence and expand the proportion and range of individuals performing SSE. In the future, new software, such as apps dedicated to confirming changes in moles, will be clinically validated and introduced to support SSE.

Physician-Based Total-Body Skin Examination

Periodic total-body examination remains mandatory for early detection of melanoma in high-risk patients because early melanoma may be difficult to recognize by SSE. In a review of studies of digital follow-up, patients monitored because of atypical mole syndrome were not aware of any change in their melanomas detected during follow-up.[47] In the past few decades, in patients with low mole numbers, dermatologists in Australia and New Zealand devised a strategy consisting of TBP of every single mole by a nurse and review of the images by a physician experienced in dermoscopy (Moletech).

Clinical Comparative Approach: Ugly Duckling Sign

In the context patients with multiple melanocytic lesions, the clinical information should consider age, skin type, location, changes, and genetic background.

In the physical examination of patient lesions, a comparative analysis approach is advocated to detect an ugly duckling lesion.[48] According to this strategy, melanocytic lesions in patients tend to follow a predominant pattern of colors and size. The ugly duckling lesion differs from other patient lesions. Because melanoma is a malignant tumor, the growth of the lesion is different from common and atypical nevi. This strategy has been postulated as more efficient for detection of melanoma in patients with multiple nevi with respect to the analytical approach of the ABCD (asymmetry, border irregularity, color variegation, diameter greater than 6 mm) rule.[49] Unfortunately, the ugly duckling sign is not always sufficient to discriminate an early melanoma in the context of patients with many atypical looking moles. Melanoma in these patients may be similar to other lesions, and the correlation of the clinical atypia with histopathologic atypia or even melanoma is low. Melanoma can be a less atypical lesion in patients with multiple nevi with the so-called Little Red Riding Hood sign.[50]

Dermoscopic Examination

Dermoscopy (also called dermatoscopy) is a technique that increases the accuracy of melanoma diagnosis in approximately 27% compared with examination with the naked eye, improving the clinical decision making of dermatologists.

Dermoscopy has been shown to increase accuracy in detecting inconspicuous malignant melanoma in clinically equivocal lesions in 3 meta-analyses.[4,23] The specific dermoscopic melanoma features are well established and the evidence strongly recommends its use for examining patients with skin tumors and, at the present, is included in most of the international melanoma guidelines.

Based on the most common dermoscopic patterns associated with melanocytic nevi, a recently proposed nevus classification includes 4 main categories: globular, reticular, starburst, and homogeneous blue nevi.[51] In this classification, the globular category includes small congenital nevi, compound nevi, and dermal nevi grouped together based on their common dermoscopic-histopathologic features (globules correspond to predominantly dermal nests of melanocytes). The reticular nevi correspond typically to junctional or lentiginous nevi with the exception of congenital nevi of the lower extremities. A third category of nevi is defined by the starburst nevus that includes both pigmented Reed nevi and Spitz nevi. Finally, the fourth group incorporates the spectrum of blue nevi. This is defined dermoscopically by homogeneous structureless blue pigmentation without additional dermoscopic features.

Even though atypical melanocytic proliferations may exhibit each of the 4 dermoscopic patterns, either alone or in combination, their patterns and pigment distribution tend to exhibit more complexity and asymmetry than those of common nevi. A dermoscopic classification of Clark nevi introduced several patterns and distribution of pigment in these complex lesions.[52]

The axiom, "the more structures, the more colors, the more suspect," in atypical melanocytic lesions may be also useful in patients with multiple nevi to identify melanoma. Regarding the distribution of dermoscopic pigmentation, in previous studies, it has been suggested that when a lesion shows eccentric hyperpigmentation or multifocal pigmentation there is a higher probability of it being melanoma.[53,54] In a more recent study in a series of melanomas and nevi, the presence of eccentric hyperpigmentation or multifocal pigmentation patterns was associated with additional melanoma-specific dermoscopic features, allowing the correct diagnosis independent to the pigment distribution in 92% of all melanomas.[55] For this reason, the investigators of this study conclude that, in the absence of another melanoma-specific pattern, lesions with these pigmentation patterns do not require closer observation than other nevi.

Dermoscopic Comparative Approach

In patients with multiple atypical moles, early melanomas cannot always be distinguished with accuracy, even with the use of dermoscopy by experienced dermatologists. This is because in these patients, early melanoma may be clinically and dermoscopically difficult to distinguish from nevi. In addition, in the early stages, melanomas may exhibit few malignancy criteria. In these cases, a dermoscopic comparative approach has been postulated. One or 2 predominant dermoscopic patterns can be found in patients with many moles.[52,56] According to this concept, the key point in the examination of individuals with multiple nevi is the identification of their predominant nevus pattern (defined as the pattern observed in more than 30% of all melanocytic lesions), which then allows the recognition of atypical lesions that deviate from this pattern.[57] An additional consideration in patients with high risk for malignant melanoma is that the predominant nevus pattern of patients with melanoma seems to differ from that of the healthy population.[58,59] In recent studies, a dermoscopic complex pattern (defined in melanocytic lesions exhibiting both network and globules, with or without structureless areas) was found significantly more frequently in melanoma patients than in controls, who usually have nevi with uniform dermoscopic patterns (ie, reticular pattern). Further studies are needed to confirm the concept of the complex dermoscopic pattern, but it is probable that individuals with multiple nevi exhibiting these patterns may benefit from closer surveillance than individuals with melanocytic lesions exhibiting uniform patterns.

The 4 × 4 × 6 Rule: Combination of Dermoscopic and Clinical Information

In the evaluation of pigmented melanocytic nevi, the clinical factors of patients should be considered to optimize the clinical management of these patients (**Table 1**). The 4 × 4 × 6 rule has been proposed to guide clinicians in the management of melanocytic lesions with a combination of basic dermoscopic nevi criteria and patient-related factors influencing their patterns.[60] According to this rule, the dermoscopic diagnosis of nevi relies on 4 criteria (each of which is characterized by 4 variables): (1) color (black, brown, gray, and blue); (2) pattern (globular, reticular, starburst, and homogeneous blue pattern); (3) pigment distribution (multifocal, central, eccentric, and uniform); and (4) special sites (face, acral areas, nail, and mucosa). In addition, 6 factors related to patients might influence the dermoscopy pattern: age, skin type, history of melanoma, UV exposure, pregnancy, and growth dynamics.

Table 1
The 4 × 4 × 6 rule. The combination of dermoscopic information of the lesion (4 colors, 4 patterns, and 4 pigment distributions) with location (4 special sites) and 6 clinical factors related to the patient has to be considered in the evaluation of a melanocytic lesion in patients with multiple nevi

Four dermoscopic factors	
4 Colors	Black, brown, gray, and blue
4 Patterns	Globular, reticular, starburst, and homogeneous blue pattern
4 Pigment distributions	Multifocal, central, eccentric, and uniform
4 Special sites	Face, acral areas, nail, and mucosa
Six clinical factors related to the patient	
Age, skin type, history of melanoma, UV exposure, pregnancy, and growth dynamics	

Adapted from Zalaudek I, Docimo G, Argenziano G. Using dermoscopic criteria and patient-related factors for the management of pigmented melanocytic nevi. Arch Dermatol 2009;145(7):816–26. Available at: http://www.pubmedcentral.nih.gov/articlerender.fcgi?artid=2856040&tool=pmcentrez&rendertype=abstract.

DIGITAL FOLLOW-UP: TOTAL-BODY PHOTOGRAPHY PLUS DIGITAL DERMOSCOPY

Several studies, including a recent meta-analysis, have demonstrated the benefit of DFU in the context of patients with atypical mole syndrome.[47] In patients at high risk for melanoma with atypical mole syndrome, DFU is one of the most efficient strategies to detect early melanomas while minimizing unnecessary excisions.[61] Several studies have shown that benign melanocytic lesions in patients with atypical mole syndrome tend to remain stable under short-term and long-term monitoring (3–6 months) whereas melanomas tend to change over time. With this assumption, different follow-up strategies with the introduction of photographic monitoring have been recommended. Moreover, in the past few years, the development of new instruments dedicated to TBP and digital monitoring has facilitated the introduction of this method in the clinical setting. DFU allows the identification of melanomas that may lack distinct dermoscopic features at baseline.[62]

Methods of Digital Follow-Up

Digital monitoring can be distinguished between TBP and DD. DD is distinguished between short term and médium/long term follow-up.

Whereas TBP allows the detection of new lesions and macroscopic changes in preexisting moles, DD allows the precise detection of changes in structures and colors of the most atypical lesions. In many of the protocols of digital monitoring, a combination of both strategies is used. In a recent study with 10 years of follow-up, a combination of TBP and DD was superior to one method alone.[14]

DD is distinguished between short-term follow-up (3 months), devoted to few lesions, and medium/long-term follow-up, designed to monitor many lesions over time every 6 to 12 months. Short-term and medium/long-term follow up strategies may be used independently or in combination depending on the context of the patient.

Short-Term Versus Medium/Long-Term DFU

Medium-term and long-term follow-up focuses on monitoring multiple lesions in patients with numerous lesions whereas short-term follow-up is oriented toward assessment of single melanocytic lesions. In most centers, a combination of both methods is used in patients with multiple atypical lesions.[14] When 1 or few lesions are more equivocal than the others, short-term follow-up is used to confirm their stability. If the lesions are stable under short-term follow-up, they are not excised and are included in medium/long-term follow-up with the other atypical lesions of the patient.

Differences in the results of the 2 modalities of DD have been analyzed. The mean number of lesions monitored per patient (from 1 lesion in short-term follow-up to 14 lesions in medium/long-term follow-up) is the main difference between both DD strategies. In the 2 strategies of follow-up, the mean numbers of lesions needed to monitor to detect 1 melanoma are different— 33 lesions in short-term follow-up and 169 lesions in medium/long-term follow-up. In short-term modality, the percentage of melanoma in excised lesions is 16.2% whereas in medium/long-term follow-up is 7.6% and the percentage of monitored lesions excised in short-term follow-up is 18.5% compared to 7.7% in medium/long-term follow-up. Using short-term follow-up, the melanoma/benign lesion ratio is lower (1:5) than dermoscopy alone (1:12).

Reliable comparison of short-term follow-up and medium/long-term follow-up is not possible because of the great differences in the reported studies in terms of excised lesions and melanomas detected, monitored lesions, and number of patients included. The main characteristics of short-term versus medium/long-term monitoring are given in **Table 2**.

Patients to be Included in DFU

The inclusion criteria for digital monitoring are not well standardized and may vary between centers. The efficacy of digital monitoring is associated with the patient risk and can be stratified according to clinical factors. When low-risk patients were included, no melanoma was detected in this subgroup; in one of the studies, no biopsy was performed.[12] In most DD studies, the main criterion was the existence of atypical mole syndrome, but this entity was considered according to different definitions. In some studies, clinical risk factors were considered in addition to atypical mole syndrome (personal or familiar melanoma, number of lesions, and number of atypical lesions). These findings are consistent with the concept that the probability of detection of early melanoma during DFU depends on the selection of high-risk individuals.

Some clinical characteristics may influence the efficacy of the digital monitoring. Older age at inclusion and higher number of lesions excised during follow-up were the variables more associated with melanoma diagnosis during DFU[14]: male gender and previous melanoma or the presence of mutation CDKN2A were also associated with melanoma during follow-up with no statistically significant differences.

Interval and Duration of Follow-up

The interval of dermoscopic follow-up varies from 3 to 6 to 12 months[63–67] (short-term, medium-term, and long-term follow-up). In short-term DFU, the interval of follow-up was 1.5 and 3 months in a study by Altamura and colleagues[68] and 3 months in a study by Menzies and colleagues.[13] Both studies focused only on short-term DFU, but in the study by Menzies and

Table 2
Short-term versus medium/long-term DFU

	DFU Strategy	
	Short-term FU	Medium/long-term FU
Mean number of patients per study (range)	1052 (245–1859)	334.8 (100–688)
Mean number of lesions per study (range)	1460 (318–2602)	4529 (272–11,396)
Mean number of lesions per patient (range)	1	14 (2–35)
Mean number of melanomas detected per study (range)	44 (7–81)	27 (0–98)
Percentage of in situ MM (%)	68	50.5
Mean number of excised lesions per study	270	350
Number of excisions out of monitored lesions (%)	18.5	7.7
Ratio of melanoma:benign lesion	1:5	1:12
Mean patients diagnosed with MM during the period of study	41.5	23.8

Adapted form Salerni G, Terán T, Puig S, et al. Meta-analysis of digital dermoscopy follow-up of melanocytic skin lesions: a study on behalf of the International Dermoscopy Society. J Eur Acad Dermatol Venereol 2013. http://dx.doi.org/10.1111/jdv.12032.

coworkers it was reported the outcome of short-term DFU of suspicious or changing atypical melanocytic lesions,[13] whereas the study by Altamura and coworkers aimed to determine whether 6 weeks could replace 3 months for short-term DFU of suspicious melanocytic lesions.[68]

The median reported length of follow-up in digital dermoscopic monitoring is 29.6 months (range 3–96 months). This duration of DFU influences the number of melanomas excised and the ratio of benign to malignant lesions excised. The number of melanomas detected during follow-up correlates with the median length of follow-up and the chance of detecting a melanoma during monitoring increases with the time of follow-up. The 2 studies published with the longest follow-up period showed the highest melanoma detection rate.[14,67] In DFU, 1 additional melanoma is detected for every additional month of monitoring. According to this evidence, it is recommended that because new melanomas are detected during the period of long-term DFU over time, the monitoring should probably be maintained almost over the whole lifetime.

Criteria for Lesions to be Monitored or Excised

The percentage of monitored lesions excised during follow-up ranges from 1.3% to 18.7% according to different studies. One of the main benefits of DFU is the low number of excisions that are needed in atypical mole syndrome patients who were previously submitted to a great number of biopsies. A mean of less than 1 lesion was excised per patient during the surveillance period in recent meta-analyses.[47]

During follow-up, 383 early melanomas were detected (mean, 29 per study). The number of lesions to monitor to detect 1 melanoma ranged from 31 to 1008, with a mean of 348 among eligible studies. The studies with a higher rate of excisions also had a higher melanoma rate among monitored lesions.

Criteria to Excise Lesions During Digital Dermoscopic Monitoring

In DFU, any lesion showing the following changes detected by DD are considered for excision and histopathologic diagnosis: (1) asymmetric enlargement in size, (2) changes in dermoscopic structures (variation in shape; expansion or decrease of pigment network; variation in the distribution or number of dots/globules; modification of depigmented areas or regression structures; and appearance of streaks, scar-like areas, blue-whitish veil, and atypical vessels), (3) increase in the number of colors, (4) regression features affecting more than 50% of the lesion, and (5) focal pigment modifications.[11,62]

In most of the DFU studies, all new or previously unregistered lesions observed during follow-up and exhibiting atypical features but no criteria for melanoma are registered and included in follow-up whereas lesions displaying dermoscopic criteria for melanoma should be removed.

Characteristics of Melanomas Detected During Digital Dermoscopic Follow-up

DD follow-up of melanocytic skin lesions with DD demonstrated the early detection of melanomas with a low rate of excisions. Using DD follow-up, the proportion of in situ melanoma and thin melanomas are higher than expected in the general population. According to available data of the melanomas detected in studies using DD follow-up, 209 (54.6%) were in situ melanomas and 174 (45.4%) were invasive melanomas, all invasive melanomas of less than 1 mm of thickness.[47]

Compliance of Patients in DFU

Compliance of patients in DFU is mandatory to assure that changing lesions are detected. In one study, a reduction of sensitivity was seen in DFU with respect to non-DFU with an increase of specificity in the first case.[61] The risk of missing a melanoma that was similar to other lesions is assumed in this strategy. The reduction of the number of lesions needed to treat and the possibility of detecting early melanomas in DFU are the main justifications for this approach. Patients need to understand the importance of compliance and adherence to the schedule similar to other clinical situations in populations at high risk for cancer.[12,63] One of the main rules of DFU is to avoid the monitoring of atypical melanocytic lesions that are not flat. This reduces the risk of missing a fast-growing melanoma with diminished prognosis in cases of delayed excision in 3 to 6 months.

COMPUTER-ASSISTED DIAGNOSIS AND OTHER METHODS

With enhancements in imaging and computer technologies as well as image-processing software for the detection of melanoma in patients with multiple nevi, the method of the future is high-resolution 3-D mapping of the entire body as a periodic screening tool. Ideally, the photographic imaging technique would be coupled with dermoscopy and possibly with another more quantitative diagnostic technique.

Commercial systems for assessment of melanocytic lesions using digital photography already exist; however, their clinical use is not widespread. Any commercial system that attempts to be implemented in the diagnosis of skin cancer needs extensive and expensive validation in clinical trials to obtain approval by official agencies. There are several algorithms and methods to aid clinicians in the diagnosis of melanoma. Some are based on the automated identification of the ABCDE (asymmetry, border irregularity, color variegation, diameter greater than 6 mm, evolution) diagnostic criteria by computer, with limited success because of the diversity and complexity of lesions.

Several emerging technologies are currently being investigated to determine their ability to diagnose melanoma. Some use multispectral information acquired and analyzed both in the spatial domain (detector measures radiation intensity at a particular point or region) and the spectral domain (detector captures radiation intensity as function of wavelength—spectrum—for the selected point or domain). These methods hold the promise of offering quantitative criteria for melanoma diagnosis.

Over the past decade, one of the most known efforts in the introduction of computerized assessment of equivocal melanocytic lesions has been the development of the MelaFind[69] technology by Mela Sciences, approved for sale since 2011 in the United States and Europe.[70] This instrument classifies skin lesions by assessment of the degree of disorganization of the lesion. The handheld component of the imaging system consists of a radiation source (illuminator) with 10 wavelengths of light, including near-infrared bands and visible light. Multispectral data are captured from a region up to 2.5 mm deep into the skin, and they provide 3-D information regarding the morphologic organization of the lesion. The information collected by the detector is analyzed by automatic data analysis algorithms. Inclusion criteria of the lesions suitable for MelaFind evaluation are summarized in **Box 1**. In the future it is probable that improved technologies of computerized assessment of melanocytic lesions will be incorporated in the screening of patients with multiple melanocytic lesions.

Another method for evaluation of equivocal melanocytic lesions uses electrical bioimpedance to assess cutaneous lesions.[71–75] Electrical impedance of cancer cells and healthy cells are different because cancer cells have a different shape, size, and orientation—criteria equivalent to those used in histopathologic evaluation. Measurements of suspicious melanocytic lesions are made with an electrical impedance spectrometer over both the

> **Box 1**
> **Characteristics of the melanocytic lesions assessed by MelaFind**
>
> 1. Lesions that are sufficiently pigmented to be clearly discerned from the surrounding normal skin using automated image-processing tools
> 2. Diameter in the range between 2 mm and 22 mm; this dimension determined by the imaging optics
> 3. Accessibility by the handheld component
> 4. Not suitable for acral, palmar, plantar, mucosal, or subungual areas as well as near the eyes
> 5. Intact skin without scars, fibrosis, or foreign matter

center of the lesion as well as an ipsilateral reference skin site.

Newer models of electrical impedance have a digital camera along with an automated software analysis. Electrical impedance in phase II studies has shown a high sensitivity for thin melanomas.[76]

A completely different approach is the use of RNA analyses obtained in the upper skin by stripping. In a study of this technique, 312 genes were differentially expressed between melanomas, nevi, and normal skin specimens. These genes are involved in melanocyte development and physiology, melanoma, cancer, and cell growth control. From this panel of genes, 17 were extracted to hierarchical clustering of melanomas and nevi. In a preliminary study, the classifier discerned in situ and invasive melanomas from nevi with 100% sensitivity and 88% specificity.[77] Results of a validation study with this technology are waiting to be submitted.

SUMMARY/DISCUSSION

Patients with multiple nevi have an increased risk of developing melanoma. According to clinical information (ie, number of nevi, atypical mole syndrome, and history of melanoma) and genetic background, a stratification of risk grades can be assessed.

In cases of atypical mole syndrome, many lesions have features associated with early melanoma. This characteristic makes accurate detection of malignant lesions with reduced number of excisions difficult; thus, clinical information associated with dermoscopy and DFU is used in this context. These complex patients benefit from periodic total-body skin examination by experienced physicians with the use of technologies devoted to the detection of melanoma.

Dermatoscopy should be used in combination with clinical information (4 × 4 × 6 rule) and comparative analyses (ugly duckling sign of dermoscopy and clinical examination). Patients with multiple nevi and complex patterns are postulated to have a higher risk compared with those with uniform patterns in their melanocytic lesions (ie, reticular pattern).

Short-term and medium-term or long-term DFU with TBP allow early detection of melanoma in patients difficult to monitor. In a recent meta-analysis of DFU studies, it was shown that in the monitoring of high-risk patients, a low number of excisions is needed (less than 1 lesion per patient). Using these methods a high ratio of melanoma diagnosis was achieved. This results are influenced by factors, such as age, number of lesions, and duration of follow-up. Therefore, low-risk patients do not benefit from this method. Because the detection of new melanomas is continued over time, long-term monitoring is needed in atypical mole patients.

In recent years, several strategies based on computer analyses of images or physical properties of tumors have been developed. Some of these technologies have advanced clinical validation with approval for complementary assessment by a dermatologist in equivocal preselected melanocytic lesions.

In the future, a combination of 3-D TBP with DD and other quantitative methods will be incorporated in the armamentarium of dermatologic management of high-risk patients. These new methods will need to be accompanied by basic strategies based on SSE or patient-based SSE with the support of images and different types of software available for patients to be used at home.

REFERENCES

1. Breitbart EW, Waldmann A, Nolte S, et al. Systematic skin cancer screening in Northern Germany. J Am Acad Dermatol 2012;66(2):201–11. http://dx.doi.org/10.1016/j.jaad.2010.11.016.
2. Bafounta ML, Beauchet A, Aegerter P, et al. Is dermoscopy (epiluminescence microscopy) useful for the diagnosis of melanoma? Results of a meta-analysis using techniques adapted to the evaluation of diagnostic tests. Arch Dermatol 2001;137(10):1343–50.
3. Kittler H, Pehamberger H, Wolff K, et al. Diagnostic accuracy of dermoscopy. Lancet Oncol 2002;3(3):159–65.
4. Vestergaard ME, Macaskill P, Holt PE, et al. Dermoscopy compared with naked eye examination for the diagnosis of primary melanoma: a meta-analysis of studies performed in a clinical setting. Br J Dermatol 2008;159(3):669–76. http://dx.doi.org/10.1111/j.1365-2133.2008.08713.x.
5. Puig S, Argenziano G, Zalaudek I, et al. Melanomas that failed dermoscopic detection: a combined clinicodermoscopic approach for not missing melanoma. Dermatol Surg 2007;33(10):1262–73. http://dx.doi.org/10.1111/j.1524-4725.2007.33264.x.
6. Carli P, De Giorgi V, Nardini P, et al. Melanoma detection rate and concordance between self-skin examination and clinical evaluation in patients attending a pigmented lesion clinic in Italy. Br J Dermatol 2002;146(2):261–6.
7. Robinson JK, Fisher SG, Turrisi RJ. Predictors of skin self-examination performance. Cancer 2002;95(1):135–46.
8. Nehal KS, Oliveria SA, Marghoob AA, et al. Use of and beliefs about baseline photography in the management of patients with pigmented lesions: a survey of dermatology residency programmes in the United States. Melanoma Res 2002;12(2):161–7.
9. Shriner DL, Wagner RF, Glowczwski JR. Photography for the early diagnosis of malignant melanoma in patients with atypical moles. Cutis 1992;50(5):358–62.
10. Kopf AW, Salopek TG, Slade J, et al. Techniques of cutaneous examination for the detection of skin cancer. Cancer 1995;75(Suppl 2):684–90.
11. Kittler H, Pehamberger H, Wolff K, et al. Follow-up of melanocytic skin lesions with digital epiluminescence microscopy: patterns of modifications observed in early melanoma, atypical nevi, and common nevi. J Am Acad Dermatol 2000;43(3):467–76.
12. Schiffner R, Schiffner-Rohe J, Landthaler M, et al. Long-term dermoscopic follow-up of melanocytic naevi: clinical outcome and patient compliance. Br J Dermatol 2003;149(1):79–86.
13. Menzies SW, Gutenev A, Avramidis M, et al. Short-term digital surface microscopic monitoring of atypical or changing melanocytic lesions. Arch Dermatol 2001;137(12):1583–9.
14. Salerni G, Carrera C, Lovatto L, et al. Benefits of total body photography and digital dermatoscopy ("two-step method of digital follow-up") in the early diagnosis of melanoma in patients at high risk for melanoma. J Am Acad Dermatol 2011. http://dx.doi.org/10.1016/j.jaad.2011.04.008.
15. Malvehy J, Puig S. Follow-up of melanocytic skin lesions with digital total-body photography and digital dermoscopy: a two-step method. Clin Dermatol 2002;20(3):297–304.
16. Green WH, Wang SQ, Cognetta AB. Total-body cutaneous examination, total-body photography, and dermoscopy in the care of a patient with xeroderma pigmentosum and multiple melanomas. Arch Dermatol 2009;145(8):910–5.

17. Malvehy J, Puig S. Dermoscopy of skin lesions in two patients with xeroderma pigmentosum. Br J Dermatol 2005;152(2):271–8. http://dx.doi.org/10.1111/J.1365-2133.2004.06332.X.

18. Salerni G, Lovatto L, Carrera C, et al. Melanomas detected in a follow-up program compared with melanomas referred to a melanoma unit. Arch Dermatol 2011;147(5):549–55. http://dx.doi.org/10.1001/archdermatol.2010.430.

19. Green A, MacLennan R, Siskind V. Common acquired naevi and the risk of malignant melanoma. Int J Cancer 1985;35(3):297–300.

20. Swerdlow AJ, English J, MacKie RM, et al. Benign melanocytic naevi as a risk factor for malignant melanoma. Br Med J (Clin Res Ed) 1986;292(6535):1555–9.

21. Ródenas JM, Delgado-Rodríguez M, Farinas-Alvarez C, et al. Melanocytic nevi and risk of cutaneous malignant melanoma in southern Spain. Am J Epidemiol 1997;145(11):1020–9.

22. Bataille V, Grulich A, Sasieni P, et al. The association between naevi and melanoma in populations with different levels of sun exposure: a joint case-control study of melanoma in the UK and Australia. Br J Cancer 1998;77(3):505–10.

23. Chang Y, Newton-Bishop JA, Bishop DT, et al. A pooled analysis of melanocytic nevus phenotype and the risk of cutaneous melanoma at different latitudes. Int J Cancer 2009;124(2):420–8.

24. Gandini S, Sera F, Cattaruzza MS, et al. Meta-analysis of risk factors for cutaneous melanoma: I. Common and atypical naevi. Eur J Cancer 2005;41(1):28–44.

25. Rhodes AR. Public education and cancer of the skin. What do people need to know about melanoma and nonmelanoma skin cancer? Cancer 1995;75(Suppl 2):613–36.

26. Rhodes AR, Weinstock MA, Fitzpatrick TB, et al. Risk factors for cutaneous melanoma. A practical method of recognizing predisposed individuals. JAMA 1987;258(21):3146–54.

27. Clark WH, Reimer RR, Greene M, et al. Origin of familial malignant melanomas from heritable melanocytic lesions. "The B-K mole syndrome". Arch Dermatol 1978;114(5):732–8.

28. Greene MH, Clark WH, Tucker MA, et al. High risk of malignant melanoma in melanoma-prone families with dysplastic nevi. Ann Intern Med 1985;102(4):458–65.

29. Carli P, Massi D, Santucci M, et al. Cutaneous melanoma histologically associated with a nevus and melanoma de novo have a different profile of risk: results from a case-control study. J Am Acad Dermatol 1999;40(4):549–57.

30. Piepkorn M. Melanoma genetics: an update with focus on the CDKN2A(p16)/ARF tumor suppressors. J Am Acad Dermatol 2000;42(5 Pt 1):705–22.

31. Soufir N, Avril MF, Chompret A, et al. Prevalence of p16 and CDK4 germline mutations in 48 melanoma-prone families in France. The French Familial Melanoma Study Group. Hum Mol Genet 1998;7(2):209–16.

32. Goldstein AM, Chan M, Harland M, et al. High-risk melanoma susceptibility genes and pancreatic cancer, neural system tumors, and uveal melanoma across GenoMEL. Cancer Res 2006;66(20):9818–28. http://dx.doi.org/10.1158/0008-5472.CAN-06-0494.

33. Goldstein AM, Chan M, Harland M, et al. Features associated with germline CDKN2A mutations: a GenoMEL study of melanoma-prone families from three continents. J Med Genet 2007;44(2):99–106. http://dx.doi.org/10.1136/jmg.2006.043802.

34. Puig S, Ruiz A, Castel T, et al. Inherited susceptibility to several cancers but absence of linkage between dysplastic nevus syndrome and CDKN2A in a melanoma family with a mutation in the CDKN2A (P16INK4A) gene. Hum Genet 1997;101(3):359–64.

35. Ruiz A, Puig S, Malvehy J, et al. CDKN2A mutations in Spanish cutaneous malignant melanoma families and patients with multiple melanomas and other neoplasia. J Med Genet 1999;36(6):490–3.

36. Puig S, Malvehy J, Badenas C, et al. Role of the CDKN2A locus in patients with multiple primary melanomas. J Clin Oncol 2005;23(13):3043–51. http://dx.doi.org/10.1200/JCO.2005.08.034.

37. Larre Borges A, Cuéllar F, Puig-Butillé JA, et al. CDKN2A mutations in melanoma families from Uruguay. Br J Dermatol 2009;161(3):536–41.

38. Ward KA, Lazovich D, Hordinsky MK. Germline melanoma susceptibility and prognostic genes: a review of the literature. J Am Acad Dermatol 2012;67(5):1055–67. http://dx.doi.org/10.1016/j.jaad.2012.02.042.

39. Bataille V, Kato BS, Falchi M, et al. Nevus size and number are associated with telomere length and represent potential markers of a decreased senescence in vivo. Cancer Epidemiol Biomarkers Prev 2007;16(7):1499–502.

40. Falchi M, Spector TD, Perks U, et al. Genome-wide search for nevus density shows linkage to two melanoma loci on chromosome 9 and identifies a new QTL on 5q31 in an adult twin cohort. Hum Mol Genet 2006;15(20):2975–9.

41. Pujana MA, Ruiz A, Badenas C, et al. Molecular characterization of a t(9;12)(p21;q13) balanced chromosome translocation in combination with integrative genomics analysis identifies C9orf14 as a candidate tumor-suppressor. Genes Chromosomes Cancer 2007;46(2):155–62. http://dx.doi.org/10.1002/gcc.20396.

42. Geller AC, O'Riordan DL, Oliveria SA, et al. Overcoming obstacles to skin cancer examinations

and prevention counseling for high-risk patients: results of a national survey of primary care physicians. J Am Board Fam Pract 2004;17(6):416–23.

43. Hamidi R, Peng D, Cockburn M. Efficacy of skin self-examination for the early detection of melanoma. Int J Dermatol 2010;49(2):126–34.

44. Stratigos AJ, Katsambas AD. The value of screening in melanoma. Clin Dermatol 2009; 27(1):10–25.

45. Oliveria SA, Chau D, Christos PJ, et al. Diagnostic accuracy of patients in performing skin self-examination and the impact of photography. Arch Dermatol 2004;140:57–62.

46. Phelan DL, Oliveria SA, Halpern AC. Patient experiences with photo books in monthly skin self-examinations. Dermatol Nurs 2005;17(2):109–14.

47. Salerni G, Terán T, Puig S, et al. Meta-analysis of digital dermoscopy follow-up of melanocytic skin lesions: a study on behalf of the International Dermoscopy Society. J Eur Acad Dermatol Venereol 2013. http://dx.doi.org/10.1111/jdv.12032.

48. Grob JJ, Bonerandi JJ. The "ugly duckling" sign: identification of the common characteristics of nevi in an individual as a basis for melanoma screening. Arch Dermatol 1998;134(1):103–4.

49. Gachon J, Beaulieu P, Sei JF, et al. First prospective study of the recognition process of melanoma in dermatological practice. Arch Dermatol 2005; 141(4):434–8.

50. Mascaro JM Jr, Mascaro JM. The dermatologist's position concerning nevi: a vision ranging from "the ugly duckling" to "little red riding hood". Arch Dermatol 1998;134(11):1484–5.

51. Argenziano G, Zalaudek I, Ferrara G, et al. Proposal of a new classification system for melanocytic naevi. Br J Dermatol 2007;157(2):217–27.

52. Hofmann-Wellenhof R, Blum A, Wolf IH, et al. Dermoscopic classification of Clark's nevi (atypical melanocytic nevi). Clin Dermatol 2001;20(3):255–8.

53. Blum A, Soyer HP, Garbe C, et al. The dermoscopic classification of atypical melanocytic naevi (Clark naevi) is useful to discriminate benign from malignant melanocytic lesions. Br J Dermatol 2003; 149(6):1159–64.

54. Fikrle T, Pizinger K. Dermatoscopic differences between atypical melanocytic naevi and thin malignant melanomas. Melanoma Res 2006;16(1): 45–50.

55. Arevalo A, Altamura D, Avramidis M, et al. The significance of eccentric and central hyperpigmentation, multifocal hyper/hypopigmentation, and the multicomponent pattern in melanocytic lesions lacking specific dermoscopic features of melanoma. Arch Dermatol 2008;144(11):1440–4.

56. Scope A, Dusza SW, Halpern AC, et al. The "ugly duckling" sign: agreement between observers. Arch Dermatol 2008;144(1):58–64.

57. Roesch A, Burgdorf W, Stolz W, et al. Dermatoscopy of "dysplastic nevi": a beacon in diagnostic darkness. Eur J Dermatol 2006;16(5):479–93.

58. Lipoff JB, Scope A, Dusza SW, et al. Complex dermoscopic pattern: a potential risk marker for melanoma. Br J Dermatol 2008;158(4):821–4.

59. Morales-Callaghan AM, Castrodeza-Sanz J, Martínez-García G, et al. Correlation between clinical, dermatoscopic, and histopathologic variables in atypical melanocytic nevi. Actas Dermosifiliogr 2008;99(5):380–9.

60. Zalaudek I, Docimo G, Argenziano G. Using dermoscopic criteria and patient-related factors for the management of pigmented melanocytic nevi. Arch Dermatol 2009;145(7):816–26.

61. Kittler H, Binder M. Risks and benefits of sequential imaging of melanocytic skin lesions in patients with multiple atypical nevi. Arch Dermatol 2001;137(12): 1590–5.

62. Salerni G, Carrera C, Lovatto L, et al. Characterization of 1152 lesions excised over 10 years using total-body photography and digital dermatoscopy in the surveillance of patients at high risk for melanoma. J Am Acad Dermatol 2012. http://dx.doi.org/10.1016/j.jaad.2012.01.028.

63. Argenziano G, Mordente I, Ferrara G, et al. Dermoscopic monitoring of melanocytic skin lesions: clinical outcome and patient compliance vary according to follow-up protocols. Br J Dermatol 2008;159(2):331–6.

64. Haenssle HA, Krueger U, Vente C, et al. Results from an observational trial: digital epiluminescence microscopy follow-up of atypical nevi increases the sensitivity and the chance of success of conventional dermoscopy in detecting melanoma. J Invest Dermatol 2006;126(5):980–5.

65. Haenssle HA, Vente C, Bertsch HP, et al. Results of a surveillance programme for patients at high risk of malignant melanoma using digital and conventional dermoscopy. Eur J Cancer Prev 2004;13(2):133–8.

66. Haenssle HA, Korpas B, Hansen-Hagge C, et al. Seven-point checklist for dermatoscopy: performance during 10 years of prospective surveillance of patients at increased melanoma risk. J Am Acad Dermatol 2010;62(5):785–93.

67. Haenssle HA, Korpas B, Hansen-Hagge C, et al. Selection of patients for long-term surveillance with digital dermoscopy by assessment of melanoma risk factors. Arch Dermatol 2010;146(3): 257–64.

68. Altamura D, Avramidis M, Menzies SW. Assessment of the optimal interval for and sensitivity of short-term sequential digital dermoscopy monitoring for the diagnosis of melanoma. Arch Dermatol 2008;144(4):502–6.

69. Gutkowicz-Krusin D, Elbaum M, Jacobs A, et al. Precision of automatic measurements of pigmented

skin lesion parameters with a MelaFind(TM) multi-spectral digital dermoscope. Melanoma Res 2000; 10(6):563–70.

70. Monheit G, Cognetta AB, Ferris L, et al. The performance of MelaFind: a prospective multi-center study. Arch Dermatol 2011;147:188–94.

71. Wilkinson BA, Smallwood RH, Keshtar A, et al. Electrical impedance spectroscopy and the diagnosis of bladder pathology: a pilot study. J Urol 2002; 168(4 Pt 1):1563–7.

72. Zou Y, Guo Z. A review of electrical impedance techniques for breast cancer detection. Med Eng Phys 2003;25(2):79–90.

73. Brown BH, Tidy JA, Boston K, et al. Relation between tissue structure and imposed electrical current flow in cervical neoplasia. Lancet 2000; 355(9207):892–5.

74. Aberg P, Nicander I, Hansson J, et al. Skin cancer identification using multifrequency electrical impedance-a potential screening tool. IEEE Trans Biomed Eng 2004;51:2097–102. http://dx.doi.org/10.1109/TBME.2004.836523.

75. Blad B, Baldetorp B. Impedance spectra of tumour tissue in comparison with normal tissue; a possible clinical application for electrical impedance tomography. Physiol Meas 1996;17(Suppl 4):A105–15 (0967-3334 (Print)).

76. Har-Shai Y, Glickman YA, Siller G, et al. Electrical impedance scanning for melanoma diagnosis: a validation study. Plast Reconstr Surg 2005;116(3): 782–90.

77. Wachsman W, Morhenn V, Palmer T, et al. Noninvasive genomic detection of melanoma. Br J Dermatol 2011;164(4):797–806.

Dysplastic Nevus
Why This Term Should be Abandoned in Dermatoscopy

Harald Kittler, MD*, Philipp Tschandl, MD

KEYWORDS

• Melanoma • Dysplastic • Congenital • Follow-up • Nevi • Dermatoscopy • Dermatopathology

KEY POINTS

- The hypothesis that the "dysplastic" nevus is a precursor of melanoma has not been supported by empiric data. The term "dysplastic nevus" is a misnomer because in pathology "dysplasia" describes an intermediate state between a benign and a malignant neoplasm.
- The statement that the diagnosis of a dysplastic nevus is based only on histopathologic criteria and does not correlate with clinical criteria is a clever way to immunize the concept against falsification.
- The strong correlation between melanoma risk and the phenotype of large and numerous nevi has erroneously been interpreted as a causal relationship.
- The terms "dysplastic" and "atypical" nevus are often used by clinicians and pathologists to express their diagnostic uncertainty but it has nothing to do with biologic uncertainty.
- There are parts of a melanoma that may look like a nevus clinically, dermatoscopically, and histopathologically, which led to the unjustified assumption that the inconspicuous part of the melanoma is a precursor nevus.

INTRODUCTION

From the outset the concept of the "dysplastic" nevus encompassed 2 different hypotheses: (1) that the dysplastic nevus is a precursor of melanoma,[1–3] and (2) that the dysplastic nevus is a marker of melanoma risk.[4–6] The first hypothesis makes a prognosis pertaining to individual lesions; the second is related to the prognosis of individuals. Although there is good evidence that the presence of multiple large nevi is indeed a marker of melanoma risk, the precursor hypothesis has been falsified by empiric data.[7,8] Both hypotheses were set forth by Wallace H Clark Jr more than 30 years ago. The first hypothesis was described in Clark's own words, as follows: "Six evident lesional steps of tumor progression form the neoplastic system that affects the human epidermal melanocyte: (1) the common acquired melanocytic nevus; (2) a melanocytic nevus with lentiginous melanocytic hyperplasia, ie, aberrant differentiation; (3) a melanocytic nevus with aberrant differentiation and melanocytic nuclear atypia, ie, melanocytic dysplasia; (4) the radial growth phase of primary melanoma; (5) the vertical growth phase of primary melanoma; and (6) metastatic melanoma."[2] This model of Clark's became accepted universally by dermatologists and dermatopathologists, attaining the status of paradigm.[9] Despite refutation of the hypothesis that the dysplastic nevus is a precursor of melanoma, the term "dysplasia" has not been abandoned.[10] It is a misnomer because in pathology "dysplasia" describes an intermediate state between a benign and a malignant neoplasm, which the dysplastic nevus is not. This article is aims to explore why the term "dysplastic nevus" has not been dropped and why this term is dispensable from a

Department of Dermatology, Medical University of Vienna, Währinger Gürtel 18-20, Vienna 1090, Austria
* Corresponding author.
E-mail address: harald.kittler@meduniwien.ac.at

Dermatol Clin 31 (2013) 579–588
http://dx.doi.org/10.1016/j.det.2013.06.009
0733-8635/13/$ – see front matter © 2013 Elsevier Inc. All rights reserved.

dermatoscopic point of view. The most important reasons the term "dysplastic nevus" has not vanished despite its inadequacy are as follows: (1) the successful attempts to immunize the concept of dysplasia against falsification, (2) the confusion of correlation with causal relationship with regard to the dysplastic nevus syndrome, (3) the confusion of diagnostic uncertainty with biologic uncertainty, (4) the confusion of portions of melanoma that look like nevi with portions of nevi that look like melanoma, (5) the term "dysplastic nevus," although inadequate, served clinicians, pathologists, and patients well, and (6) the partition into 2 different camps of doctors, believers and nonbelievers, that did not bring forward a productive, scientific discussion based on critical arguments but an unfruitful vendetta in which each side took up rigid positions.

SUCCESSFUL ATTEMPTS TO IMMUNIZE THE CONCEPT OF DYSPLASIA AGAINST FALSIFICATION

It has often been stated that the diagnosis of a dysplastic nevus is based on histopathologic criteria and does not correlate with clinical or dermatoscopic criteria. This argument is often used to refute clinical or dermatoscopic data that contradict the precursor hypothesis[7,8,11–14] and it is a clever way to immunize the concept against falsification. If clinical and dermatoscopic atypia would not in some way correlate with histopathologic "dysplasia," in other words, if there were no clinical or dermatoscopic criteria for the dysplastic nevus, it could not be diagnosed by clinicians and dermatoscopists. It could only be diagnosed by dermatopathologists. This is not the case for any other type of nevus. Even Spitz nevi can be diagnosed clinically and dermatoscopically with some specificity,[15,16] although cytologic features are so important for their diagnosis. If a nevus has to be excised to see dysplasia, then any attempts to verify or falsify the hypothesis that the dysplastic nevus is a precursor lesion are doomed to fail. Once the lesion is excised, its future remains unclear forever and, for this reason, the opinion that the dysplastic nevus can only be diagnosed histopathologically immunizes the concept of dysplasia against falsification, which is not comparable to the situation of precursors of epithelial skin cancer, for example, actinic keratoses. From original clinical observations, it is known that the proportion of actinic keratoses that will progress to invasive squamous cell carcinoma within a certain period of time is relevant.[17,18] In the case of actinic keratosis there is empiric evidence that some of them will progress to squamous cell carcinoma. On the other hand thousands of atypical nevi were monitored in patients with the dysplastic nevus syndrome with digital dermatoscopy but a transformation to melanoma was not observed.[19–21] Practically no melanomas were detected arising in those nevi. Most if not all of the small number of melanomas detected during follow-up were melanomas from the outset and showed no associated nevus histopathologically.[22]

If the dysplastic nevus could only be diagnosed histopathologically, it would also be difficult to explain why so many nevi that are excised for diagnostic reasons are diagnosed as dysplastic nevi histopathologically. If they are picked only by chance, then they must be very common, more common than common nevi! It cannot be both ways. Either nevi referred to as being "atypical" by clinicians are likely to be dysplastic on pathology and then it must be accepted that most atypical/dysplastic nevi never progress to melanoma or clinicians and dermatoscopists pick dysplastic nevi only by chance. The question then remains as to why dysplastic nevi are so common among excised lesions.

Other reasons the concept of dysplasia is difficult to falsify are that the histopathologic criteria used to diagnose a dysplastic nevus are vague and subjective and that the criteria are not used in a consistent way. The interobserver agreement for grading dysplasia is low because terms like nuclear atypia are highly subjective.[23] Another issue is that what currently is depicted in leading textbooks of dermatology and dermatopathology as dysplastic nevus in some instances represents a variant of a congenital nevus, in other instances, a Clark nevus.[24] These 2 nevi are fundamentally different and can be distinguished by dermatoscopy.[16] In other words, what has been termed "dysplastic nevus" is not one type of nevus (**Figs. 1** and **2**). From a dermatoscopic point of view, nevi with different patterns can be differentiated.[16] The most important patterns in this regard are the reticular pattern, the pattern of clods (globular pattern), the radial pattern (starburst pattern), and the structureless pattern. It is known that each of these patterns has different biologic significance. Nevi with a pattern of clods predominate in children; nevi with a reticular pattern predominate in adults.[25] Nevi with a radial pattern grow rapidly; nevi with a reticular pattern grow slowly.[26] Nevi with a hyperpigmented structureless pattern in the center and reticular lines at the periphery are different from nevi with a raised hypopigmented center or nevi with a pattern of clods. These nevi are different from a clinical, dermatoscopic, and biologic point of view and should not be summarized under the inadequate generic

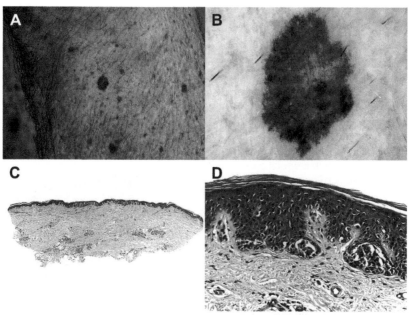

Fig. 1. Clinical (*A*) and dermatoscopic (*B*) image of a clinically "atypical" lesion, histopathologically reported as "dysplastic nevus." (*C*) and (*D*) Dermatopathologic images, revealing nests of melanocytes within tips of the rete ridges, corresponding to reticular lines seen in dermatoscopy (hematoxylin eosin, original magnification ×20). Clinical, dermatoscopic, and histopathologic appearance of this nevus is different from the lesions shown in **Fig. 2**. Integrating all information, the specific diagnosis should be Clark nevus and not dysplastic nevus.

term "dysplastic nevus" that does not capture these differences.

THE DYSPLASTIC NEVUS SYNDROME AND THE CONFUSION OF CORRELATION WITH CAUSE

The strong correlation between melanoma risk and the phenotype of large and numerous nevi[1] has erroneously been interpreted as a causal relationship. It was thought that the large nevi of these individuals are the precursors of their melanomas.[2] Although some melanomas may start in preexisting nevi, it is the exception and not the rule.[7] Most melanomas start de novo and not in a preexisting nevus of any type, and if they start in a preexisting nevus, it is often a completely inconspicuous nevus and not a large dysplastic one.[27] The risk of melanoma and the phenotype of large and numerous nevi are correlated because there is a common genetic background that is associated with both conditions. Some of the genes involved have been identified. It is known that some melanoma families with the dysplastic nevus syndrome bear mutations in the CDKN2A or in the CDK4 locus.[28–32] The cause for the increased risk to develop melanoma is genetically determined and one cannot decrease that risk by removing the nevi. That the dysplastic nevus syndrome is

genetically determined is supported by the fact that many so-called dysplastic nevi are actually congenital.[24] Many patients with the dysplastic nevus syndrome have multiple small congenital nevi with an increased number of terminal hairs (**Fig. 3**). If investigated dermatoscopically, they show a combination of pattern of clods (globular pattern), reticular lines, and brown structureless areas (see **Fig. 3**). It is known that they are congenital (although most of them were not present at birth) because some of them present with terminal hairs, which identify them as hamartomas. Other nevi in the same patients have the same dermatoscopic pattern and, although they have no increase in the number of terminal hairs, it is likely that they are also congenital. The point thatis demonstrated by dermatoscopy is that at least some patients with the so-called dysplastic nevus syndrome actually have a congenital nevus syndrome. A high number of nevi of patients with the dysplastic nevus syndrome were monitored with digital dermatoscopy but practically none of them transformed into melanoma as suggested by the precursor hypothesis. Most if not all of the small number of melanomas detected during follow-up developed on normal skin and not in a preexisting nevus or were melanomas from the outset and showed no associated nevus histopathologically,[21,22] which is how digital dermatoscopy falsified the precursor hypothesis.

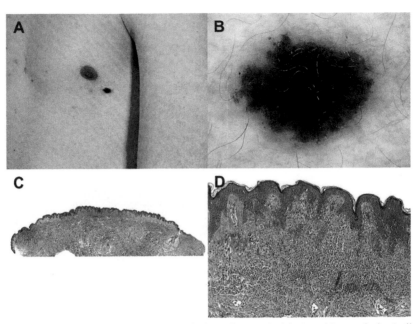

Fig. 2. Clinical (*A*) and dermatoscopic (*B*) image of clinically atypical lesion, histopathologically reported as dysplastic nevus. (*C*) and (*D*) Dermatopathologic images of the lesion, revealing a large but well-circumscribed proliferation of melanocytes within the dermis, corresponding to a brown structureless area in dermatoscopy (hematoxylin eosin, original magnification ×40). The clinical, dermatoscopic, and histopathologic appearance of this nevus is different from the lesions shown in **Fig. 1**. Integrating all information, the specific diagnosis should be superficial and deep congenital nevus and not dysplastic nevus.

THE CONFUSION OF DIAGNOSTIC UNCERTAINTY WITH BIOLOGIC UNCERTAINTY

The terms "dysplastic" and "atypical" nevus are often used by clinicians to express their diagnostic uncertainty. "Atypical" or "dysplastic" nevi share some clinical and dermatoscopic features with melanoma and are contrasted with so-called common nevi that are usually not confused with melanoma. This zone of morphologic overlap between nevi and melanoma has been interpreted

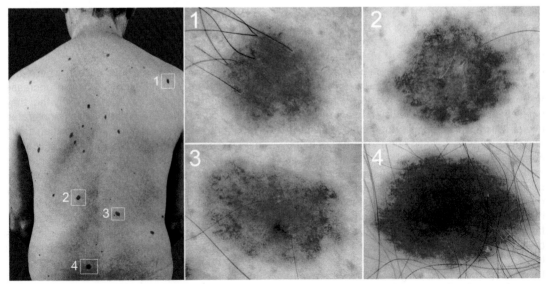

Fig. 3. Left: Clinical image of a patient with dysplastic nevus syndrome. Dermatoscopically (*1–4*) it can be seen that some of the large dysplastic nevi are congenital nevi by the presence of terminal hairs.

as biologic overlap. This analogy is a logical fallacy and not justified. A so-called dysplastic or atypical nevus has a higher chance to be a melanoma but not a higher chance to become a melanoma. Diagnostic uncertainty[23] must not be confused with biologic uncertainty. In **Fig. 4** dermatoscopy images of two nevi are shown. The left one is flat and has a reticular pattern and asymmetry of color; the right one is slightly raised, has a pattern of clods (globular pattern) and symmetry of pattern and color. Which one is more atypical/dysplastic? Most will say the left one because the probability that this lesion is a melanoma is higher. However, if this lesion is excised and the unequivocal diagnosis of nevus has been made, pathologically there is no justification to think that this lesion would have had a higher chance to transform into a melanoma than the lesion on the right. This is a logical fallacy. If a melanoma starts in a nevus, it most often starts in a nevus that looks like the nevus on the right (**Fig. 5**)![7,12,33]

Another example to demonstrate the fallacy that morphology predicts biologic behavior is given in **Fig. 6**. Here the baseline images of 4 pigmented lesions of the some patient with "dysplastic nevus syndrome" are shown. All 4 lesions were monitored with digital dermatoscopy. Only one turned out to be a melanoma. Can you predict which one will turn out to be the melanoma by morphology? The lesions that turned out to be a melanoma during follow-up did not appear more dysplastic or more atypical at baseline than the other nevi that did not change, at least from a dermatoscopic point of view (**Fig. 7**).

In analogy to the use of the term "atypical nevus" by clinicians and dermatoscopists, the term "dysplastic nevus" is used by some pathologists to express their diagnostic uncertainty. In this instance, the term "severe dysplasia" is used to capture the possibility that the lesion actually is a

melanoma and not a nevus. For practical purposes, the lower grades of "dysplasia," like "moderate or minimal dysplasia," do not convey this meaning; in fact, their practical meaning (ie, their diagnostic or biologic significance) is completely unclear.

THE CONFUSION OF PORTIONS OF MELANOMA THAT LOOK LIKE NEVI WITH PORTIONS OF NEVI THAT LOOK LIKE MELANOMA

There are parts of a melanoma that may look like a nevus clinically, dermatoscopically, and histopathologically. Flat melanomas especially may have inconspicuous parts that may lack melanoma clues, which often led to the assumption that the inconspicuous part of the melanoma is a precursor nevus. This assumption is not justified. The realization of criteria used by dermatoscopists and dermatopathologists to diagnose melanomas may vary from classic over weak to absent. The absence of criteria in certain parts of the lesion does not eliminate the possibility that the whole lesion is a melanoma. The lesion shown in **Figs. 8** and **9** demonstrates this concept with regard to the example of the dermatoscopic feature of the pigment network ("reticular pattern"). An atypical or irregular pigment network like the one shown in the dermatoscopic image in **Fig. 9** is considered to be a strong clue to melanoma. The irregular network means that the network looks differently in different parts of the lesion. In some parts the lines are gray and thick and in others the lines are thin and light brown. One is tempted to assume that the thin and light brown parts correspond to a nevus and the thick and gray parts correspond to a melanoma. However, on dermatopathology (**Fig. 10**) it is evident that the entire lesion is a melanoma in situ. The misinterpretation of portions of melanoma as "dysplastic nevus" is not restricted to dermatoscopy; it is

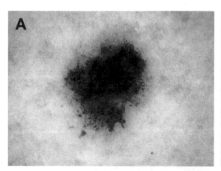
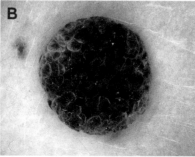

Fig. 4. Dermatoscopic images of 2 melanocytic nevi. (*A*) A flat Clark's nevus showing brown reticular lines and clods, with patterns and colors arranged asymmetrically. (*B*) A slightly raised dermal nevus (Unna nevus) dermatoscopically showing a pattern of clods with symmetrically arranged pattern and color.

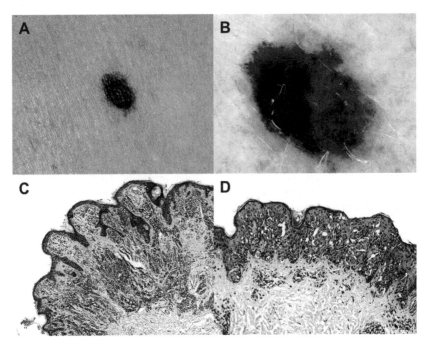

Fig. 5. Clinical (*A*), dermatoscopic (*B*), and histopathologic (*C, D*) images of a melanoma (*D*) arising within an otherwise inconspicuous dermal nevus with a pattern of clods (*C*) (hematoxylin eosin, original magnification ×100).

also common in dermatopathology. Parts of a melanoma may resemble a nevus on dermatopathology. This phenomenon is well known by dermatopathologists under the term "nevoid" melanoma, which is a melanoma that as a whole looks like nevus.

THE TERM "DYSPLASTIC NEVUS," ALTHOUGH INADEQUATE, SERVED CLINICIANS, PATHOLOGISTS, AND PATIENTS WELL

Although inadequate, the term "dysplastic nevus" served dermatologists and dermatopathologists

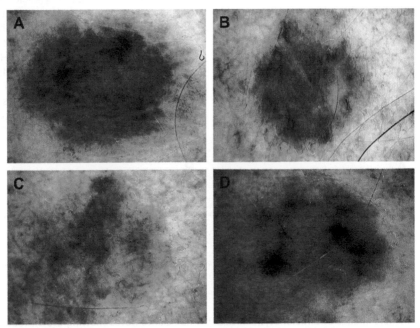

Fig. 6. (*A–D*) Four atypical melanocytic lesions on the same patient, documented by dermatoscopic follow-up. Although all lesions show atypia, only the lesion on the lower right (*D*) was a melanoma.

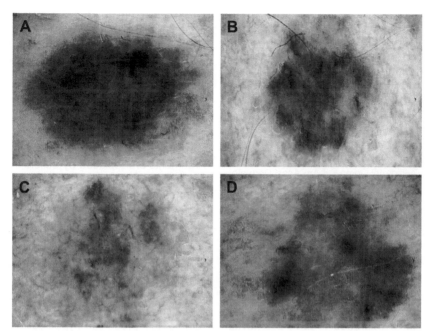

Fig. 7. Dermatoscopic follow-up images of lesions corresponding to those shown in **Fig. 6**, imaged 6 months after baseline. Only the melanoma (*D*) changed significantly; the other atypical nevi (*A–C*) did not change during follow-up.

well in the past for various reasons. First, the concept of stepwise tumor progression is appealing and plausible and the dysplastic nevus fills the gap between a benign lesion and a malignant lesion. When melanomas are small and flat, they are difficult to diagnose clinically and dermatoscopically. They look like nevi. From a dermatologist's point of view it is appealing to assume that the phase when melanoma is still inconspicuous is a benign precursor stage of malignancy but not yet malignant. This averts to confess the inability to diagnose small and flat melanoma with certainty. The same limits that pertain to clinicians and dermatoscopists pertain to dermatopathologists. Melanomas are rarely diagnosed when they are smaller than 5 mm, although they exist. Second, there is a certain fear of doctors that diagnostic uncertainty will be misinterpreted as incompetence. From the point of view of a dermatopathologist, it may be easier to call a lesion a severely dysplastic nevus than to admit that he does not know for sure whether this lesion is a melanoma in situ or a Clark nevus. There is an understandable need to paraphrase diagnostic uncertainty. The terms "dysplastic nevus" and "atypical nevus" fulfill this purpose. Third, removal of a nevus for diagnostic reasons is associated with morbidity and is not a pleasure to the patients. It costs them time and money; it may leave scars, and there may be complications including bleeding and infection. If the removed nevus turns out to be just an "ordinary" nevus, patients may view the efforts and risks taken into account to have it removed under a different light as compared with

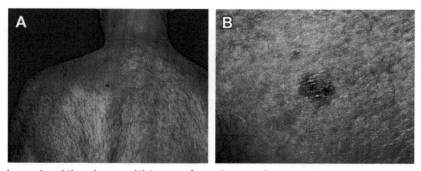

Fig. 8. Clinical overview (*A*) and macro (*B*) image of a melanoma shown in **Figs. 9** and **10**.

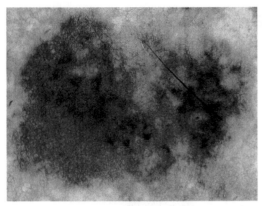

Fig. 9. Dermatoscopic image of the melanoma shown in **Fig. 8.** Inconspicuous reticular lines on the lower left coexist with an atypical pigment network within the rest of the lesion.

the situation if the removed nevus turns out to be a more "dangerous " dysplastic nevus. By mentioning that "it was good to have this nevus removed because it might have been on the way to something malignant" it sanctifies our decisions in retrospect. Last, it has to be admitted that the phenotype of multiple large nevi commonly known as "dysplastic nevus syndrome" is associated with an increased risk to develop melanoma. Although the fate of a single lesion cannot be predicted, neither by clinical nor by dermatoscopic examination, it is known that these patients need lifelong

surveillance of their skin by skilled dermatologists to detect melanomas as early as possible and to remove them when they are still small and flat so that the patient is cured by simple excision.

TWO DIFFERENT CAMPS: BELIEVERS AND NONBELIEVERS

Unfortunately, some disputes in dermatology and dermatopathology are not solved by arguments. Arguments are replaced by beliefs and critique is not tolerated or ignored. Sometimes 2 or more camps are forming that are centered on charismatic persons and the camp with more followers and more visibility prevails. The camp of the critics of the "dysplastic nevus" was led by A Bernard Ackerman, one of the most distinguished and charismatic figures in dermatology and dermatopathology of the last century. He was the first to express significant doubts with regard to the existence and relevance of the dysplastic nevus and refuted the precursor hypothesis.[34] During the past years the controversy of the dysplastic nevus has not been solved. The positions of believers and critics of the dysplastic nevus eventually become so entrenched, especially in dermatopathology, that any open and critical discussions stopped. This is where dermatoscopy comes into play. Dermatoscopy may create a new momentum and supply the dermatologic community with new arguments that may lead to fresh and surprising

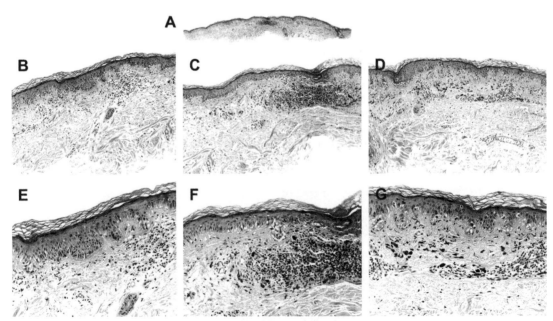

Fig. 10. Overview (A) and close-up (B–G) histopathologic images of the melanoma shown in **Fig. 9.** Nests of melanocytes confined to the rete ridges (D, G) coexist with confluent single melanocytes at the dermoepidermal junction (C, F) (hematoxylin eosin, original magnification ×100).

solutions of an old problem. The problem of the dysplastic nevus in particular and the unsolved problem of the classification of nevi cannot be solved by pathology alone but only by clinical-dermatoscopic-biologic-pathologic correlation.

SUMMARY

The term "dysplastic nevus" is a misnomer and should be abandoned. The generic term "dysplastic nevus" is not just a name, it is the root of the concept that histomorphology (or any morphologic examination including dermatoscopy) is able to predict the fate of a benign melanocytic proliferation. There is no evidence that this hypothesis is true but there are observations that falsify it. This does not necessarily mean that the concept of stepwise tumor progression is not valid; it means that the accumulation of mutations that is necessary to induce malignancy does not express itself as a morphologic spectrum that spans from common nevus over dysplastic nevus to melanoma in situ.

From a dermatoscopic point, the diagnosis of atypia or dysplasia describes diagnostic uncertainty and not an entity (ie, a specific type of nevus). In contrast to the histomorphologic criteria of dysplasia, the patterns observed by dermatoscopy are reproducible and robust and can be used to classify nevi without the need to excise them except when there is diagnostic uncertainty. The use of the generic terms "dysplastic nevus" and "atypical nevus" for nevi with chaotic arrangement of colors or patterns (morphologic characteristics that are correlated with diagnostic uncertainty) is discouraged. Preferably a specific diagnosis should be made based on dermatoscopic pattern (for example, Spitz nevus, Reed nevus, Clark nevus, or congenital nevus) and if this is not possible on clinical or dermatoscopic grounds alone the term "nevus, not otherwise specified" should be used.

REFERENCES

1. Clark WH Jr, Reimer RR, Greene M, et al. Origin of familial malignant melanomas from heritable melanocytic lesions. 'The B-K mole syndrome'. Arch Dermatol 1978;114:732–8.
2. Clark WH Jr, Elder DE, Guerry D, et al. A study of tumor progression: the precursor lesions of superficial spreading and nodular melanoma. Hum Pathol 1984;15:1147–65.
3. Greene MH, Clark WH Jr, Tucker MA, et al. Acquired precursors of cutaneous malignant melanoma. The familial dysplastic nevus syndrome. N Engl J Med 1985;312:91–7.
4. Lynch HT, Frichot BC 3rd, Lynch JF. Familial atypical multiple mole-melanoma syndrome. J Med Genet 1978;15:352–6.
5. Kraemer KH, Greene MH, Tarone R, et al. Dysplastic naevi and cutaneous melanoma risk. Lancet 1983;2:1076–7.
6. Arumi-Uria M, McNutt NS, Finnerty B. Grading of atypia in nevi: correlation with melanoma risk. Mod Pathol 2003;16:764–71.
7. Bevona C, Goggins W, Quinn T, et al. Cutaneous melanomas associated with nevi. Arch Dermatol 2003;139:1620–4 [discussion: 1624].
8. Tsao H, Bevona C, Goggins W, et al. The transformation rate of moles (melanocytic nevi) into cutaneous melanoma: a population-based estimate. Arch Dermatol 2003;139:282–8.
9. Miller AJ, Mihm MC Jr. Melanoma. N Engl J Med 2006;355:51–65.
10. Duffy K, Grossman D. The dysplastic nevus: from historical perspective to management in the modern era: part I. Historical, histologic, and clinical aspects. J Am Acad Dermatol 2012;67(1):e1–16 [quiz: 17–8].
11. Hastrup N, Osterlind A, Drzewiecki KT, et al. The presence of dysplastic nevus remnants in malignant melanomas. A population-based study of 551 malignant melanomas. Am J Dermatopathol 1991;13:378–85.
12. Sagebiel RW. Melanocytic nevi in histologic association with primary cutaneous melanoma of superficial spreading and nodular types: effect of tumor thickness. J Invest Dermatol 1993;100:322S–5S.
13. Tucker MA, Fraser MC, Goldstein AM, et al. A natural history of melanomas and dysplastic nevi: an atlas of lesions in melanoma-prone families. Cancer 2002;94:3192–209.
14. Decarlo K, Yang S, Emley A, et al. Oncogenic BRAF-positive dysplastic nevi and the tumor suppressor IGFBP7–challenging the concept of dysplastic nevi as precursor lesions? Hum Pathol 2010;41:886–94.
15. Bär M, Tschandl P, Kittler H. Differentiation of pigmented Spitz nevi and Reed nevi by integration of dermatopathologic and dermatoscopic findings. Dermatol Pract Concept 2011;2:3.
16. Kittler H, Rosendahl C, Cameron A, et al. Dermatoscopy - an algorithmic method based on pattern analysis. Facultas.wuv; 2011. p. 334.
17. Criscione VD, Weinstock MA, Naylor MF, et al. Actinic keratoses: natural history and risk of malignant transformation in the Veterans Affairs Topical Tretinoin Chemoprevention Trial. Cancer 2009;115:2523–30.
18. Glogau RG. The risk of progression to invasive disease. J Am Acad Dermatol 2000;42:23–4.
19. Kittler H, Pehamberger H, Wolff K, et al. Follow-up of melanocytic skin lesions with digital epiluminescence microscopy: patterns of modifications

observed in early melanoma, atypical nevi, and common nevi. J Am Acad Dermatol 2000;43:467–76.

20. Kittler H, Seltenheim M, Dawid M, et al. Frequency and characteristics of enlarging common melanocytic nevi. Arch Dermatol 2000;136:316–20.

21. Fuller SR, Bowen GM, Tanner B, et al. Digital dermoscopic monitoring of atypical nevi in patients at risk for melanoma. Dermatol Surg 2007;33:1198–206 [discussion: 1205–6].

22. Salerni G, Carrera C, Lovatto L, et al. Characterization of 1152 lesions excised over 10 years using total-body photography and digital dermatoscopy in the surveillance of patients at high risk for melanoma. J Am Acad Dermatol 2012;67:836–45.

23. Meyer LJ, Piepkorn M, Goldgar DE, et al. Interobserver concordance in discriminating clinical atypia of melanocytic nevi, and correlations with histologic atypia. J Am Acad Dermatol 1996;34:618–25.

24. Ackerman A. Gentle word of advice: atypical melanocytic nevi. Available at: Derm101.com. Accessed July 15, 2013.

25. Zalaudek I, Grinschgl S, Argenziano G, et al. Age-related prevalence of dermoscopy patterns in acquired melanocytic naevi. Br J Dermatol 2006; 154:299–304.

26. Beer J, Xu L, Tschandl P, et al. Growth rate of melanoma in vivo and correlation with dermatoscopic and dermatopathologic findings. Dermatol Pract Concept 2011;1(1):13.

27. Marks R, Dorevitch AP, Mason G. Do all melanomas come from "moles"? A study of the histological association between melanocytic naevi and melanoma. Australas J Dermatol 1990;31:77–80.

28. Hussussian CJ, Struewing JP, Goldstein AM, et al. Germline p16 mutations in familial melanoma. Nat Genet 1994;8:15–21.

29. Kamb A, Gruis NA, Weaver-Feldhaus J, et al. A cell cycle regulator potentially involved in genesis of many tumor types. Science 1994;264:436–40.

30. Zuo L, Weger J, Yang Q, et al. Germline mutations in the p16INK4a binding domain of CDK4 in familial melanoma. Nat Genet 1996;12:97–9.

31. Molven A, Grimstvedt MB, Steine SJ, et al. A large Norwegian family with inherited malignant melanoma, multiple atypical nevi, and CDK4 mutation. Genes Chromosomes Cancer 2005;44: 10–8.

32. Gast A, Scherer D, Chen B, et al. Somatic alterations in the melanoma genome: a high-resolution array-based comparative genomic hybridization study. Genes Chromosomes Cancer 2010;49:733–45.

33. Goodson AG, Florell SR, Boucher KM, et al. A decade of melanomas: identification of factors associated with delayed detection in an academic group practice. Dermatol Surg 2011;37:1620–30.

34. Ackerman A, Nierlsen T, Massi D. Dysplastic nevus: atypical mole or typical myth? Ardor Scribendi; 1999.

Spitz Nevus, Spitz Tumor, and Spitzoid Melanoma
A Comprehensive Clinicopathologic Overview

Gerardo Ferrara, MD[a],*, Raffaele Gianotti, MD[b],
Stefano Cavicchini, MD[c], Tiziana Salviato, MD[d],
Iris Zalaudek, MD[e,f], Giuseppe Argenziano, MD[f]

KEYWORDS

- Dermoscopy • Histopathology • Spitz nevus • Atypical Spitz nevus • Spitz tumor
- Spitzoid melanoma

KEY POINTS

- A classification of spitzoid melanocytic lesions into tumors (without or with atypical features) and melanoma has been recently proposed, thereby underlining the existence of a morphobiologic spectrum of lesions, ranging from benignity to full-blown malignancy. However, only in rare instances are spitzoid lesions clinically tumors (ie, cutaneous elevations [nodules] exceeding the size of a cherry [>2 cm]).
- Dermoscopy has demonstrated that the pigmented (brown-black) variant of Spitz nevus is more common than the classical (pink-red) variant; the main dermoscopic patterns are defined as globular, starburst, and multicomponent (atypical, melanoma-like). In clinicopathologic studies the classical (pink-red) variant of Spitz nevus, dermoscopically typified by dotted vessels and white network, is surprisingly rare and is an atypical Spitz nevus or a Spitz tumor with a greater probability than a brown-black plaque.
- A grading system for atypical spitzoid lesions is desirable to avoid overtreatment, mainly in prepubescent patients. We propose a distinction between atypical Spitz nevus and (atypical) Spitz tumor, based on the presence of tumorigenic features (ulceration, dermal sheets of cells, numerous, or deep-sited mitoses) solely in the latter.
- Pediatric spitzoid melanoma is genetically different from its adult counterpart and has very peculiar clinicopathologic features, namely the presence of an overtly malignant nonspitzoid morphologic clone arising in the context of a spitzoid lesion. Such a highly unusual occurrence can be detected even clinically and dermoscopically.
- No single clinicodermoscopic feature can allow reliable differentiation of Spitz nevus from melanoma. In patients up to 12 years of age, small (up to 1 cm) and dermoscopically typical spitzoid lesions can be submitted to follow-up with controls every 3 to 6 months; conversely, all spitzoid lesions must be excised in patients older than 12 years.

Funding Sources: None.
Conflicts of Interest: None.

[a] Anatomic Pathology Unit, Department of Oncology, 'Gaetano Rummo' General Hospital, Via dell'Angelo 1, Benevento I-82100, Italy; [b] Department of Pathophysiology and Transplantation, University of Milan, Via Pace 9, Milan I-20122, Italy; [c] Dermatology Unit, Fondazione IRCCS Ca' Granda Ospedale Maggiore Policlinico, Via Pace 9, Milan I-20122, Italy; [d] Anatomic Pathology Unit, Department of Laboratory Medicine, 'Santa Maria degli Angeli' General Hospital, Via Montereale 24, Pordenone I-33170, Italy; [e] Department of Dermatology, Medical University of Graz, Auenbruggerplatz 1, Graz A-8036, Austria; [f] Dermatology and Skin Cancer Unit, Department of Dermatology, Arcispedale Santa Maria Nuova IRCCS, Viale Risorgimento 80, Reggio Emilia I-42100, Italy
* Corresponding author.
E-mail address: gerardo.ferrara@libero.it

derm.theclinics.com

INTRODUCTION

The clinicopathologic classification, diagnosis, and management of spitzoid melanocytic lesions are some of the most problematic topics in dermatopathology. This is because of the efforts in terms of time and attention they require and the potential medicolegal implications, as a result of under and over diagnosis of melanoma.

After earlier anecdotal reports[1,2] the history of these controversial lesions began in 1948 when Sophie Spitz described 13 cases of what she called "juvenile melanoma," underlining its presumably good prognosis because only one case of her series had proved fatal.[3] During the following 40 years, the entity described by Sophie Spitz was thought to be completely benign, with metastasizing cases being intuitively considered as cases of melanomas simulating Spitz nevus (spitzoid melanoma).[4] In 1989, Smith and coworkers described the so-called Spitz nevus with atypia and metastasis or malignant Spitz nevus (ie, a kind of Spitz lesion showing histopathologic features insufficient for a diagnosis of malignancy, yet capable of nodal metastasis, usually with no further dissemination).[5] This apparently contradictory concept was then set forth by Barnhill with the diagnostic category of metastasizing Spitz tumor[6] or atypical Spitz nevus/tumor.[7] To date, although Ackerman and his fellows maintain that there are only two diagnostic categories (nevus and melanoma), and that every abnormal behavior is simply a diagnostic mistake,[8] others suggest that spitzoid lesions are indeed a morphobiologic spectrum ranging from benignity to full-blown malignancy,[9] with the intermediate lesions requiring a diagnostic approach based on different (peculiar) taxonomic and diagnostic criteria.[10] As an extreme consequence of this view, every spitzoid lesion actually could be intermediate and thereby designated as tumors (without or with atypical features)[11]: this implies that all spitzoid lesions could be virtually nonbenign and that the new dichotomic approach could be tumor versus melanoma. This article argues against old and new dichotomic diagnostic approaches.

A NEW CLINICAL STEREOTYPE OF SPITZ NEVUS

A classification of spitzoid lesions into Spitz tumors without atypical features, atypical Spitz tumors, and spitzoid melanoma[11] is not easily accepted; nor is it in keeping with existing clinicopathologic terminology, because clinical dermatology literally defines tumors as cutaneous elevations (nodules) exceeding the size of a cherry (ie, generally >2 cm),[12,13] and this is seldom the case for spitzoid lesions.

The increasing use of dermoscopy (dermatoscopy, skin surface microscopy) in the preoperative evaluation of cutaneous lesions will dramatically change the view of these lesions. Before dermoscopy (or without dermoscopy), Spitz nevus could be mainly identified by clinicians as a red nodule of the face and extremities of children; in addition, histopathologists previously stated that about one-fourth of Spitz nevi could be found in patients older than 14 years and that some cases could also present as tan-brown or black macules or plaques.[14] Such a pigmented variant of Spitz nevus was thoroughly described pathologically, albeit with a few exceptions,[15] as composed of spindle cells (pigmented spindle cell Spitz nevus), but was poorly characterized on clinical grounds. Moreover, its histopathologic recognition raised the issue of the nosologic autonomy, if any, of pigmented spindle cell Spitz nevus[14,16] from Reed nevus.[17] In a recent histopathologic review on a large series of Spitz nevi, Requena and colleagues[18] embraced the largely adopted theory that considers Reed nevus as belonging to the morphologic spectrum of Spitz nevus.[16,19,20] Requena and colleagues[18] stated that Reed nevus is the most common variant of Spitz nevus (64 out of 349 cases in their series). In agreement with the findings of Requena and colleagues,[18] we have previously found that a histopathologic distinction between pigmented spindle cell Spitz nevus and Reed nevus is not feasible.[19] In addition, and even more importantly, such a distinction has no clinical relevance: clinically, pigmented spindle cell Spitz nevus and Reed nevus are commonly medium-sized (mean size in our series, 4.9 mm[19]) brown to black macules or plaques; these lesions are not tumors inasmuch as they are (relatively) small and flat or only slightly raised. Dermoscopically, pigmented spindle cell Spitz nevus and Reed nevus are more or less heavily pigmented, with three main global patterns: (1) globular; (2) starburst; and (3) multicomponent (atypical, melanoma-like).[19] In these frankly pigmented lesions, globules are brown to black, large, and regularly distributed at the periphery (**Fig. 1**A). When peripheral globules are fused with the central body of the lesion, regular, "on focus" radial projections (so-called streaks) are found in the so-called starburst pattern (see **Fig. 1**B). In a minority of cases, a heavy pigmentation also gives rise to a regular black network, which lies superficially (in the stratum corneum) and can be removed by tape stripping (ie, superficial black network; see **Fig. 1**C).[20] Several of these features can be simultaneously present or

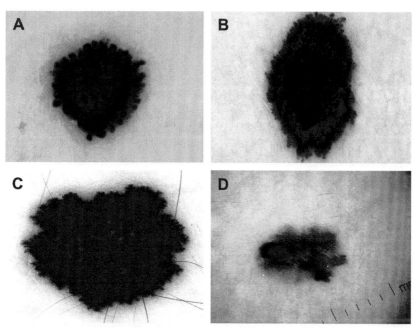

Fig. 1. Dermoscopic view of a Spitz/Reed nevus with a globular pattern (*A*), starburst pattern (*B*), starburst pattern with superficial black network (*C*), and atypical multicomponent pattern (*D*).

irregularly and asymmetrically distributed within a given lesion, thus giving a multicomponent, atypical, or melanoma-like pattern (see **Fig. 1**D). Dermoscopic atypia is also increased by the presence of a blue whitish veil, which results from deep dermal pigmentation with an overlying epidermal hyperplasia.

Histopathologically, these heavily pigmented lesions are plaque-shaped, well circumscribed, and mostly composed of sharply demarcated melanocytic nests within a more or less hyperplastic epidermis (**Fig. 2**A). Spindle or epithelioid melanocytes are arranged perpendicular and parallel to the skin surface (see **Fig. 2**B); they are highly cohesive and do not destroy the nearby keratinocytes; therefore, a semilunar cleavage is often evident around nests (capping) and even around the few single intraepidermal melanocytes (microcapping) (see **Fig. 2**C). Transepidermal elimination of nests is common and can be responsible for the complete involution of these lesions.[21] Melanin pigment is present mainly within spindle cells, dermal melanophages (often arranged in a band-like fashion), and single intraepidermal dendritic melanocytes[22]; pigmented parakeratosis can be present in a tidy skip fashion, thereby accounting for the presence of a superficial black network.[20] When a sizable dermal component is present, the lesion becomes dome-shaped, with regularly spaced dermal nests and cords of cells; maturation is at least focally seen; mitoses may be easily

found, but virtually never in large number and never close to the base of the lesion. Overall, ulceration, dermal sheets of cells, and significant mitotic activity are lacking: therefore, these lesions are not tumors.

In clinicodermoscopic-pathologic studies, pink-red Spitz nevi with a monomorphic dotted vascular pattern, often associated with regularly intersecting white lines (the so-called reticular depigmentation or white network),[23] are surprisingly rare (4.8% in our series[19]). Therefore, dermoscopy seems to allow clinicians to increasingly identify and excise pigmented spindle cell Spitz nevus/Reed nevus, to such an extent that the previously poorly defined tan or black Spitz nevus is surprisingly becoming the most common Spitz nevus encountered in clinicodermoscopic-pathologic studies.

ATYPICAL SPITZ NEVUS OR TUMOR: DOES THE CLINICAL PICTURE MATTER?

Once a typical Spitz nevus is redefined, we should define the atypical categories. At present, an unequivocal and reproducible definition for atypical Spitz nevus and (atypical) Spitz tumor is probably lacking. In general, these diagnostic categories can be used for lesions showing some distinctly abnormal characteristics commonly absent in conventional spitzoid lesions.

In 2005, Urso[10] performed a review of 19 papers reporting 62 spitzoid neoplasms showing an

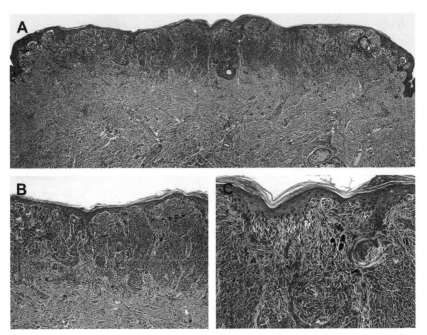

Fig. 2. Histopathologic picture of the lesion shown in **Fig. 1**B, removed from the thigh of a 28-year-old woman. A medium-sized, sharply circumscribed, symmetric plaque (*A*; hematoxylin and eosin, original magnification ×40) composed of fascicles of spindle cells (*B*; hematoxylin and eosin, original magnification ×100); these are highly monomorphic and cohesive, with evidence of microcapping (*C*; hematoxylin and eosin, original magnification ×250).

aggressive biologic behavior despite histopathologic features that were insufficient for a diagnosis of clear-cut malignancy. Nine criteria were thus found to be predictive of metastatic potential: notably, such criteria were not the same as for conventional melanoma and, most importantly, they had to be used in a completely different manner, because even the presence of one criterion could be virtually incompatible with benignity. Urso's[10] criteria are listed in **Table 1**, along with their expected clinicodermoscopic counterpart. By accepting Urso's approach[10] atypical (possibly malignant) spitzoid neoplasms could be clinically outlined as medium to large, papulonodular lesions lacking brownish to black pigmentation. Pink-red, papulonodular lesions, previously considered as the classical Spitz nevus, could be histopathologically atypical and possibly biologically malignant with a greater probability than tan-black macules and plaques of pigmented spindle cell Spitz nevus/Reed nevus (see previous paragraph).

A major problem, however, is raised by Urso's diagnostic approach,[10] namely the introduction of a low threshold for potential (but relatively unlikely) malignant behavior with the implementation of relatively few diagnostic criteria. Because many atypical spitzoid neoplasms are found in the

prepubertal age-group, in which melanoma is exceedingly rare,[24] this approach can result in a consistent overtreatment of patients.[25] This is the main consideration that should point toward a grading system for spitzoid lesions. In 1999, Spatz and colleagues[26] proposed approaching pediatric cases of atypical spitzoid lesions according to a grading system (ie, low, intermediate, and high-risk categories) based on patient age, lesion diameter, presence of ulceration, involvement of the subcutis, and mitotic count. However, this system has never been validated in a larger series, nor has it ever been extended to adult cases. In our view the gamut of spitzoid lesions comprises a spectrum from typical (overtly benign) Spitz nevus; to atypical Spitz nevus (benign, with atypical histopathologic features); to (atypical) Spitz tumor (potential low-grade melanoma); then finally to frankly malignant spitzoid melanoma (ie, melanoma with spitzoid features). This schema probably reflects a progressive accumulation of genetic alterations in the spitzoid lesion, which places any given lesion at a certain point in the spectrum ranging from nevus to melanoma. It is noteworthy that molecular morphology techniques (immunohistochemistry and fluorescence in situ hybridization) can disclose additional atypical features and, instead of assisting in formulating a

Table 1
Histomorphologic criteria for metastasizing atypical Spitz nevi/tumors with their clinicodermoscopic correlates

Histopathologic Features	Clinicodermoscopic Correlates
Expansile dermal nodule	(Large) nodule
Deep extension	(Large) nodule
Deep mitoses	Nodule
Abundant melanin at depth	Brown-black pigmentation absent; bluish hue possible
Great nuclear pleomorphism	No correlate
Asymmetry	Asymmetry (when superficial)
Necrosis	No correlate
Epidermal atrophy	Prominent vascular pattern, ulceration
Cells within the lymph vessels	No correlate

Data from Urso C. A new perspective for Spitz tumors? Am J Dermatopathol 2005;27:364–6.

clear-cut differential diagnosis between benignity and malignancy, they seem to give further evidence for the existence of a spectrum of lesions ranging from benignity to full-blown malignancy.[27] **Fig. 3** compares our four-tiered classification system of spitzoid lesions with previously proposed diagnostic categories. **Table 2** summarizes our proposal regarding the histopathologic criteria that may be used to differentiate atypical Spitz nevus and (atypical) Spitz tumor. It should be noted briefly that a Spitz tumor is by literal definition not only atypical but also tumorigenic (and potentially a type of low-grade melanocytic malignancy), that is, it is characterized by a nodular silhouette made by confluent sheets of cells in the dermis without intervening collagen, or (nontraumatic) ulceration or high mitotic rate.

The relationship between dermoscopic and histopathologic atypia is not absolute, inasmuch as dermoscopically atypical lesions are not necessarily histopathologically atypical: we have already demonstrated that about 27% of dermoscopically atypical (melanoma-like) Spitz nevi are not histopathologically atypical as one would expect.[19] However, when a given spitzoid lesion is histopathologically atypical but its grading (ie, atypical

Spitz nevus vs tumor) is uncertain, the presence of clinical/dermoscopic features of significant atypia could point toward its management as a tumor (ie, potential low-grade melanoma) instead of an atypical Spitz nevus (see later). An example of such is provided in **Fig. 4**.

Whether (atypical) Spitz tumors represent a merely morphologic or also a biologic intermediate category is still under debate. We regard these neoplasms as potentially representing a kind of low-grade malignant melanocytic tumor (different from conventional melanoma), partly based on the results of a dermatopathology tutorial held in 2008 in Graz, Austria. The tutorial was aimed at evaluating 57 melanocytic tumors of uncertain malignant potential, 35 of which were (atypical) Spitz tumors of Breslow depth 1.1 to 9.4 mm. Fifteen Spitz tumors had an unfavorable behavior, with the onset of distant metastasis or large metastatic deposits in the lymph nodes or disease-related death. A panel of expert histopathologists was unable to differentiate cases with favorable and unfavorable behavior based on morphologic grounds. Consequently, it was concluded that the cases were all malignant, albeit clearly different from conventional melanoma because of a great

Diagnostic system	Diagnostic categories			
Ackerman's two-tiered [8]	Spitz nevus		Spitzoid melanoma	
Barnhill's two-tiered [11]	Spitz tumor		Spitzoid melanoma	
Barnhill's three-tiered [7]	Spitz nevus	Atypical Spitz nevus/tumor		Spitzoid melanoma
Da Forno's four-tiered [34]	Spitz nevus	Atypical Spitz nevus	Atypical Spitz tumor	Spitzoid melanoma

Fig. 3. A comparison of the different diagnostic approaches to spitzoid lesions, as set forth over time. The four-tiered classification system best reflects the existence of a morphobiologic spectrum encompassing intermediate (*gray*) lesions placed in between complete benignity (*white*) and full-blown malignancy (*black*).

Table 2
Proposed histopathologic criteria for the differential diagnosis between atypical Spitz nevus and Spitz tumor

Microscopic Features	Atypical Spitz Nevus	Atypical Spitz Tumor (possible low-grade melanoma)
Size	7–10 mm	>10 mm
Tumorigenicity (ie, nodule)	−	++
Asymmetry	Superficial	Deep ± superficial
Sharp circumscription, intraepidermal	±	±
Sharp circumscription, lateral dermal	−	±
Sharp circumscription, deep dermal	−	+/++
Epidermal atrophy	±	+/++
Ulceration	−	±
Large dermal nests	Superficial	Deep ± superficial
Dermal sheets of cells	−	+/++
Deep extension	−	+
Melanin in the deep portion of the lesion	−	±
Cytologic atypia	Focal (random)	Widespread
Maturation	+	−
Inflammation	± (uniformly distributed)	−/++ (patchy, irregular)
Mitotic figures	Few	Numerous or close to the base

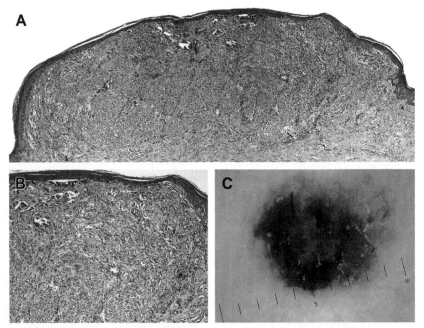

Fig. 4. A spitzoid neoplasm removed from the thigh of a 19-year-old woman. The lesion is dome-shaped with slight and superficial asymmetry (*A*; hematoxylin and eosin, original magnification ×40); there is epidermal atrophy with some tendency to confluence of the dermal nests (*B*; hematoxylin and eosin, original magnification ×100). Overall, the lesion is histopathologically within the spectrum between an atypical Spitz nevus and atypical Spitz tumor. Dermoscopy shows an asymmetrically pigmented lesion with structureless brown to bluish color and an atypical vascular pattern. Based on these atypical dermoscopic features the lesion was managed as a Spitz tumor. The re-excision and sentinel node biopsy specimens showed no microscopic disease.

thickness associated with a low metastatic rate.[28] The term "melanocytoma" has been recently proposed for putatively low-grade melanocytic malignancies that seem capable of metastasis to regional lymph nodes but have limited potential for distant spread.[29] In our opinion, (atypical) Spitz tumor may represent one member of the melanocytoma family.

SPITZOID MELANOMA: LESSONS FROM DERMOSCOPY

Ongoing molecular genetic studies on spitzoid neoplasms seem to be a promising diagnostic tool. HRAS mutations and amplifications have been detected in 11.8% of Spitz nevi,[30] whereas BRAF and NRAS mutations, which are frequently found in melanoma on skin without chronic sun damage (ie, intermittently sun-exposed sites),[31] are rare in Spitz nevi.[32] Indeed, when evaluating the reported frequency of BRAF and NRAS mutations, at a first glance it seems that Spitz nevi are different from typical acquired nevi, whereas spitzoid melanoma genetically resembles common (ie, conventional) melanoma.[33] However, if more stringent morphologic criteria are used,[34] and if

investigation is restricted to lesions removed from children aged less than or equal to 10 years, it becomes evident that, like classical Spitz nevus, spitzoid melanoma does not harbor BRAF or NRAS activating mutations.[35] Notably, Da Forno and colleagues[34] have argued that studies in which the genetic signature of spitzoid melanoma is demonstrated to be different from conventional melanoma have a lower mean age of patients[35,36] than studies in which BRAF or NRAS mutations are found also in spitzoid melanoma.[33] Thus, Da Forno and colleagues[34] conclude that age could have some bearing on the likelihood of BRAF or NRAS mutation in a spitzoid lesion. In other words, pediatric spitzoid melanoma might be a peculiar entity, biologically different from adult-type spitzoid melanoma and from common melanoma.

Our clinicopathologic experience, based on a limited number of cases, mirrors these recent molecular findings: adult spitzoid melanoma is often clinically and dermoscopically indistinguishable from conventional melanoma, whereas pediatric spitzoid melanoma shows peculiar clinicopathologic features. Indeed, it differs from atypical Spitz nevus or Spitz tumor by showing a nonspitzoid cytomorphologic clone arising in the context of a

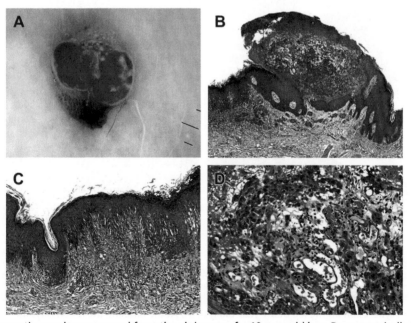

Fig. 5. A melanocytic neoplasm removed from the abdomen of a 10-year-old boy. Dermoscopically (A) the lesion is composed of two distinctive portions: a larger reddish papular part, typified by polymorphic vessels; and a smaller flat part, with reticular depigmentation and a structureless brown pigmentation. Histopathologically the neoplasm is strikingly asymmetric, polypoid, and ulcerated (B; hematoxylin and eosin, original magnification ×25); the shoulder is consistent with a junctional spindle cell Spitz nevus (C; hematoxylin and eosin, original magnification ×100); conversely, the exophytic portion is composed of pleomorpic epithelioid cells (D; hematoxylin and eosin, original magnification ×250), which are morphologically distinct from the junctional lateral component and represent an overtly malignant component.

spitzoid lesion. Such a highly unusual occurrence can be detected even clinically and dermoscopically. In **Fig. 5** the overtly malignant clone is the red nodule with an atypical vascular pattern, which is histopathologically composed of pleomorphic epithelioid cells that are strikingly different from the monomorphic spindle cells of the shoulder of the neoplasm (consistent with a junctional spindle cell Spitz nevus). In **Fig. 6** the clone is the deeply pigmented eccentric peripheral island[37] detected during dermoscopic digital follow-up and histopathologically corresponding to an atypical epithelioid proliferation in a pagetoid configuration (ie, melanoma) arising in the background of a spindle cell Spitz nevus. These cases also suggest that a (spitzoid) melanoma can arise in the background of a Spitz nevus, just as has been reported for melanoma arising in a Spitz tumor.[38]

GUIDELINES FOR MANAGEMENT

As a general rule, Spitz nevi can be considered as potentially showing all the dermoscopic features

of melanoma, but in a more or less regular fashion. However, the occurrence of an atypical dermoscopic pattern in Spitz nevi is well recognized,[19] as is the occurrence of melanomas showing very few or no dermoscopic features suggestive of malignancy but exhibiting instead either the globular or the starburst pattern typical of Spitz nevi.[39]

Based on these considerations, a classical or pigmented Spitz nevus appearing up to the age of 12 years can be readily diagnosed and managed conservatively if it is relatively small (up to 1 cm) and shows no atypical clinical and dermoscopic features. Under these circumstances, a follow-up can be scheduled with controls every 3 to 6 months.[40] In the absence of dramatic changes in color, shape, or size, such a follow-up protocol can be continued until the appearance of a homogeneous pattern; thereafter, a 1-year follow-up can be used.

Large (>1 cm), nodular, ulcerated, rapidly growing or changing, or otherwise atypical spitzoid lesions of childhood must be excised. Surgical excision is also recommended when spitzoid

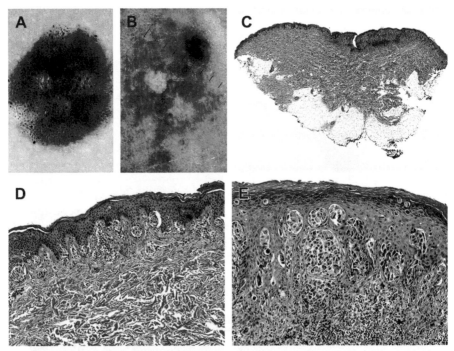

Fig. 6. A melanocytic lesion on the leg of a 1-year-old girl. (*A*) At the baseline the lesion is typified by a symmetric globular pattern. After 37 months follow-up, there is evidence of widespread involution[21] associated with the presence of a peripheral eccentric hyperpigmented area (*B*; dermoscopic island).[35] Histopathologically the lesion is very broad, with an asymmetric lichenoid band (*C*; hematoxylin and eosin, original magnification ×25); the cytoarchitectural features are largely consistent with a junctional spindle cell Spitz nevus, also with evidence of capping (*D*; hematoxylin and eosin, original magnification ×100); however, the area with the lichenoid lymphocytic infiltrate is characterized by pleomorphic epithelioid cells in a clear-cut pagetoid pattern, featuring an early melanoma (*E*; hematoxylin and eosin, original magnification ×250). The atypical area corresponds to the recently detected dermoscopic island.

lesions appear in adulthood, regardless of the presence of atypical clinical or dermoscopic features.

The management of patients with a histopathologic diagnosis of atypical Spitz nevus or tumor should be decided with a multidisciplinary approach and on an informed consent basis. Re-excision can be considered for atypical Spitz nevi and (atypical) Spitz tumors, and must be recommended for all incompletely excised lesions. The opportunity of a sentinel node biopsy for (atypical) Spitz tumors should be evaluated case by case. The decision must be made by preliminarily considering that in Spitz tumors the presence of isolated tumor cells in the sentinel node may not be an unequivocal sign of malignancy[41] and is not an indication to completion lymphadenectomy, based on the ambiguity of the primary. If this is true, an echotomographic monitoring of the regional nodes (and echotomography-guided fine-needle aspiration biopsy cytology) might even replace sentinel node biopsy, because it is effective in detecting massive replacement of the nodes by neoplastic cells, thereby directing selected patients to election lymphadenectomy.[25] Such a follow-up protocol is probably the best choice in patients younger than 10 years, especially for lesions located in the head and neck area, a region in which surgical procedures are aesthetically relevant and are hampered by a sizable failure rate.[42]

Current management of spitzoid melanoma is the same as for conventional melanoma, with wider re-excision of the primary lesion guided by tumor depth, ancillary work-up, or medical treatment, as directed by a multidisciplinary team.

SUMMARY

The introduction of dermoscopy has significantly changed the clinical diorama of spitzoid lesions. Because there are still many controversial points in the histopathologic categorization of these lesions, clinicopathologic correlation must be the mainstay for their diagnosis and proper management.

REFERENCES

1. Darier FJ, Civatte A. Naevus ou naevo-carcinoma chez on nourisson? Bull Soc Franc Dermatol Syphilol 1910;21:61–3.
2. Pack GT. Pre-pubertal melanoma of the skin. Surg Gynecol Obstet 1948;86:374–5.
3. Spitz S. Melanoma of childhood. Am J Pathol 1948; 24:591–609.
4. Kernen JA, Ackerman LV. Spindle cell nevi and epithelioid cell nevi (so-called juvenile melanomas) in children and adults: a clinicopathologic study of 27 cases. Cancer 1960;13:612–25.
5. Smith KJ, Barrett TL, Skelton HG, et al. Spindle cell and epithelioid cell nevi with atypia and metastasis (malignant Spitz nevus). Am J Surg Pathol 1989; 13:931–9.
6. Barnhill RL, Flotte TJ, Fleischli M, et al. Cutaneous melanoma and atypical Spitz tumors in children. Cancer 1995;76:1833–45.
7. Barnhill RL, Argenyi ZB, From L, et al. Atypical Spitz nevi/tumor: lack of consensus for diagnosis, discrimination from melanoma, and prediction of outcome. Hum Pathol 1999;30:513–20.
8. Mones JM, Ackerman AB. "Atypical" Spitz's nevus, "malignant" Spitz's nevus, and "metastasizing" Spitz's nevus: a critique in historical perspective of three concepts flawed fatally. Am J Dermatopathol 2004;26:310–33.
9. Casso EM, Grin-Jorgensen CM, Grant-Kels JM. Spitz nevi. J Am Acad Dermatol 1992;27:901–13.
10. Urso C. A new perspective for Spitz tumors? Am J Dermatopathol 2005;27:364–5.
11. Barnhill RL. The spitzoid lesion: the importance of atypical variants and risk assessment. Am J Dermatopathol 2006;28:75–83.
12. Dearborn FM. Diseases of the skin with illustrations. New Delhi: B. Jain Publishers; 2002.
13. Ackerman AB, Kerl H, Sanchez J, et al. A clinical atlas of 101 common skin diseases: with histopathologic correlation. 2nd edition. New York: Ardor Scribendi; Available at: https://derm101.com/content/4711. Accessed June 9, 2013.
14. Lever WF, Schamburg-Lever G. Histopathology of the skin. 6th edition. Philadelphia: JB Lippincott; 1983. p. 766–9.
15. Choi JH, Sung KJ, Koh JK. Pigmented epithelioid cell naevus: a variant of Spitz naevus? J Am Acad Dermatol 1993;28:497–8.
16. Paniago-Pereira C, Maize JC, Ackerman AB. Nevus of large spindle and/or epithelioid cell (Spitz's nevus). Arch Dermatol 1978;114:1811–23.
17. Reed RJ, Ichinose H, Clark WH, et al. Common and uncommon melanocytic nevi and borderline melanomas. Semin Oncol 1975;2:119–47.
18. Requena C, Requena L, Kutzner H, et al. Spitz nevus: a clinicopathological study of 349 cases. Am J Dermatopathol 2009;31:107–16.
19. Ferrara G, Argenziano G, Soyer HP, et al. The spectrum of Spitz nevi: a clinicopathologic study of 83 cases. Arch Dermatol 2005;141:1381–7.
20. Argenziano G, Soyer HP, Ferrara G, et al. Superficial black network: an additional dermoscopic clue for the diagnosis of spinal and/or epithelioid cell nevus. Dermatology 2001;203:333–5.
21. Argenziano G, Zalaudek I, Ferrara G, et al. Involution: the natural evolution of pigmented Spitz and Reed nevi? Arch Dermatol 2007;143:549–51.

22. Ferrara G, Crisman G, Soyer HP, et al. Intraepidermal dendritic melanocytes in spitzoid neoplasms. Am J Dermatopathol 2006;28:449–50.

23. Zalaudek I, Kittler H, Hofmann-Wellenhof R, et al. 'White network' in Spitz nevi and early melanomas lacking significant pigmentation. J Am Acad Dermatol 2013;69(1):56–60.

24. Moscarella E, Zalaudek I, Cerroni L, et al. Excised melanocytic lesions in children and adolescents: a 10-year survey. Br J Dermatol 2012;167:368–73.

25. Ferrara G, Errico ME, Donofrio V, et al. Melanocytic tumors of uncertain malignant potential in childhood: do we really need sentinel node biopsy? J Cutan Pathol 2012;39:1049–51.

26. Spatz A, Calonje E, Handfield-Jones S, et al. Spitz tumors in children. A grading system for risk stratification. Arch Dermatol 1999;135:282–5.

27. Ferrara G, Misciali C, Brenn T, et al. The impact of molecular morphology techniques on the expert diagnosis in melanocytic skin neoplasms. Int J Surg Pathol 2013.. [E-pub ahead of print].

28. Cerroni L, Barnhill R, Elder D, et al. Melanocytic tumors of uncertain malignant potential: results of a tutorial held at the XXIX Symposium of the International Society of Dermatopathology in Graz, October 2008. Am J Surg Pathol 2010;34:314–26.

29. Zembowicz A, Scolyer RA. Nevus/melanocytoma/melanoma: an emerging paradigm for classification of melanocytic neoplasms? Arch Pathol Lab Med 2011;135:300–6.

30. Bastian BC, LeBoit PE, Pinkel D. Mutations and copy number increase of HRAS in Spitz nevi with distinctive histopathological features. Am J Pathol 2000;157:967–72.

31. Curtin JA, Fridlyand J, Kageshita T, et al. Distinct sets of genetic alterations in melanoma. N Engl J Med 2005;353:2135–47.

32. Palmedo G, Hantschke M, Ruetten A, et al. The T1796A mutation of the BRAF gene is absent in Spitz nevi. J Cutan Pathol 2004;31:266–70.

33. Van Dijk MC, Bernsen MR, Ruiter DJ. Analysis of mutations in B-RAF, N-RAS, and H-RAS genes in the differential diagnosis of Spitz nevus and spitzoid melanoma. Am J Surg Pathol 2005;29:1145–51.

34. Da Forno PD, Fletcher A, Pringle JY, et al. Understanding spitzoid tumours: new insights from molecular pathology. Br J Dermatol 2008;158:4–14.

35. Gill M, Cohen J, Renwick N, et al. Genetic similarities between Spitz nevus and spitzoid melanoma in children. Cancer 2004;101:2636–40.

36. Lee DA, Cohen JA, Twaddel WS, et al. Are all melanomas the same? Spitzoid melanoma is a distinct subtype of melanoma. Cancer 2006;106:907–13.

37. Borsari S, Longo C, Ferrari C, et al. Dermoscopic island: a new descriptor for thin melanoma. Arch Dermatol 2010;146:1257–62.

38. Magro CM, Yaniv S, Mihm MC. The superficial atypical Spitz tumor and malignant melanoma of the superficial spreading type arising in association with the superficial atypical Spitz tumor: a distinct form of dysplastic spitzoid nevomelanocytic proliferation. J Am Acad Dermatol 2009;60:814–23.

39. Argenziano G, Scalvenzi M, Staibano S, et al. Dermatoscopic pitfalls in differentiating pigmented Spitz nevi from cutaneous melanomas. Br J Dermatol 1999;141:788–93.

40. Brunetti B, Nino M, Sammarco E, et al. Spitz naevus: a proposal for management. J Eur Acad Dermatol Venereol 2005;19:391.

41. LeBoit PE. What do these cells prove? Am J Dermatopathol 2003;25:355–6.

42. Jones EL, Jones TS, Pearlman NW, et al. Long-term follow-up and survival of patients following a recurrence of melanoma after a negative sentinel node biopsy result. JAMA Surg 2013;148:456–61.

The Morphologic Universe of Melanoma

Natalia Jaimes, MD[a],*, Ashfaq A. Marghoob, MD[b]

KEYWORDS

- Dermoscopy • Melanoma • Melanoma specific-structures • Non-glabrous skin • Lentigo maligna
- Nail melanoma • Acral melanoma • Mucosal melanoma

KEY POINTS

- Melanomas usually display an asymmetric and chaotic dermoscopic morphology.
- Most melanomas will reveal at least one of the following melanoma-specific structures: atypical network, negative network, streaks, crystalline structures, atypical dots/globules, irregular blotch, blue-white veil, regression structures, atypical vessels, and peripheral tan structureless areas.
- Melanomas located on the face and on chronically sun-damaged skin are associated with polygonal lines. In addition, melanomas located on the face can also reveal annular-granular pattern with perifollicular granularity, asymmetric perifollicular openings, and rhomboidal structures.
- Melanomas on volar skin are associated with a parallel-ridge pattern or homogeneous pigment involving both the ridges and furrows, and melanomas of the nail unit may reveal a micro-Hutchinson sign and are linked with irregular bands with disruption of parallelism.
- Melanomas on mucosal surfaces are associated with blue, gray, or white colors.
- Featureless melanomas can be identified via digital surveillance (short-term digital dermoscopic monitoring).

Dermoscopy is recognized as a useful tool for the evaluation of skin lesions by increasing diagnostic accuracy by up to 30% above that of the unaided eye examination. However, this level of improvement is contingent on gaining expertise in its use.[1–4] Dermoscopy increases not only sensitivity but also specificity for the diagnosis of skin cancer in general and melanoma in particular.[2,5,6] In other words, dermoscopy allows one to detect more melanomas at an early stage, while reducing the number of unnecessary biopsies of benign lesions. This in turn results in an improved malignant-to-benign biopsy ratio.[4,7–11]

One of the main objectives of dermoscopy remains differentiating atypical or dysplastic nevi (DN) from melanoma.[12] To accomplish this task, it is important to recognize the benign patterns commonly seen in DN. Studies have demonstrated that nevi and DN tend to manifest 1 of the 10 benign patterns, all of which exhibit symmetry in their dermoscopic colors and structures (Fig. 1). In contrast, melanomas tend to manifest patterns that deviate from the benign nevus patterns. In fact, melanomas manifest a wide gamut of dermoscopic characteristics, and these can vary depending on factors such as the histopathological subtype, anatomic location, tumor thickness, and possibly even the specific genetic mutations present within the tumor. It should thus be intuitively obvious that the patterns

---

The authors have no conflict of interest to declare.

Funding Sources: None.

[a] Dermatology Service, Aurora Skin Cancer Center and Universidad Pontificia Bolivariana, Cra. 25 # 1 A Sur 155, Ed. Platinum Superior. CS 342, Medellín, Colombia; [b] Dermatology Service, Department of Dermatology, Memorial Sloan-Kettering Cancer Center, 160 East 53rd street, New York, NY 10022, USA

* Corresponding author.

E-mail address: njaimeslo@gmail.com

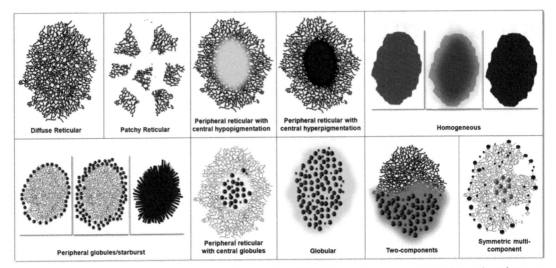

Diffuse Reticular | Patchy Reticular | Peripheral reticular with central hypopigmentation | Peripheral reticular with central hyperpigmentation | Homogeneous

Peripheral globules/starburst | Peripheral reticular with central globules | Globular | Two-components | Symmetric multi-component

Fig. 1. The most common patterns encountered in acquired "Clark" nevi, blue nevi, some Spitz nevi, and congenital nevi. (© Ashfaq A. Marghoob and Natalia Jaimes.)

expressed by melanoma are, in essence, infinite. With that said, what many melanomas have in common is that they deviate from the benign patterns shown in **Fig. 1**, and they often reveal at least one of the melanoma-specific structures listed in **Table 1**.[13–15] Unfortunately, there still remain melanomas that are featureless and these lesions may be missed, especially at the time of the first evaluation. Fortunately, periodic surveillance with the use of digital imaging can help identify these featureless melanomas while they are still thin. Toward this end, digital surveillance of suspicious melanocytic lesions with total body photography and dermoscopy has proven to be quite effective in identifying these melanomas.[16–21]

This article provides an overview of the different dermoscopic morphologies of melanoma as a function of the anatomic location of the lesion.

MELANOMA ON NONGLABROUS SKIN

Melanomas on nonglabrous skin may manifest a wide range of clinical and dermoscopic characteristics. These features will depend to some degree on the histologic subtype (ie, superficial spreading, nodular, lentigo maligna), anatomic location, thickness, and growth phase of the tumor. With that said, most melanomas developing on nonglabrous skin are of the superficial spreading subtype (SSM). In general, these melanomas tend to reveal 3 or more colors and at least 1 of the 10 melanoma-specific structures listed in **Table 1** (**Fig. 2**A, B). Colors may range from brown to black with red, white, and/or blue-gray also present to varying degrees. The melanoma-specific structures are those

dermoscopic structures that have a documented heightened odds ratio for melanoma (see **Table 1**; **Table 2**). The 10 melanoma-specific structures often seen in melanomas located on nonglabrous skin are listed in **Table 1** (see **Fig. 2**A, B).

Although 1 or more of these 10 melanoma-specific structures are usually seen in melanomas on nonglabrous skin, there are yet some melanomas that are structureless/featureless.[16–19] Because of this, all featureless lesions, especially if they are outliers, should raise suspicion for melanoma. These featureless lesions can be biopsied or, if flat, can be subjected to digital surveillance. Flat lesions lend themselves to monitoring because even if they are early melanomas, they tend to grow slowly enough that a 3-month to 4-month delay will not have any detrimental prognostic implications.[17,19,22] Monitoring of such lesions can be effectively accomplished via short-term digital dermoscopic monitoring (STM).[17,19,23–26] STM is based on comparing dermoscopic images of the same lesion taken 3 to 4 months apart. STM should be performed only on flat lesions (nodular lesions should never be subjected to STM), and by those with experience in using the technique.[25] The rationale behind STM is that stable lesions are considered biologically indolent and benign, whereas changing lesions are biologically dynamic, and approximately 11% to 18%[19,26] of these will prove to be melanoma.[19,25,26] Thus, in general, lesions found to have any morphologic change on STM, with the exception of changes in the overall global color or in the number of millialike cysts, should be biopsied to rule out a melanoma.[19]

Table 1
Melanoma-specific structures

Dermoscopic Structure	Definition	Schematic Illustration
Atypical pigment network	Increased variability in the width of the network lines, their color and distribution. The hole sizes also have increased variability, and may end abruptly at the periphery.[47]	
Negative pigment network	Serpiginous interconnecting hypopigmented lines, which surround irregularly shaped pigmented structures resembling elongated curvilinear globules. It can be seen diffusely and asymmetrically throughout the lesion or focally located.	
Streaks (pseudopods or radial streaming)	Radial projections located at the periphery of the lesion, extending from the tumor toward the surrounding normal skin. The presence of irregularly, asymmetric, and focally distributed streaks are highly suggestive of melanoma.[48] *Pseudopods* are fingerlike projections with small knobs at their tips, whereas *radial streaming* indicates the same structures without the knobs.	
Crystalline structures	Shiny white linear streaks that are often oriented parallel or orthogonal to each other.[49] Also known as shiny white streaks or lines.	
Atypical dots or globules	*Dots* are small, round structures that may be black, brown, and/or blue-gray. In melanoma, dots vary in size, color, and distribution; tend to be located at the periphery of the lesion; and are not associated with the pigmented network. *Globules* consist of 3 to 5 or more clustered, well-demarcated, round to oval structures that may be brown, black, blue and white, larger than dots. In melanoma they are usually multiple, and of different size, shape, and color, which may be asymmetrically and/or focally distributed within the lesion.	
Off-center blotch or multiple asymmetrically located blotches	Dark-brown to black, usually homogeneous areas of pigment that obscure visualization of any other structures. In melanoma, blotches are asymmetrically and/or focally located at the periphery of the lesion or can present as multiple blotches. Eccentric peripheral hyperpigmentation is often found in melanoma.[14]	

(continued on next page)

Table 1
(*continued*)

Dermoscopic Structure	Definition	Schematic Illustration
Regression structures (white scarlike depigmentation and/or blue-gray granularity or peppering overlying macular areas and not associated with vessels)	Consist of granularity (also known as peppering) and scarlike areas. When both are present together, it gives the appearance of a blue-white veil over a macular area.[50] In melanoma, they tend to be asymmetrically located and often involve more than 50% of the lesion.	
Blue-white veil overlaying raised areas	Confluent blue pigmentation with an overlying white "ground glass" haze, which tends to be asymmetrically located or diffuse throughout the lesion, and with different hues or shades.	
Atypical vascular structures	• Dotted vessels: Over milky-red background suggests melanoma/Spitz. • Serpentine (linear irregular) vessels • Polymorphous vessels: two or more vessel morphologies within the same lesion. • Corkscrew vessels: usually seen in nodular or desmoplastic melanoma, and melanoma metastases	
Peripheral tan structureless areas	Structureless light-brown area, located at the periphery of the lesion, larger than 10% of a lesion.[51]	

© Ashfaq A. Marghoob and Natalia Jaimes.

MELANOMA ON FACIAL SKIN

With the exception of acrolentiginous melanoma, melanoma of any histologic subtype can be located on facial skin and can manifest any of the melanoma-specific structures mentioned previously (see **Table 1**). However, the most common subtype of melanoma presenting on the face is lentigo maligna (LM) and LM characteristically displays a different set of dermoscopic structures than those listed in **Table 1** (see **Fig. 2**C, D). Early clinical recognition of LM on the face is challenging, especially in the presence of numerous solar lentigines, which often have clinical morphology features overlapping with early LM. Fortunately, dermoscopy has proven to help in the differentiation of these 2 entities. Schiffner and colleagues[27] described the dermoscopic features of LM and created a progression model for LM that may help explain the evolution of this

cancer from a morphologic perspective. The investigators suggested that slate-gray dots/granules surrounding adnexal openings and pigment, especially when gray in color, surrounding follicular openings in an asymmetric fashion are early features of LM. As the LM progresses, the pigment invades the interfollicular space, creating polygonal lines, rhomboidal structures, and homogeneous darkly pigmented areas in which the ostial openings can still be observed. Finally, in the last stage, the ostial openings within the homogeneous pigmented areas can no longer be seen (see **Fig. 2**C, D, **Table 3**).[27,28] In addition, Cognetta and colleagues[29] described an additional dermoscopic structure for LM consisting of fine concentric pigmented rings encircling each other. This structure, named concentric isobar pattern (also known as circle within a circle) is another dermoscopic clue for the diagnosis of LM (see **Fig. 2**C).[29] Although the aforementioned features

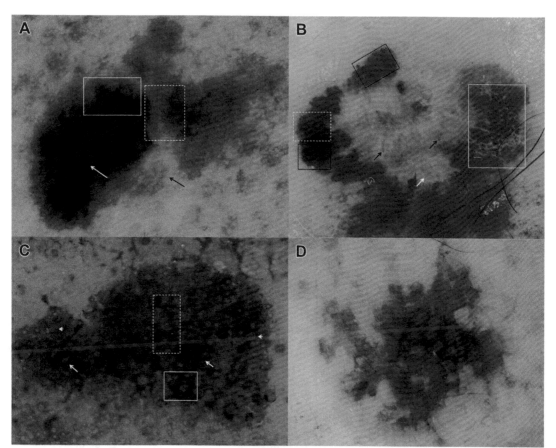

Fig. 2. (*A*) Dermoscopic image of a melanoma on the lower back with the following melanoma-specific structures: atypical network (*solid box*), regression structures (*dashed box*), off-center blotch (*white arrow*), peripheral tan structureless area (*black arrow*). (*B*) Dermoscopic image of a melanoma located on the abdomen, with atypical network (*black solid boxes*), atypical globules (*dashed box*), negative network (*white solid box*), scarlike areas (*white arrow*), and atypical vessels, including serpentine, dotted, and irregular hairpin vessels (*black arrows*). (*C*) Dermoscopic image of a lentigo maligna located on the nose with perifollicular granularity and asymmetric gray perifollicular openings (*solid box*), polygonal structures (*dashed box*), rhomboidal structures (*solid arrows*), and circle within a circle (*arrowheads*). (*D*) Lentigo maligna on sun-damaged skin of the shoulder that on dermoscopy revealing prominent polygonal lines. (© Ashfaq A. Marghoob and Natalia Jaimes.)

are commonly seen in LM on the face, many of the same structures can also be seen in melanomas located on chronically sun-damaged skin of the torso and extremities (see **Fig. 2**D).

When evaluating a pigmented lesion on the face, it is important to first assess the lesion for the presence of any of the 10 melanoma-specific structures seen on nonglabrous skin (see **Table 1**). The presence of any one of these structures should raise concern that the lesion being evaluated may be a melanoma. If none of the melanoma-specific structures listed in **Table 1** are present, the lesion needs to be evaluated further for specific structures associated with facial LM (and with melanomas located on chronically sun-damaged skin), which are listed in **Table 3**.

Macular pigmented lesions on the face that do not have any diagnostic features, akin to structureless melanomas on nonglabrous skin, can be subjected to dermoscopic digital monitoring. Similar to melanomas on nonglabrous skin (usually SSM subtype), LM will usually reveal changes within 3 months of monitoring. However, unlike SSM, up to 25% of LMs (including melanomas located on chronically sun-damaged skin) grow slowly and thus it is recommended that the monitoring interval be extended for these lesions.[26] In other words, if, at the 3-month monitoring interval, no dermoscopic changes are observed, then the lesion should be monitored again at the 6-month to 12-month interval before dismissing the lesion as benign.[26] Besides digital monitoring, other

Table 2
Melanoma-specific structures

Melanoma-Specific Structure	Sensitivity (%)		Specificity (%)	PPV (%)	NPV (%)	OR
	Amelanotic Melanoma	Pigmented Melanoma				
1. Atypical network	21[52]	35–82[47,51,54-57]	62–89[47,51,52,55-57]	18[56], 42[47], 67[51]	71[47]; 75[51]; 88[56]	1.1[48], 1.8[47], 2.0[52], 2.2[47,58], 4.3[59], 5.2[60], 9[12]
2. Peripheral streaks (Pseudopods and radial streaming)	5[52]	9–23[6,51,54-56], 32[47]	77[47]; 93–99[6,51,52,55-57]	39[47]; 22[56], 77[51]	71[47]; 86[56], 54[51]	1.6[47]; 2.9[48]; 3.0[60]; 3.9[52]; 5.8[12]
3. Negative pigment network	—					
Asymmetrically located and disordered	—	22[55]	95[55]	—	—	1.8[61]
4. Blotch (off-centered)	—	—	—	—	—	4.1[12], 4.9[60]
5. Atypical dots and/or globules	24[52]	25[56], 40[51]	74–92[51,52,56]	13[56], 79[51]	61[51], 86[56]	2.9[60], 3.2[51], 4.8[12]
6. Regression structures						
Scarlike areas	23[52]	17[47,54], 36[55]	93–99[47,52,54,55]	89[47]	70[47]	4.4[52], 18.3[47]
Peppering	22[52]	85[50]	93[52], 99[50]	27[50]	99[50]	3.5[52]
Scarlike areas + peppering	—	22[52], 42[51]	93[52], 97–99[51,52,55]	78[51]	—	3.9[60], 5.4[12], 7.8[51]
BWV overlying macular areas + scarlike areas + peppering	—		—	44[a,62]	91[b,62]	3.1[58], 8.7[59]

7. Blue-white veil overlying raised areas	11[52]	17[51]; 29[47]; 51[54,55]; 75[57]	86[47]; 94[51,57]; 97[54,55]; 99[52]	52[47]; 73[51]	55[51]; 70[47]	2.5[47]; 2.9[12]; 11[60]; 13[52]
8. Atypical vascular structures[63-65]	63[52]	9.4[51]	54[52]; 96[51]	69[51]	53[51]	1.5–1.9[12,48]; 2.0[52]; 7.4[60]
Dotted + serpentine	30[52]	—	85[52]	—	—	2.3[52]
Serpentine vessels	34[52]	—	80[52]	68[66]	—	2.1[52]
Polymorphous vessels	—	—	—	68[66]	—	2.1[52]
Milky-red areas	51[52]	—	71[52]	77.8[66]	—	2.5[52]
Red globules	21[52]	—	88[52]		—	2.0[52]
Corkscrew vessels	—	—	—	—	—	—
9. Crystalline structures (also known as shiny white streaks)	—	—	—	—	—	9.7[67]
10. Brown peripheral structureless areas	19[52]	63[51]	93–96[51,52]	94[51]	73[51]	2.9[52]; 28[51]

ORs shown in Table 2 are statistically significant for differentiation between melanoma and nonmelanoma, as 95% confidence interval does not include the unit.

Abbreviations: BWV, Blue-White Veil; NPV, negative predictive value; OR, odds ratio; PPV, positive predictive value.

a When involving >50% of the lesion.

b When involving <50% of the lesion.

Data from Refs.[13,52–54]

Table 3
Melanoma structures seen in facial and sun-damaged skin

Dermoscopic structure	Perifollicular granularity	Asymmetric gray perifollicular openings	Polygonal structures (zig-zag lines)	Rhomboidal structures	Follicle obliteration	Circle within a circle (isobar pattern)
Definition	Dots aggregated around hair follicles.[27]	Dots aggregated around hair follicles in an asymmetric fashion.[27]	Brown to bluish gray dots and lines arranged in an angulated linear pattern.[68]	Hyperpigmented brown and gray streaks surrounding hair follicles.[27]	Rhomboidal structures become broader, obliterating hair follicles.[27]	Concentric pigmented rings encircling each other.[29]
Schematic illustration						

© Ashfaq A. Marghoob and Natalia Jaimes.

diagnostic alternatives for these structureless lesions include a skin biopsy, or confocal microscopy.[30]

ACRAL MELANOMA

Acral melanomas include those melanomas located on volar surfaces of the palms and soles. Although in theory any histologic subtype of melanoma can present at these locations, the most frequent melanoma subtype to be diagnosed on volar skin is the acrolentiginous type.

Evaluation of melanocytic lesions on palms or soles requires understanding of the anatomy associated with volar skin. The rete ridges on the palms and soles create furrows and ridges, which in turn are responsible for the unique dermatoglyphic pattern present in an individual person. The ducts of the eccrine glands open on the surface of the skin overlying the ridges. Thus, the dermatoglyphic ridges can be identified on dermoscopy by the fact that they are wider than the furrows and that the eccrine duct openings can be seen on their surface as tiny white dots aligned in rows. However, at times it may be difficult to differentiate the ridges from the furrows and in such instances the ink test published by Braun and colleagues[31] and Uhara and colleagues[32] can prove useful. Why is it important to be able to isolate the furrows from the ridges on volar skin viewed with dermoscopy? Because pigment localized to the ridges (ie, parallel ridge pattern) is highly suggestive of melanoma (Fig. 3A, B, Table 4). In fact, the presence of a parallel ridge pattern carries with it a diagnostic accuracy of 82% for melanoma, with a sensitivity of 86%, specificity of

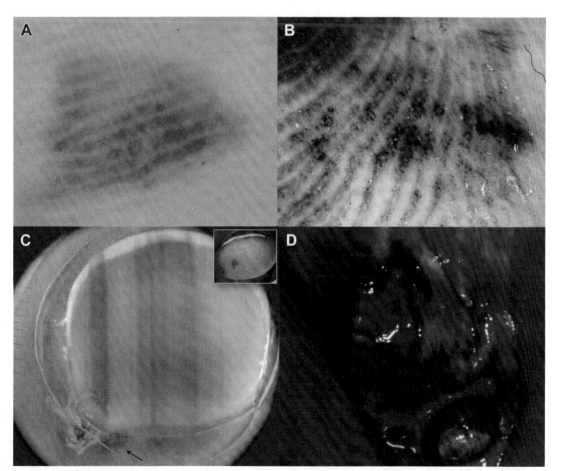

Fig. 3. (A, B) Dermoscopic image of melanomas located on the soles with parallel ridge pattern. (C) Dermoscopic image of a 0.6-mm melanoma involving the nail unit with multiple, longitudinal irregular brown bands with irregular spacing and thickness, micro-Hutchinson sign (black arrow). Also present is irregular pigmentation on the hyponychium (clinical image at the top right corner). (D) Dermoscopic image of a vaginal melanoma, demonstrating the presence of blue, gray, and white colors within the lesion, and a multicomponent pattern composed by irregular brown-black globules and blue-white veil. (© Ashfaq A. Marghoob and Natalia Jaimes.)

Table 4
Melanoma structures in acral melanoma

Dermoscopic Structure	Definition	Schematic Illustration
Parallel ridge pattern	Pigmentation on ridges of palms and soles[33]	
Irregular diffuse pigmentation	Irregular diffuse pigmentation with different shades of tan, brown, black, and gray[33]	
Irregular fibrillar pattern	Any fibrillar pattern on palms, or fibrillar pattern on soles with an increased variability of line thickness or colors, or colors other than brown.	
Large-diameter lesion	New, acquired lesion greater than 7–10 mm, especially in a 50-year-old person	

© Ashfaq A. Marghoob and Natalia Jaimes.

99%, a positive predictive value of 94%, and a negative predictive value of 98%.[33,34] In contrast, nevi rarely manifest a parallel ridge pattern, revealing most often a pattern with pigment located predominantly in the furrows (ie, parallel furrow and latticelike patterns). It is not completely clear as to why nevi frequently have pigment in the furrows and melanomas often have pigment on the ridges. It was initially believed that nevomelanocytic nests have a tendency to cluster around the rete ridge of the crista limitans, which corresponds to the dermatoglyphic furrows, and melanoma cells cluster around the crista intermedia, which corresponds to the dermatoglyphic ridges. However, Saida and colleagues[35] have shown that nevomelanocytes may in fact be located both near the crista limitans and crista intermedia, but for reasons that have yet to be elucidated, only the nevomelanocytes associated with the crista limitans have the ability to transfer melanin to the epidermis, thereby resulting in the dermoscopic observation of pigment concentrated along the furrows. The reason for why melanomas often display a ridge pattern remains unknown; however, some have posited that the melanocytic stem cell giving rise to acral melanoma may reside near the crista intermedia or near the eccrine ducts. Others have postulated that early acral melanomas may simply prefer, for biochemical environmental reasons, to reside in the environment near the crista intermedia.

In addition to the parallel ridge pattern, melanomas on volar skin can have a homogeneous pattern displaying multiple shades of brown and/or other colors, such as black, red, white, gray, and blue (see **Table 4**).[33,36] Moreover, any lesion on the palms that reveals a fibrillar pattern should be viewed with suspicion. In contrast, the fibrillar pattern is quite common in melanocytic neoplasms on the soles; however, in nevi on the soles, this fibrillar pattern tends to be brown in color with thin and regular lines, whereas in melanoma the lines tend to have increased variability in thickness, spacing, and colors.[37] Last, any acquired lesion on volar skin that is larger than 7 to 10 mm should raise concern for melanoma (see **Table 4**).[38]

Similar to the dermoscopic evaluation of melanocytic lesions on other anatomic locations, the observer should begin by assessing the lesion for any of the 10 melanoma-specific structures listed in **Table 1**. If none of these melanoma-specific structures are seen, the lesion needs to be further evaluated for the presence of the additional melanoma-specific structures peculiar to acral volar skin listed in **Table 4**.[30,33,34,36] If none of these features are seen, then the observer should determine if the lesion has one of the classic benign acral volar patterns (ie, furrow, lattice, or typical fibrillar patterns); and if seen, the physician can reassure the patient that the lesion is benign. If, on the other hand, the acquired lesion does not reveal any diagnostic features, management will need to rely on the maximal diameter of the lesion. Lesions larger than 7 to 10 mm in diameter should be considered for biopsy, especially in patients older than 50 years, whereas lesions smaller than 7 to 10 mm in diameter can be either biopsied or digitally monitored as previously described.[38]

MELANOMA INVOLVING THE NAIL UNIT

Evaluating melanonychia striata requires inspection of the nail plate, cuticle, paranychium, and hyponychium. Pigment found on the cuticle, or paronychial or hyponychial area in association with acquired melanonychia striata is highly suggestive of melanoma (see **Fig. 3**C). At times, pigment within the skin of the cuticle is visible only after being viewed with dermoscopy: the so-called micro-Hutchinson sign (see **Fig. 3**C). This micro-Hutchinson sign needs to be differentiated from the pseudo-Hutchinson sign, which simply reflects the presence of pigment in the nail matrix that is visible through the relatively translucent cuticular skin, and it has no diagnostic significance. Pigment on the hyponychium should be evaluated in the same manner as for acral/volar melanoma, as described previously. For example, pigmentation with a parallel ridge pattern on the hyponychium would be highly suggestive for melanoma. Once the skin surrounding the nail plate has been examined, our attention should turn to the melanonychia striata on the nail plate. It should be remembered that the actual lesion, which is located in the nail matrix, cannot be visualized directly. Although some have suggested applying dermoscopy directly to the nail matrix and nail bed after nail avulsion,[39] this is not a practical means for the routine evaluation of melanonychia striata. Instead, dermoscopic examination of the pigmented nail band can provide valuable clues, albeit indirect, regarding the nature of the lesion residing in the nail matrix. Examination should start by measuring the width of the pigmented band at the proximal end of the nail plate and comparing it to the width of the band at the distal end of the nail plate. In rapidly growing tumors, such as in some melanomas, it can be observed that there is a wider diameter at the proximal end as compared with the distal end of the band, resulting in a somewhat triangular shape of the melanonychia striata.[36] Next, dermoscopy should be used to evaluate the individual striations/bands that are present within the melanonychia striata.

Benign lesions are characterized by a regular pattern consisting of parallel lines spaced at regular intervals with minimal variation in their color or thickness. The color of the lines tends to get lighter toward the lateral edges, creating an overall symmetric-appearing dermoscopic pattern. In contrast, melanomas are associated with an irregular pattern consisting of multiple longitudinal bands, of different colors (ie, brown, black, gray) and thickness, with irregular spacing and disruption of parallelism (see **Fig. 3**C).[36] In melanomas that are in advanced stages, nail plate dystrophy or destruction can be observed.[36] Melanoma-specific structures of the nail unit are listed in **Table 5**.

MUCOSAL MELANOMA

Mucosal melanomas include those located on the glabrous portion of the lips, oral cavity, and anogenital areas. The primary differential diagnosis for pigmented lesions on mucosal surfaces are melanosis versus nonmelanoma.[40] Although clinically it may prove impossible to distinguish between these two entities, dermoscopy can provide assistance. It has been shown that mucosal melanomas often reveal a multicomponent pattern composed of irregular brown-black dots, blue-white veil, atypical vessels, and/or negative network (see **Fig. 3**D).[41] Other dermoscopic structures described in mucosal melanomas include focal areas of pigment network, globules, parallel structures (linear streaks of pigment, also known as "hyphae" structures), or ringlike structures (arciform structures or incomplete circles, also known as "fish-scalelike structures"). It has been suggested that the presence of multiple patterns and colors are associated with more advanced melanomas, whereas structureless areas and gray color are more frequently seen in early melanomas.[42] However, in the largest study to date regarding the dermoscopic morphology of mucosal melanoma, the investigators concluded that the most sensitive and specific feature to help distinguish melanoma from nonmelanoma was not any specific structure but rather the colors expressed by the lesion.[42] The investigators found that the strongest factors that facilitated the differentiation between malignant and benign lesions was the presence of blue, gray, or white color within the lesion; with a sensitivity of 100% and a specificity of 64% for melanoma (see **Fig. 3**D). In addition, structureless areas were also shown to be significantly associated with malignant lesions. In fact, the combination of 1 of the 3 aforementioned colors and structureless areas were found to be highly predictive of melanoma, with a sensitivity of 100% and a specificity of 82%.[42]

As shown previously, the dermoscopic structures seen in melanoma are a function of the anatomic location of the tumor. However, other factors can also influence the structures seen in melanoma, including the subtype, tumor thickness, and skin type.[22,27,28,33,34,43–46] Some preliminary evidence is even suggesting that the mutational profile of the melanoma may have an impact on its morphologic appearance with darkly pigmented lesions with streaks often harboring Kit mutations; we all watch with interest as this translational story unfolds.

Table 5
Melanoma-specific structures of the nail unit

Dermoscopic Structure	Definition	Schematic Illustration
Hyponychial pigment with any features described in **Table 4**	Irregular pigmentation on the distal periungual skin, with any of the features associated with melanomas on acral skin.	
Hutchinson or micro-Hutchinson sign	Pigmentation of the proximal nail fold that can be seen with the naked eye (Hutchinson) or only under dermoscopy (micro-Hutchinson).	
Triangular shape	Width of the band is wider at the proximal end.	
Irregular pattern	Multiple, longitudinal irregular bands, of different colors (ie, black, brown, and gray) with irregular spacing, thickness, and disruption of parallelism.	
Nail dystrophy	Complete or partial nail destruction, and/or absence of the nail plate.	

© Ashfaq A. Marghoob and Natalia Jaimes.

ACKNOWLEDGMENTS

We thank Dr Ralph P. Braun for the dermoscopic and clinical image of the nail melanoma.

REFERENCES

1. Braun RP, Rabinovitz H, Oliviero M, et al. Dermoscopy of pigmented skin lesions. J Am Acad Dermatol 2005;52:109–21.
2. Kittler H, Pehamberger H, Wolff K, et al. Diagnostic accuracy of dermoscopy. Lancet Oncol 2002;3: 159–65.
3. Pehamberger H, Steiner A, Wolff K. In vivo epiluminescence microscopy of pigmented skin lesions. I. Pattern analysis of pigmented skin lesions. J Am Acad Dermatol 1987;17:571–83.
4. Benvenuto-Andrade C, Marghoob AA. Ten reasons why dermoscopy is beneficial for the evaluation of skin lesions. Exp REv Dermatol 2006;1: 369–74.
5. Bafounta ML, Beauchet A, Aegerter P, et al. Is dermoscopy (epiluminescence microscopy) useful for the diagnosis of melanoma? Results of a meta-analysis using techniques adapted to the evaluation of diagnostic tests. Arch Dermatol 2001;137:1343–50.
6. Dal Pozzo V, Benelli C, Roscetti E. The seven features for melanoma: a new dermoscopic algorithm for the diagnosis of malignant melanoma. Eur J Dermatol 1999;9:303–8.
7. Noor O 2nd, Nanda A, Rao BK. A dermoscopy survey to assess who is using it and why it is or is not being used. Int J Dermatol 2009;48:951–2.
8. Carli P, de Giorgi V, Chiarugi A, et al. Addition of dermoscopy to conventional naked-eye examination in

melanoma screening: a randomized study. J Am Acad Dermatol 2004;50:683–9.

9. Argenziano G, Puig S, Zalaudek I, et al. Dermoscopy improves accuracy of primary care physicians to triage lesions suggestive of skin cancer. J Clin Oncol 2006;24:1877–82.

10. Carli P, Mannone F, De Giorgi V, et al. The problem of false-positive diagnosis in melanoma screening: the impact of dermoscopy. Melanoma Res 2003; 13:179–82.

11. Carli P, De Giorgi V, Crocetti E, Mannone F, et al. Improvement of malignant/benign ratio in excised melanocytic lesions in the "dermoscopy era": a retrospective study 1997-2001. Br J Dermatol 2004;150:687–92.

12. Argenziano G, Soyer HP, Chimenti S, et al. Dermoscopy of pigmented skin lesions: results of a consensus meeting via the Internet. J Am Acad Dermatol 2003;48:679–93.

13. Marghoob AA, Korzenko AJ, Changchien L, et al. The beauty and the beast sign in dermoscopy. Dermatol Surg 2007;33:1388–91.

14. Hofmann-Wellenhof R, Blum A, Wolf IH, et al. Dermoscopic classification of atypical melanocytic nevi (Clark nevi). Arch Dermatol 2001;137:1575–80.

15. Hofmann-Wellenhof R, Blum A, Wolf IH, et al. Dermoscopic classification of Clark's nevi (atypical melanocytic nevi). Clin Dermatol 2002;20:255–8.

16. Kittler H, Binder M. Follow-up of melanocytic skin lesions with digital dermoscopy: risks and benefits. Arch Dermatol 2002;138:1379.

17. Kittler H, Guitera P, Riedl E, et al. Identification of clinically featureless incipient melanoma using sequential dermoscopy imaging. Arch Dermatol 2006;142:1113–9.

18. Skvara H, Teban L, Fiebiger M, et al. Limitations of dermoscopy in the recognition of melanoma. Arch Dermatol 2005;141:155–60.

19. Menzies SW, Gutenev A, Avramidis M, et al. Short-term digital surface microscopic monitoring of atypical or changing melanocytic lesions. Arch Dermatol 2001;137:1583–9.

20. Salerni G, Teran T, Puig S, et al. Meta-analysis of digital dermoscopy follow-up of melanocytic skin lesions: a study on behalf of the International Dermoscopy Society. J Eur Acad Dermatol Venereol 2013;27:805–14.

21. Salerni G, Carrera C, Lovatto L, et al. Benefits of total body photography and digital dermatoscopy ("two-step method of digital follow-up") in the early diagnosis of melanoma in patients at high risk for melanoma. J Am Acad Dermatol 2012; 67:e17–27.

22. Liu W, Dowling JP, Murray WK, et al. Rate of growth in melanomas: characteristics and associations of rapidly growing melanomas. Arch Dermatol 2006; 142:1551–8.

23. Kittler H, Pehamberger H, Wolff K, et al. Follow-up of melanocytic skin lesions with digital epiluminescence microscopy: patterns of modifications observed in early melanoma, atypical nevi, and common nevi. J Am Acad Dermatol 2000;43: 467–76.

24. Robinson JK, Nickoloff BJ. Digital epiluminescence microscopy monitoring of high-risk patients. Arch Dermatol 2004;140:49–56.

25. Argenziano G, Mordente I, Ferrara G, et al. Dermoscopic monitoring of melanocytic skin lesions: clinical outcome and patient compliance vary according to follow-up protocols. Br J Dermatol 2008;159:331–6.

26. Altamura D, Avramidis M, Menzies SW. Assessment of the optimal interval for and sensitivity of short-term sequential digital dermoscopy monitoring for the diagnosis of melanoma. Arch Dermatol 2008;144:502–6.

27. Schiffner R, Schiffner-Rohe J, Vogt T, et al. Improvement of early recognition of lentigo maligna using dermatoscopy. J Am Acad Dermatol 2000; 42:25–32.

28. Schiffner R, Perusquia AM, Stolz W. One-year follow-up of a lentigo maligna: first dermoscopic signs of growth. Br J Dermatol 2004;151:1087–9.

29. Cognetta AB Jr, Stolz W, Katz B, et al. Dermatoscopy of lentigo maligna. Dermatol Clin 2001;19: 307–18.

30. Guitera P, Pellacani G, Crotty KA, et al. The impact of in vivo reflectance confocal microscopy on the diagnostic accuracy of lentigo maligna and equivocal pigmented and nonpigmented macules of the face. J Invest Dermatol 2010;130:2080–91.

31. Braun RP, Thomas L, Kolm I, et al. The furrow ink test: a clue for the dermoscopic diagnosis of acral melanoma vs nevus. Arch Dermatol 2008;144: 1618–20.

32. Uhara H, Koga H, Takata M, et al. The whiteboard marker as a useful tool for the dermoscopic "furrow ink test". Arch Dermatol 2009;145:1331–2.

33. Saida T, Miyazaki A, Oguchi S, et al. Significance of dermoscopic patterns in detecting malignant melanoma on acral volar skin: results of a multicenter study in Japan. Arch Dermatol 2004;140:1233–8.

34. Saida T, Oguchi S, Miyazaki A. Dermoscopy for acral pigmented skin lesions. Clin Dermatol 2002; 20:279–85.

35. Saida T, Koga H, Goto Y, et al. Characteristic distribution of melanin columns in the cornified layer of acquired acral nevus: an important clue for histopathologic differentiation from early acral melanoma. Am J Dermatopathol 2011;33:468–73.

36. Phan A, Dalle S, Touzet S, et al. Dermoscopic features of acral lentiginous melanoma in a large series of 110 cases in a white population. Br J Dermatol 2010;162:765–71.

37. Altamura D, Altobelli E, Micantonio T, et al. Dermoscopic patterns of acral melanocytic nevi and melanomas in a white population in central Italy. Arch Dermatol 2006;142:1123–8.

38. Koga H, Saida T. Revised 3-step dermoscopic algorithm for the management of acral melanocytic lesions. Arch Dermatol 2011;147:741–3.

39. Hirata SH, Yamada S, Enokihara MY, et al. Patterns of nail matrix and bed of longitudinal melanonychia by intraoperative dermatoscopy. J Am Acad Dermatol 2011;65:297–303.

40. Jaimes N, Halpern AC. Practice gaps. Examination of genital area: comment on "dermoscopy of pigmented lesions of the mucosa and the mucocutaneous junction." Arch Dermatol 2011;147:1187–8.

41. Ferrari A, Zalaudek I, Argenziano G, et al. Dermoscopy of pigmented lesions of the vulva: a retrospective morphological study. Dermatology 2011;222:157–66.

42. Blum A, Simionescu O, Argenziano G, et al. Dermoscopy of pigmented lesions of the mucosa and the mucocutaneous junction: results of a multicenter study by the International Dermoscopy Society (IDS). Arch Dermatol 2011;147:1181–7.

43. Jaimes N, Chen L, Dusza SW, et al. Clinical and dermoscopic characteristics of desmoplastic melanomas. JAMA Dermatol 2013;149:413–21.

44. Kalkhoran S, Milne O, Zalaudek I, et al. Historical, clinical, and dermoscopic characteristics of thin nodular melanoma. Arch Dermatol 2010;146:311–8.

45. Argenziano G, Kittler H, Ferrara G, et al. Slow-growing melanoma: a dermoscopy follow-up study. Br J Dermatol 2010;162:267–73.

46. Cuellar F, Puig S, Kolm I, et al. Dermoscopic features of melanomas associated with MC1R variants in Spanish CDKN2A mutation carriers. Br J Dermatol 2009;160:48–53.

47. Salopek TG, Kopf AW, Stefanato CM, et al. Differentiation of atypical moles (dysplastic nevi) from early melanomas by dermoscopy. Dermatol Clin 2001;19:337–45.

48. Pizzichetta MA, Stanganelli I, Bono R, et al. Dermoscopic features of difficult melanoma. Dermatol Surg 2007;33:91–9.

49. Marghoob AA, Cowell L, Kopf AW, et al. Observation of chrysalis structures with polarized dermoscopy. Arch Dermatol 2009;145:618.

50. Braun RP, Gaide O, Oliviero M, et al. The significance of multiple blue-grey dots (granularity) for the dermoscopic diagnosis of melanoma. Br J Dermatol 2007;157:907–13.

51. Annessi G, Bono R, Sampogna F, et al. Sensitivity, specificity, and diagnostic accuracy of three dermoscopic algorithmic methods in the diagnosis of doubtful melanocytic lesions: the importance of light brown structureless areas in differentiating atypical melanocytic nevi from thin melanomas. J Am Acad Dermatol 2007;56:759–67.

52. Menzies SW, Kreusch J, Byth K, et al. Dermoscopic evaluation of amelanotic and hypomelanotic melanoma. Arch Dermatol 2008;144:1120–7.

53. Stoecker WV, Stolz W. Dermoscopy and the diagnostic challenge of amelanotic and hypomelanotic melanoma. Arch Dermatol 2008;144:1207–10.

54. Soyer HP, Smolle J, Leitinger G, et al. Diagnostic reliability of dermoscopic criteria for detecting malignant melanoma. Dermatology 1995;190:25–30.

55. Menzies SW, Ingvar C, McCarthy WH. A sensitivity and specificity analysis of the surface microscopy features of invasive melanoma. Melanoma Res 1996;6:55–62.

56. Haenssle HA, Korpas B, Hansen-Hagge C, et al. Seven-point checklist for dermatoscopy: performance during 10 years of prospective surveillance of patients at increased melanoma risk. J Am Acad Dermatol 2010;62:785–93.

57. Kenet RO, Kang S, Kenet BJ, et al. Clinical diagnosis of pigmented lesions using digital epiluminescence microscopy. Grading protocol and atlas. Arch Dermatol 1993;129:157–74.

58. Soyer HP, Argenziano G, Zalaudek I, et al. Three-point checklist of dermoscopy. A new screening method for early detection of melanoma. Dermatology 2004;208:27–31.

59. Zalaudek I, Argenziano G, Soyer HP, et al. Three-point checklist of dermoscopy: an open Internet study. Br J Dermatol 2006;154:431–7.

60. Argenziano G, Fabbrocini G, Carli P, et al. Epiluminescence microscopy for the diagnosis of doubtful melanocytic skin lesions. Comparison of the ABCD rule of dermatoscopy and a new 7-point checklist based on pattern analysis. Arch Dermatol 1998;134:1563–70.

61. Pizzichetta MA, Talamini R, Marghoob AA, et al. Negative pigment network: an additional dermoscopic feature for the diagnosis of melanoma. J Am Acad Dermatol 2012;68:552–9.

62. Zalaudek I, Argenziano G, Ferrara G, et al. Clinically equivocal melanocytic skin lesions with features of regression: a dermoscopic-pathological study. Br J Dermatol 2004;150:64–71.

63. Bono A, Maurichi A, Moglia D, et al. Clinical and dermatoscopic diagnosis of early amelanotic melanoma. Melanoma Res 2001;11:491–4.

64. Pizzichetta MA, Talamini R, Stanganelli I, et al. Amelanotic/hypomelanotic melanoma: clinical and dermoscopic features. Br J Dermatol 2004;150:1117–24.

65. Puig S, Argenziano G, Zalaudek I, et al. Melanomas that failed dermoscopic detection: a combined clinicodermoscopic approach for not missing melanoma. Dermatol Surg 2007;33:1262–73.

66. Argenziano G, Zalaudek I, Corona R, et al. Vascular structures in skin tumors: a dermoscopy study. Arch Dermatol 2004;140:1485–9.

67. Balagula Y, Braun RP, Rabinovitz HS, et al. The significance of crystalline/chrysalis structures in the diagnosis of melanocytic and nonmelanocytic lesions. J Am Acad Dermatol 2012;67: 194.e1–8.

68. Slutsky JB, Marghoob AA. The zig-zag pattern of lentigo maligna. Arch Dermatol 2010;146:1444.

Special Locations Dermoscopy
Facial, Acral, and Nail

Luc Thomas, MD, PhD*, Alice Phan, MD, PhD,
Pauline Pralong, MD, Nicolas Poulalhon, MD,
Sébastien Debarbieux, MD, Stéphane Dalle, MD, PhD

KEYWORDS

- Dermoscopy • Melanoma • Nevus • Nail • Palm • Soles • Face • Pigmentation

KEY POINTS

- Although dermoscopy reflects the anatomy, skin anatomy is different on facial and acral skin as well as in the nail unit.
- Malignant patterns on acral sites include the parallel ridge pattern and irregular diffuse pigmentation, whose presence should lead to a biopsy.
- Malignant patterns on the face include features of follicular invasion (signet-ring images, annular-granular images, and rhomboidal structures) and atypical vessels.
- Malignant patterns on the nail unit include the micro-Hutchinson sign and irregular longitudinal lines.

INTRODUCTION

Although dermoscopy reflects anatomy, usual dermoscopic clues observed on glabrous skin do not apply on so-called special locations, namely the face, scalp, acral skin, nails, mucous membranes, and scars. In these locations the classic 2-step dermoscopic diagnostic procedure used elsewhere on skin does not apply and, with the remarkable exception of Cliff Rosendahl's "chaos and clues" training method,[1] most dermoscopy education programs consider these special locations as exceptions, with specific subchapters appearing in most dermoscopy textbooks and courses worldwide.[2]

This article focuses on 3 anatomic sites: the face, acral skin (distal to Wallace's line), and nails.

Only pigmented lesions are discussed, because unpigmented facial tumors have not been studied separately from those in other locations and because inflammatory skin diseases on the face are not usually described differently.

On the face most of the dermoscopic corpus of knowledge derives from the visionary work of Stolz and colleagues.[3] The most representative facial-specific dermoscopic features, anatomically speaking, reflect the progressive invasion of the pilo-sebaceous unit.

Similarly, most of the acral skin-specific dermoscopic diagnosis criteria for pigmented lesions have been described in the extensive contributions of Saida and colleagues.[4,5] The dermoscopic features of acral skin reflect the peculiar disposition of pigment along the dermatoglyphs.

The authors declare no potential conflict of interest with this article.

Academic work and research activity of the department of dermatology of Claude Bernard – Lyon 1 university of the Center Hospitalier Lyon Sud is supported by grants of Claude Bernard Lyon 1 university (to L. Thomas, A. Phan, and S. Dalle), of the Direction de la Recherche Clinique des Hospices Civils de Lyon (to L. Thomas), and of la Ligue Contre le Cancer du Rhône (to L. Thomas and S. Debarbieux).

Department of Dermatology, Centre Hospitalier Lyon Sud, Université Claude Bernard Lyon 1, Pierre Bénite Cedex 69495, France

* Corresponding author.

E-mail address: luc.thomas@chu-lyon.fr

The authors' group has contributed to the description of nail-specific dermoscopic features.[6-8] In this location, the originality of the observed dermoscopic features is due to the indirect signs observed on the nail plate created by the presence of nail-matrix pigmented disorders.

The high number of anatomic exceptions in the dermoscopic approach to pigmented tumors of the skin may justify the proposal for some kind of reformation in teaching methods.[9]

FACIAL DERMOSCOPY

Facial skin is characterized by its flat dermal-epidermal junction, the early presence of solar elastosis in its dermis, its relatively thinner epidermis, and the presence of larger pilo-sebaceous units. From the flattened dermal-epidermal junction derives the quasi absence of "classic" reticulation, ad from the early presence of solar elastosis the often "structureless" aspect of pigment deposits. A thinner epidermis allows better visibility of dermal structures such as blood vessels or melanophages (usually reflecting the presence of histopathologic features of regression). However, the most face-specific dermoscopic features are due to the relatively larger pilo-sebaceous units present in facial skin, interrupting the pigmentation by the creation of a broader network with round-shaped holes different from the thin, honeycomb-like network observed on glabrous extrafacial skin in cases of junctional pigmentation observed on nevi, melanomas, in the periphery of most dermatofibromas, and in supernumerary nipples. Moreover, invasion of the pilo-sebaceous unit by melanoma (mostly of the lentigo maligna type) creates, when observed with a dermoscope, relatively specific features.

On facial skin, dermoscopic diagnosis of pigmented basal cell carcinoma (in fact most pigmented basal cell carcinomas occur on sun-exposed facial skin), raised seborrheic keratosis, blue nevi and, though much more uncommon, dermatofibroma, is not made following site-specific rules. For information on these diagnoses the reader is referred to other articles elsewhere in this issue.

Nevi on the face generally belong to either the poorly pigmented or unpigmented raised type, histopathologically corresponding usually to the dermal nevi or the globular pigmented type. The first group is usually dermoscopically mainly characterized by the presence of brown globules, "comma-like" vessels, and in some cases the presence of orange-colored superficial keratin deposits. The second group is characterized by a globular (or cobblestone) pattern, the presence of a positive wobble sign and, in some cases, a squamous surface. Both types of lesion are usually dermoscopically homogeneous and geometrically symmetric. Differential diagnosis of unpigmented nevi of the face usually encompasses basal cell carcinoma, sebaceous hyperplasia, and mollusca contagiosa. Vascular morphology of these 3 entities (ie, arborizing for the first and coronal for the 2 others) is described in a specific article of this issue and differs from the comma-like (curved, irregular in size) vessels observed in amelanotic nevi.

The main problem regarding differential diagnosis of facial skin is the distinction between lentigo maligna, either invasive (lentigo maligna melanoma) or intraepidermal (lentigo maligna stricto sensu), solar lentigo, pigmented actinic keratoses, and flat pigmented seborrheic keratoses. The authors believe that lentigo maligna and lentigo maligna melanoma belong to the same evolutionary spectrum; moreover, dermoscopy is unable to accurately distinguish between the two, therefore both entities are herein described together under the name of lentigo maligna melanoma (LMM). The authors also believe that solar lentigo, flat pigmented seborrheic keratoses, and pigmented actinic keratoses closely correspond histopathologically; moreover, their dermoscopic features do not differ significantly. These entities are referred to herein as solar lentigo (SL). However, pigmented lichen planus and actinic keratoses, which represent a specific differential diagnosis problem with LMM, deserve specific description.

LMM is rarely but somewhat specifically characterized by its darkening when observed by dermoscopy. Presence of a Stolz Total Dermoscopy Score darker color[10] when observed on dermoscopy when compared with being seen by the naked eye best reflects this phenomenon (eg, the black color on dermoscopy when only dark- brown or gray was clinically observable).

Granulation (also known as peppering), 1 of the 2 dermoscopic criteria usually associated with histopathologic features of regression (melanophages),[11] is more easily visible through the thinner facial epidermis, so it is therefore not surprising that its observation is common in LMM, a slowly growing subtype of melanoma with long-lasting equilibrium between an indolent radial growth phase and immunologic host response. Often this granulation is disposed around the facial pilo-sebaceous units, producing an annular-granular pattern (**Fig. 1**). Scar-like depigmentation, the other regression-associated dermoscopic criterion, might also be observed, usually in more advanced cases.

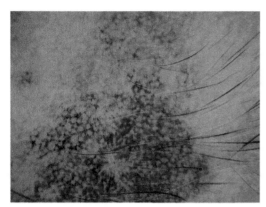

Fig. 1. Annular-granular pattern in a Clark level II, 0.35-mm thick lentigo maligna melanoma (LMM) of the eyebrow.

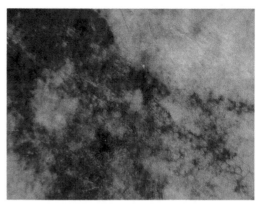

Fig. 3. Red rhomboidal structures are observed in the center of the picture of this Clark level III 0.26-mm thick forehead LMM.

For similar reasons, blood vessels are also much more visible on facial skin. Pralong and colleagues[12] described 2 diagnostically helpful features of LMM-associated vasculature: (1) their different aspect from what is observed in surrounding skin (**Fig. 2**) where erythro-rosacea is very common, and (2) the presence of lozenge-shaped vascular structures observed around the pilo-sebaceous units (also known as rhomboid red structures) (**Fig. 3**).

Stolz's group precisely described the different steps of the follicular invasion by the malignant pigmented process during LMM progression.[3] Their princeps description was confirmed by subsequent work without any addition to their visionary work.[12] The first change corresponds to the earliest invasion of the hair shaft; observed with magnification it shows a regular then irregular underlining of the follicular opening drawing O-shaped and C-shaped pigmented structures. With further invasion of the hair shaft, this initially thin underlining becomes thicker and irregular, creating signet-ring–shaped structures (**Fig. 4**). While progressing, the follicular invasion creates annular-granular structures around the hair follicles as described earlier. Thickening of these perifollicular pigmented structures creates lozenge-shaped pigmented structures in the interfollicular spaces, called pigmented rhomboidal structures (**Fig. 5**). Further progression of the follicular invasion then completely covers the follicular lumen, creating uniformly pigmented areas in which only the presence of hairs testifies to the presence of follicular structures. Within the very same lesion, in different locations the steps in progression may present under a more or less advanced feature; this adds to the global asymmetry of the lesion and indeed reinforces the diagnostic suspicion of malignancy. All the different

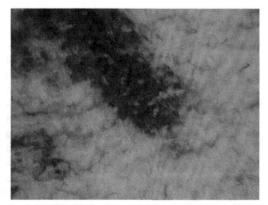

Fig. 2. A clearly different vascular pattern is observed within the lesion when compared with the erythro-rosacea of the patient in this Clark level II 0.41-mm thick cheek LMM.

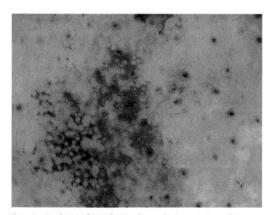

Fig. 4. O-shaped, C-shaped, and signet-ring features as well as an annular-granular pattern are seen in this Clark level III, 0.36-mm thick LMM of the nose.

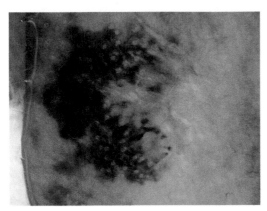

Fig. 5. Rhomboidal structures are observed in this Clark level III 0.7-mm LMM of the earlobe.

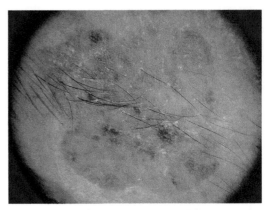

Fig. 6. Structureless pigmentation without any sign of follicular invasion and well-delineated polycyclic borders in this solar lentigo of the forehead.

steps of this follicular invasion process are observed while the lesion remains flat. Dermoscopic presence of a raised, structureless, black or blue-black or whitish-blue area also speaks in favor of the diagnosis of malignant melanoma on the face as well as anywhere on skin, but this is observed at more advanced phases of the disease progression when dermoscopy adds little more to the diagnostic accuracy of LMM.[13]

It must be borne in mind that the precise diagnosis of the surface extension of LMM is extremely difficult. Histopathologic evaluation of the limits of LMM is a tremendously difficult task by itself, and therefore from a more superficial approach cannot be expected to give accurate information. Dermoscopy certainly helps to encompass the unpigmented peripheral regression-modified areas of the lesion within the therapeutic area, but cannot give precise enough excision margins.

By contrast, SL is characterized by the (as yet unspecific) absence of darkening of the lesion on dermoscopy in comparison with examination by the naked eye. Granulation is unusual, and signs of follicular invasion are absent (**Fig. 6**).[3] No specific vascular changes are observed within the lesion area in comparison with surrounding skin. Usually the lesion is characterized dermoscopically by the presence of light- to dark-brown homogeneous areas of pigmentation with sharp polycyclic borders. Occasionally, milia-like cysts, "moth-eaten" border, and hairpin-like vessels are observed, usually in slightly raised lesions.[14]

A difficult differential diagnosis of LMM is pigmented lichen planus–like actinic keratosis (PLiPLAK). It is possible that this entity also encompasses several histopathologically close but benign conditions such as regressing actinic keratoses, traumatized flat seborrheic keratoses, and inflammatory SLs. Again dermoscopy does not allow adequate distinction (if any) between these entities, therefore they all are referred to herein as PLiPLAK. These lesions are dermoscopically characterized by the presence of granulation ("peppering") often showing, on the face, an annular-granular disposition around the follicular openings.[15] A benign PLiPLAK-associated annular-granular pattern is clearly indistinct from a malignant LMM-associated pattern; therefore, discovery of an isolated annular granula, in the case of a unique facial pigmented spot, will lead to a proposal for biopsy or, preferably, a digital follow-up.

Many other malignant conditions, such as spitzoid (pigmented or unpigmented, childhood or adulthood) melanoma,[16] squamous cell carcinoma, Bowen disease,[17] malignant blue nevus, Merkel cell carcinoma,[18] and dermatofibrosarcoma protuberans,[19] are observed on facial skin; however, their description by far exceeds the scope of this article.

ACRAL SKIN DERMOSCOPY

Acral skin is defined by its presence distal of the Wallace line that separates the glabrous skin of the limbs from the skin beyond. It is characterized by the presence of dermatoglyphs. The particular anatomy of this region leads to a peculiar disposition of the pigment in benign as well as malignant conditions. Dermatoglyphs are constituted by the parallel arrangement of ridges and furrows. The dermoscopic patterns observed on acral skin are mainly characterized by their position along the ridges and furrows, creating parallel pigmentation patterns and their variants. At times, absence of specific pigment arrangement results in diffuse (regular and, more importantly, irregular) pigmented patterns.

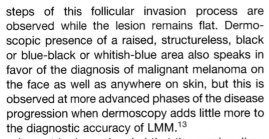

Saida and colleagues[4,5] made the princeps description of the dermoscopic pigmented parallel patterns and of the irregular diffuse pigmented pattern on acral skin. Since their outstanding initial contributions, further works have confirmed their accurate prescience.[8]

Dermoscopic examination of the area of the junction between acral and glabrous skin of the limbs shows so-called transitional patterns, which are very difficult to analyze because the association of glabrous skin patterns with acral skin patterns creates an asymmetric, worrisome assemblage of pigmentation.[20]

Unpigmented benign or malignant tumors also exist on acral skin, their diagnosis being based on the analysis of their vascular pattern[21,22]; however, the diagnostic rules about vascular patterns on acral skin do not differ from those concerning other locations. The reader is referred to the specific article elsewhere in this issue for more complete information. However, attention should be given to pigmented structures (improperly named remnant of pigmentation, because it is unknown whether pigmentation was present earlier), only observed by dermoscopy and invisible to the naked eye, in the diagnostic approach to unpigmented or hypopigmented acral tumors, so as not to miss amelanotic acral lentiginous melanoma (ALM).[23,24]

On acral skin it is usual to distinguish benign pigmented patterns and malignant pigmented patterns; however, the observer must remember that if the presence of at least 1 malignant criterion is sufficient to suggest the diagnosis of melanoma, the presence of 1 or more benign criteria is not enough to rule out this diagnosis.

The 2 malignant patterns are the parallel ridge pattern and irregular diffuse pigmentation.

The parallel ridge pattern[4,5,8] is characterized by the presence of the pigment on the dermatoglyph's ridges; however, because dermoscopy is a 2-dimensional examination technique, the slightly raised ridges are not distinguished from the furrows by their elevation but by their anatomic properties, which are 2-fold: they appear larger than the furrows and the sweat-gland openings are located in the center of the ridges (**Fig. 7**). If this is not enough to make an accurate distinction between ridges and furrows, one can use the ink test (if ink is deposited on the acral skin, after gentle clearing of the ink, its remnant stays in the furrows).[25] The presence of a parallel ridge pattern even in a small part of the lesion is enough for consideration of the diagnosis of melanoma. There are, however, a few exceptions, such as lentiginoses (Laugier-Hutziker-Baran, Peutz-Jeghers-Touraine), repetitive trauma-induced pigmentation

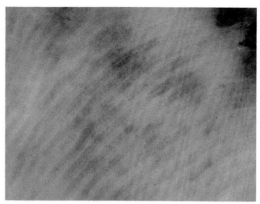

Fig. 7. Parallel ridge pattern in the periphery is observed in this Clark level IV, 1.4-mm thick acral lentiginous melanoma (ALM).

(also known as joystick fingers), congenital nevi, exogenous pigmentation, and subcorneal hemorrhages.[26–29]

Irregular diffuse pigmentation is characterized by the presence of multiple structureless areas of pigmentation of different shades of brown, gray, or black, generally arranged asymmetrically and irrespective of the dermatoglyph architecture (**Fig. 8**).[4,5,8] Again the presence of irregular diffuse pigmentation, even in a small portion of a lesion, is sufficient cause to consider the diagnosis of melanoma.

The 3 benign patterns[4,5,8] are the parallel furrow pattern and its variants, the lattice-like pattern, and the fibrillar pattern.

The parallel furrow pattern[4,5,8] is characterized by the pigmentation of the furrows; that is, the thinner component of the dermatoglyph microstructure devoid of sweat-gland openings and marked by the ink test (**Fig. 9**).[25] This aspect is best observed on the periphery of the lesion and

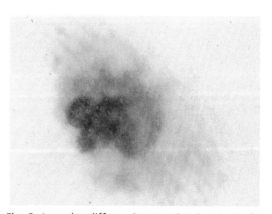

Fig. 8. Irregular diffuse pigmentation is seen in this Clark level III, 0.76-mm thick ALM of the sole.

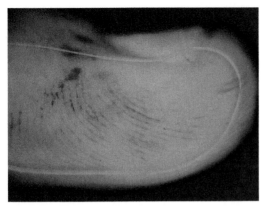

Fig. 9. Parallel furrow pattern is seen in this benign acral nevus of the second left finger. Transitional images are visible in the upper part of the picture.

is usually characterized by a linear pigmentation, but many variants of similar benign significance exist (the double-line variant, the dotted variant, and the double-line dotted variant).[4]

The lattice-like pattern[4,5,8] is characterized by a pigmentation of the furrows associated with orthogonal ridge-crossing lines. It is often associated with the parallel pattern on the periphery of the lesion.

The fibrillar pattern[4,5,8] is observed in high-pressure areas[30] and is characterized by the parallel disposition of thin-pigmented lines perpendicularly oriented toward the dermatoglyphs' general orientation (**Fig. 10**).

It is worth repeating that the presence of 1 or more of the 3 benign patterns within a pigmented multicomponent acral lesion is not sufficient to rule out melanoma.

NAIL DERMOSCOPY

Diagnosis of nail-unit melanoma is often delayed by a poor general knowledge of its clinical characteristics, and a many-year history of a misdiagnosed condition is common at a patient's first interrogation. Indeed, dermoscopy is not needed in advanced cases but does permit a very early diagnosis in paucisymptomatic cases characterized by only a longitudinal nail pigmentation (also known as melanonychia striata longitudinalis [MSL]).[8] The authors' group contributed to the definition of the dermoscopic features of MSL[6–8] and its management.[31–33]

Early pigmented nail-unit melanoma is characterized by the presence of a brown background of the pigmentation and of an irregular pattern of the longitudinal microlines, only dermoscopically visible. These lines are irregular in their color, thickness, spacing, and parallelism. Occasionally an only-dermoscopically visible periungual pigmentation (also known as the micro-Hutchinson sign) is seen on the proximal nail-fold skin; this criterion is rare but very specific (**Fig. 11**).[6–8]

In more advanced pigmented melanoma, dermoscopic features also include granulation, scar-like depigmentation, blue-black structureless areas, blood spots, prominent periungual pigmentation with a parallel ridge pattern, atypical vasculature areas, erosion of the nail plate, or ulceration of the nail bed, but the clinical naked-eye diagnosis is usually sufficient.[6–8]

Nail-matrix nevus is also characterized by brown-background pigmentation. As in melanoma, the shade of brown is much more reflective of the patient's skin type (ie, darker skin types have darker nevi or melanomas). However, the pattern of the only-dermoscopically visible longitudinal microlines is regular and composed of homogeneously colored, spaced, and thick lines (**Fig. 12**).[6–8]

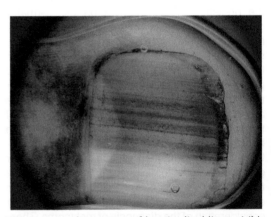

Fig. 11. Irregular pattern of longitudinal lines, visible only dermoscopically. There is brown background pigmentation and a micro-Hutchinson sign in this Clark level II, 0.18-mm thick ALM of the thumbnail.

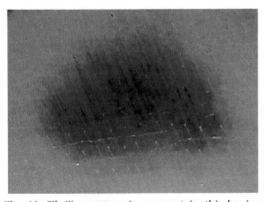

Fig. 10. Fibrillar pattern is apparent in this benign nevus of the heel.

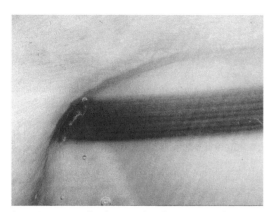

Fig. 12. Brown background coloration and regular longitudinal micro-lines are observed in this benign nevus of the second left finger.

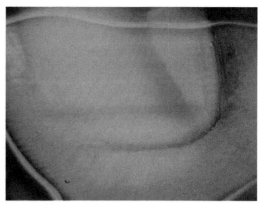

Fig. 14. Gray coloration of a benign nail-matrix lentigo of the right thumb.

Congenital or congenital-type nevi of the nail unit are very difficult to manage because most of the classically melanoma-associated criteria can be found in such cases (**Fig. 13**) (triangular shape, irregular pattern of the longitudinal lines, changes of the plate, periungual pigmentation, change over time). An international register of these cases has been compiled under the auspices of the International Dermoscopy Society (IDS). Inclusions are still ongoing. No definitive management rule for these cases can be yet defined based on the first 100 cases included; however, follow-up is highly recommended[34] as well as inclusion in the IDS register.

Nail-matrix lentigo (either isolated or included in a lentiginosis such as Laugier-Hutziker-Baran disease), drug-induced nail pigmentation, repetitive trauma-induced nail pigmentation, and ethnic-type nail pigmentation share the same dermoscopic characteristics (**Fig. 14**). The background

of the pigmentation is grayish or yellowish, and the only-dermoscopically visible longitudinal microlines are regularly spaced, colored, and thick.[6–8]

Dermoscopy can be used to diagnose amelanotic nail-unit melanoma. However, diagnostic criteria do not differ from those observed in nodular-type amelanotic melanomas observed anywhere on skin. In brief, the pattern of the vessels is atypical (linear and irregular and/or multiple-pattern [≥3] vessels and/or presence of milky-red areas), and improperly named remnants of pigmentation can be observed in places.[21,22] Regarding this peculiar location, mention should be made that amelanotic ulcerated nodular melanoma differs neither clinically nor dermoscopically from pyogenic granuloma, and that systematic histopathologic examination of every ungual or periungual pyogenic granuloma-like lesion is mandatory.

The diagnosis of subungual hemorrhage is also helped by dermoscopy, which shows the presence of blood spots characterized by their shape (and not by their color, which better reflects the age of the lesion, a recent lesion being purple or black whereas an older one is more brownish). The blood spots have a sharply demarcated round-shaped proximal limit and a more fuzzy filamentous distal edge. The presence of blood spots does not rule out the diagnosis of a malignant tumor because they are observed in 25% of subungual squamous cell carcinomas and in 60% of amelanotic melanomas, but if no other symptom is observed the patients can only be simply followed up. This follow-up, however, is mandatory to ensure that the lesion is distally progressively eliminated and that there is no underlying preexisting or coexisting malignant condition.[6–8,34]

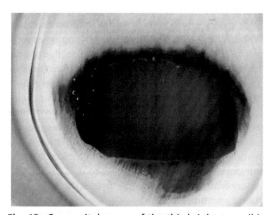

Fig. 13. Congenital nevus of the third right toenail in a 2-year-old female patient (follow-up over 8 years did not show any progression or change).

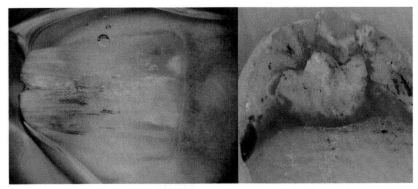

Fig. 15. Longitudinal leucoxanthonychia, splinter hemorrhages, and localized subungual hyperkeratosis on examination of dermoscopic free edge in this squamous cell carcinoma of the left thumbnail.

The early diagnosis of nail-unit squamous cell carcinoma and Bowen disease is greatly improved by dermoscopy.[34] Examination of the nail plate shows longitudinal leucoxanthonychia with, in a few cases, areas of grayish coloration. Splinter hemorrhages are also seldom seen. A localized (distally to the longitudinal abnormalities) subungual hyperkeratosis at the nail-plate free-edge dermoscopic examination (**Fig. 15**) is a key criterion for all nail-matrix keratinizing tumors, including squamous cell carcinoma and onychomatricoma.[34]

Braun and colleagues[35] have described the use of dermoscopic examination of the free edge of the nail matrix to estimate the anatomic origin of the pigmentation within the matrix. In brief, the location of the pigment in the upper half of the plate at free-edge dermoscopic examination reflects the proximal matrix origin of the pigmentation, whereas its presence in the lower half signifies that its origin is in the distal matrix.

The authors also believe that digital follow-up offers interesting perspectives in doubtful cases of longitudinal nail pigmentation.[34] These cases are rare enough to permit a personalized follow-up schedule so as not to miss an initially featureless melanoma. However, further work is needed to better determine the precise role of this technique in the management of MSL.

Perioperative nail-matrix or nail-bed dermoscopy has been described by Hirata and colleagues.[36] This approach offers interesting and accurate new information to better classify matrix pigmentation into the melanocytic hyperplasia subtype (nevi and melanomas) and the hypermelaninosis subtype (lentigos, ethnic-type, drug-induced, repetitive trauma–induced pigmentations). The authors believe that, despite encouraging preliminary data, further work in this field is needed to better establish the role of this technique in the general management of MSL.[33,34]

Onychomatricomas, (Lesort C, Poulalhon N, Phan A, et al. Dermoscopy of onychomatricoma. Submitted for publication) subungual infestations or infections,[37] blue nevi of the nail unit,[38,39] subungual glomus cell tumors,[34] subungual osteochondromas (also known as exostoses),[34] and subungual keratoacanthomas[34] can also be diagnosed by dermoscopy, but the description of these entities exceeds the scope of this review.

SUMMARY

Dermoscopic appearance of pigmented and, to a lesser extent, nonpigmented, cutaneous, or appendageal lesions, is greatly influenced by the anatomy. On facial skin the melanoma-associated features reflect the invasion of the pilo-sebaceous units. On acral skin the pigmented melanoma-associated features reflect the preferential location of malignant melanocytes at the dermal-epidermal junction and the crista intermedia, leading to preponderant ridge pigmentation, whereas benign melanocytes are more commonly located in the crista limitans, responsible for a furrow-predominant pigmentation. Moreover, the pressure-induced change on the stratum corneum explains the fibrillar pattern of some plantar lesions. Dermoscopy of the nail indirectly reflects pathologic changes in the nail matrix: regular lines observed by dermoscopy on the nail plate reflect the regular disposition on melanocytes and melanocytic nests, and in the corresponding matrix irregular lines are created by the melanoma-linked architectural disorganization of the matrix by malignant cells and nests. Longitudinal leucoxanthonychia, associated with localized subungual hyperkeratosis, reflects the presence of a nail-matrix keratinizing tumor.

In an era of analytical reappraisal of dermoscopic criteria (mandatory as a first step in the process of creation of a digital "machine vision"), it is perhaps time to reconsider the general concept of "special location dermoscopy" and to describe site-specific symptoms (preferentially in nonmetaphoric terms) as geometric, reproducible entities. Reformation of teaching methods will be needed, especially when the exceptions become as numerous as to overcome the general rule.[1,9]

REFERENCES

1. Rosendahl C, Cameron A, McColl I, et al. Dermatoscopy in routine practice—'chaos and clues'. Aust Fam Physician 2012;41(7):482–7.

2. Argenziano G, Soyer HP, Chimenti S, et al. Dermoscopy of pigmented skin lesions: results of a consensus meeting via the Internet. J Am Acad Dermatol 2003;48(5):679–93.

3. Schiffner R, Schiffner-Rohe J, Vogt T, et al. Improvement of early recognition of lentigo maligna using dermatoscopy. J Am Acad Dermatol 2000;42(1 Pt 1): 25–32.

4. Saida T, Oguchi S, Miyazaki A. Dermoscopy for acral pigmented skin lesions. Clin Dermatol 2002; 20(3):279–85.

5. Saida T, Miyazaki A, Oguchi S, et al. Significance of dermoscopic patterns in detecting malignant melanoma on acral volar skin: results of a multicenter study in Japan. Arch Dermatol 2004; 140(10):1233–8.

6. Ronger S, Touzet S, Ligeron C, et al. Dermoscopic examination of nail pigmentation. Arch Dermatol 2002;138(10):1327–33.

7. Thomas L, Dalle S. Dermoscopy provides useful information for the management of melanonychia striata. Dermatol Ther 2007;20(1):3–10.

8. Phan A, Dalle S, Touzet S, et al. Dermoscopic features of acral lentiginous melanoma in a large series of 110 cases in a white population. Br J Dermatol 2010;162(4):765–71.

9. Kittler H. Why the first step should be abandoned! Arch Dermatol 2010;146(10):1182–3.

10. Nachbar F, Stolz W, Merkle T, et al. The ABCD rule of dermatoscopy. High prospective value in the diagnosis of doubtful melanocytic skin lesions. J Am Acad Dermatol 1994;30(4):551–9.

11. Braun RP, Gaide O, Oliviero M, et al. The significance of multiple blue-grey dots (granularity) for the dermoscopic diagnosis of melanoma. Br J Dermatol 2007;157(5):907–13.

12. Pralong P, Bathelier E, Dalle S, et al. Dermoscopy of lentigo maligna melanoma: report of 125 cases. Br J Dermatol 2012;167(2):280–7.

13. Argenziano G, Longo C, Cameron A, et al. Blueblack rule: a simple dermoscopic clue to recognize pigmented nodular melanoma. Br J Dermatol 2011; 165(6):1251–5.

14. Braun RP, Rabinovitz HS, Krischer J, et al. Dermoscopy of pigmented seborrheic keratosis: a morphological study. Arch Dermatol 2002;138(12):1556–60.

15. Bugatti L, Filosa G. Dermoscopy of lichen planuslike keratosis: a model of inflammatory regression. J Eur Acad Dermatol Venereol 2007;21(10): 1392–7.

16. Argenziano G, Scalvenzi M, Staibano S, et al. Dermatoscopic pitfalls in differentiating pigmented Spitz naevi from cutaneous melanomas. Br J Dermatol 1999;141(5):788–93.

17. Zalaudek I, Argenziano G, Leinweber B, et al. Dermoscopy of Bowen's disease. Br J Dermatol 2004; 150(6):1112–6.

18. Dalle S, Parmentier L, Moscarella E, et al. Dermoscopy of Merkel cell carcinoma. Dermatology 2012;224(2):140–4.

19. Bernard J, Poulalhon N, Argenziano G, et al. Dermoscopy of dermatofibrosarcoma protuberans: a study of 15 cases. Br J Dermatol 2013;169(1): 85–90.

20. Altamura D, Altobelli E, Micantonio T, et al. Dermoscopic patterns of acral melanocytic nevi and melanomas in a white population in central Italy. Arch Dermatol 2006;142(9):1123–8.

21. Zalaudek I, Kreusch J, Giacomel J, et al. How to diagnose nonpigmented skin tumors: a review of vascular structures seen with dermoscopy: part I. Melanocytic skin tumors. J Am Acad Dermatol 2010;63(3):361–74.

22. Menzies SW, Kreusch J, Byth K, et al. Dermoscopic evaluation of amelanotic and hypomelanotic melanoma. Arch Dermatol 2008;144(9):1120–7.

23. Phan A, Touzet S, Dalle S, et al. Acral lentiginous melanoma: a clinicoprognostic study of 126 cases. Br J Dermatol 2006;155(3):561–9.

24. Phan A, Touzet S, Dalle S, et al. Acral lentiginous melanoma: histopathological prognostic features of 121 cases. Br J Dermatol 2007;157(2):311–8.

25. Braun RP, Thomas L, Kolm I, et al. The furrow ink test: a clue for the dermoscopic diagnosis of acral melanoma vs nevus. Arch Dermatol 2008;144(12): 1618–20.

26. Phan A, Dalle S, Marcilly MC, et al. Benign dermoscopic parallel ridge pattern variants. Arch Dermatol 2011;147(5):634.

27. Tanioka M. Benign acral lesions showing parallel ridge pattern on dermoscopy. J Dermatol 2011; 38(1):41–4.

28. Ko JH, Shih YC, Chiu CS, et al. Dermoscopic features in Laugier-Hunziker syndrome. J Dermatol 2011;38(1):87–90.

29. Robertson SJ, Leonard J, Chamberlain AJ. PlayStation purpura. Australas J Dermatol 2010;51(3): 220–2.

30. Miyazaki A, Saida T, Koga H, et al. Anatomical and histopathological correlates of the dermoscopic

patterns seen in melanocytic nevi on the sole: a retrospective study. J Am Acad Dermatol 2005; 53(2):230–6.

31. Braun RP, Baran R, Le Gal FA, et al. Diagnosis and management of nail pigmentations. J Am Acad Dermatol 2007;56(5):835–47.

32. Sureda N, Phan A, Poulalhon N, et al. Conservative surgical management of subungual (matrix derived) melanoma: report of seven cases and literature review. Br J Dermatol 2011;165(4):852–8.

33. Debarbieux S, Hospod V, Depaepe L, et al. Perioperative confocal microscopy of the nail matrix in the management of in situ or minimally invasive subungual melanomas. Br J Dermatol 2012;167(4):828–36.

34. Thomas L, Vaudaine M, Wortsman X, et al. Imaging the nail unit. In: Baran R, De Berker DA, Holzberg M, et al, editors. Baran and Dawber's diseases of the nail and their management. 4th edition. London: Wiley Blackwell; 2012. p. 101–82.

35. Braun RP, Baran R, Saurat JH, et al. Surgical Pearl: dermoscopy of the free edge of the nail to determine the level of nail plate pigmentation and the location of its probable origin in the proximal or distal nail matrix. J Am Acad Dermatol 2006;55(3): 512–3.

36. Hirata SH, Yamada S, Enokihara MY, et al. Patterns of nail matrix and bed of longitudinal melanonychia by intraoperative dermatoscopy. J Am Acad Dermatol 2011;65(2):297–303.

37. Zalaudek I, Giacomel J, Cabo H, et al. Entodermoscopy: a new tool for diagnosing skin infections and infestations. Dermatology 2008;216(1):14–23.

38. Dalle S, Ronger-Savle S, Cicale L, et al. A blue-gray subungual discoloration. Arch Dermatol 2007;143(7): 937–42.

39. Causeret AS, Skowron F, Viallard AM, et al. Subungual blue nevus. J Am Acad Dermatol 2003;49(2): 310–2.

Special Criteria for Special Locations 2
Scalp, Mucosal, and Milk Line

Rainer Hofmann-Wellenhof, MD

KEYWORDS

• Nevi of special site • Dermoscopy • Melanoma • Nevus • Mucosal melanosis

KEY POINTS

- The anatomic region influences the dermoscopic features of lesions, resulting in specific criteria that help make correct management decisions for lesions located on the scalp, mucosal membranes, and milk-line and in flexural locations.
- Biopsy should be performed in lesions of the scalp if atypical pigment net or pseudopigment net in association with regression areas is present, if a homogeneous blue lesion lacks a convincing subjective history of no changes, and if there is a growing nodular tumor. Regular globular pattern and reticular pattern with central hypopigmentation (eclipse nevus) are most common in melanocytic nevi on the scalp of children and young adults.
- In mucosal lesions with diameter larger than 1 cm, gray color and the presence of structureless areas are highly suggestive for mucosal melanoma, whereas one color and regular dermoscopic structures are the main criteria of benign mucosal melanosis.
- Nevi located on the milk line and in flexural locations, such as axilla, inguinal region, popliteal, and antecubal fossa, can frequently display a prominent pigment net, sometimes with bizarre lines, and large globules mimicking features of melanoma.

LESIONS ON THE SCALP

A high concentration of pilosebaceous follicles and rich vascular and lymphatic supply form the special anatomic appearance of the skin of the scalp. Scalp tumors account for approximately 2% of all skin tumors and may derive from different cell types of the pilosebaceous unit, from the interfollicular epidermis and dermis, or as cutaneous metastases from other tumors.[1,2]

The great variety of scalp tumors consists of sebaceous nevus, seborrheic keratosis, basal cell carcinoma, actinic keratosis, squamous cell carcinoma, hemangioma, angiosarcoma, and rare adnexal tumors. The dermoscopic appearance of these tumors normally does not differ from that on other body sites. Thus, this article concentrates on melanocytic lesions.

Melanocytic scalp tumors differ in some epidemiologic, morphologic, and biologic aspects from their counterparts on the trunk. For example, scalp melanoma has a poorer prognosis compared with thickness-matched melanomas of the trunk. Blue nevi are more frequently found on the scalp than on other body sites and histopathology of some melanocytic nevi may simulate melanoma.[3,4]

Melanocytic Nevi

The prevalence of nevi of the scalp in children is approximately 10%.[5] The morphology of nevi of the scalp changes according to the age of

The author does not have any conflict of interest.
Department of Dermatology, Medical University of Graz, Auenbruggerplatz 8, Graz A-8038, Austria
E-mail address: rainer.hofmann@medunigraz.at

Dermatol Clin 31 (2013) 625–636
http://dx.doi.org/10.1016/j.det.2013.07.003

patients, and older people more frequently show less pigmented papillomatous nevi.

Large congenital nevi involving the scalp should always lead to a screening for neurocutaneus melanosis. Dermoscopy is not helpful in deciding further management of congenital nevi, especially those located on the scalp. In this location, hairs make an investigation of nevi sometimes impossible. The threshold for excision should be low (**Fig. 1**).

Scalp nevi in children may be a source of anxiety for parents. Clinically, these nevi can display large size, irregular borders, and color variation. Frequently, these nevi appear in the first years of live. Because of the sometime worrisome clinical appearance and the anxiety of parents, these nevi are unnecessarily excised.[5] In their study, Tcheung and colleagues[6] described 4 different clinical patterns of scalp nevi in children: homogeneous brown (48%), solid pink (28%), eclipse (21%), and cockade (3%). The predominant dermoscopic feature was globules, which was found in 57% of scalp nevi as the only dermoscopic feature. In addition, 27% of scalp nevi showed a combination of globular and reticular patterns. Only 9% of the nevi showed solely a reticular pattern, followed by 6% showing a homogenous pattern.

Perifollicular hypopigmentation was seen in the majority of nevi. This finding was confirmed in a study by Stanganelli and colleagues.[1] In this study, the investigators studied 323 excised tumors of the scalp (including 78 melanocytic nevi and 21 blue nevi) from 315 patients (mean age 52 years; range 3–88 years); 48% of melanocytic nevi were found to display hypopigmentation, which was perifollicular in 15 cases and central in 14. Perifollicular hypopigmentation was also present at the border of lesions, resulting in an irregular shape.

Because excision was an inclusion criterion of this study, the percentage of linear irregular

vessels was surprisingly high in this sample. In the author's experience, the main vascular pattern in scalp nevi is comma vessels and dotted vessels.

Clinically, scalp nevi in children and adolescents present as macule or flat nodule with homogeneous pink or brown color. Most of the lesions on the scalp are symmetric. Dermoscopy normally reveals a globular pattern, perifollicular hypopigmentation, and central hypopigmentation (eg, eclipse nevus) (**Figs. 2** and **3**), whereas most scalp nevi in adults are usually nodular and faint pigmented or skin colored with a smooth or papillomatous surface. Comma vessels and dotted vessels are found by dermoscopy (**Figs. 4** and **5**). All these lesions can be managed conservatively, because there is no documented risk for malignant transformation.[7]

Small congenital nevi with asymmetry and multiple colors or nevi displaying melanoma-specific criteria should be excised.

Blue Nevus of the Scalp

Blue nevi are common on the scalp and may develop at any age. Clinically, blue nevi present as flat to prominent blue nodules with a smooth surface. In most cases, the diameter is smaller than 1 cm but giant congenital forms are also described. Once developed, they do not change over a long time period.[8]

The homogeneous blue pattern is the stereotypical dermoscopic pattern of blue nevi, and lesions on the scalp are not an exception (**Figs. 6** and **7**). In their study, Stanganelli and colleagues[1] included 27 blue nevi, which showed in 89% a homogenous blue pigmentation and in almost half the cases areas of hypopigmentation. In contrast to blue nevi located on other body sites, the investigators found in 8 blue nevi on the scalp an atypical vascular pattern (ie, linear irregular vessels [see

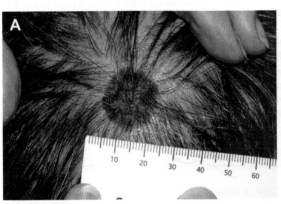
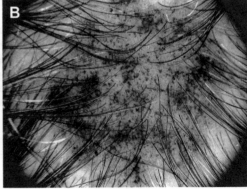

Fig. 1. (*A*) Clinical image of a congenital nevus: brown plaque with some darker areas, diameter 3.5 cm. (*B*) Dermoscopic image: cobblestone pattern with some irregular darker areas.

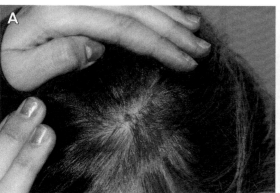
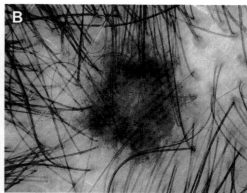

Fig. 2. (A) Clinical image of an eclipse nevus in a girl: brown solitary macule, diameter 0.6 cm. (B) Dermoscopic image: the hypopigmented center is surrounded by a brown rim, which shows a reticular pattern; notice the perifollicular hypopimentation and the irregularity of the border.

Fig. 6]). This might be due to the rich vascular supply of the scalp.

Variants of blue nevi, such as deep penetrating blue nevus and so-called malignant blue nevus, which represents a variant of nodular melanoma in the eyes of some investigators, seem more frequent on the scalp than on other body sites. In a retrospective histopathologic study of 23 malignant blue nevi, 6 tumors were located on the scalp and the prognosis did not differ from matched melanomas of the same thickness.[9]

Moreover, nodular melanoma, cutaneous metastases of melanoma, and heavily pigmented basal cell carcinoma can be indistinguishable from blue nevi. The history of change and growth is sometimes the only criterion, which can lead to the correct diagnosis of a malignant tumor. Thus, it is has been recommended to excise blue lesions on the scalp, if there is not subjective history of a stable lesion over years.[1]

Melanoma of the Scalp

Melanoma and nonmelanoma skin cancer of the scalp are most frequent in bald men aged over 65 years. Frequently, signs of chronic sun damage and previous history of skin cancer are found in patients developing a melanoma on the scalp.[1] These data support that UV irradiation plays a role in their pathogenesis.

Lentigo maligna, lentigo maligna melanomas, superficial spreading melanomas, and nodular, fast-growing melanomas can be differentiated.

Generally, the dermoscopic features of melanomas on the scalp do not differ from those on other body sites.

On bald skin, lentigo maligna and lentigo maligna melanomas display the characteristic features of asymmetric pigmented hair follicles, gray dots and globules, and occlusion of the hair follicles. The association with actinic keratosis or other nonmelanoma skin tumors can obscure the

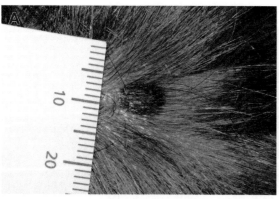
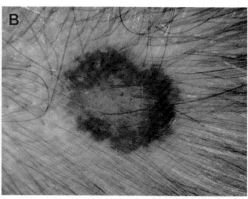

Fig. 3. (A) Clinical image of another example of an eclipse nevus: brown flat plaque with a fainter center, diameter 0.7 cm. (B) Dermoscopic image: homogenous-globular pattern with a hypopigmented structureless center; the perifollicular hypopigmentation at the periphery leads to an irregular border.

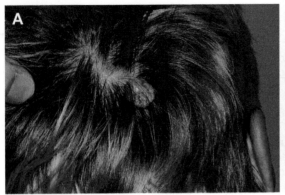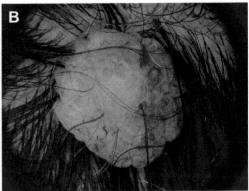

Fig. 4. (*A*) Clinical image of intradermal nevus: red papillomatous nodule, diameter 0.8 cm. (*B*) Dermoscopic image: papillomatous surface and many comma-like vessels.

diagnosis. Moreover, the differentiation of lentigo maligna from a solar lentigo may be difficult (**Fig. 8**). Brown color, sharp moth-eaten borders, and fingerprint-like structures favor the diagnosis of solar lentigo, whereas gray color, diffuse border, and asymmetric hair follicles are suggestive of lentigo maligna.

Most cases of superficial spreading melanoma on the scalp display the typical dermoscopic features of melanoma and can be diagnosed easily. Asymmetry and more than 3 colors together with melanoma-specific local criteria are found in melanomas on the scalp at a similar frequency as in melanomas on other anatomic sites. Atypical network or brown-gray pseudonetwork and regression were found predictive for thin (<1-mm) melanomas (**Fig. 9**).[1,10]

Thick, fast-growing, nodular melanoma often lacks specific dermoscopic patterns (**Fig. 10**).[11] The homogenous blue and or black nodules frequently resemble blue nevi, heavily pigmented basal cell carcinoma, or metastatic melanoma. Sometimes irregular, polymorphous vessels can

be a hint for malignancy of a given tumor. Irregular black blotches or dots over a blue background may be an important clue for diagnosis. Black blotches and dots were absent in 26 of 27 blue nevi in an International Dermoscopy Society study. Usually the history of rapid growth makes excision mandatory.[1]

Amelanotic or hypomelanotic nodular melanoma can mimic pyogenic granuloma, the main dermoscopic features of which are a white collarette and white thick lines (white rail lines).[12] When pyogenic granuloma is removed, histology is obligatory to exclude melanoma.

Summary: Melanocytic Lesions on the Scalp

Total body skin examination should include the scalp.

Melanocytic nevi of the scalp show age-related changes in the their dermoscopic appearance. While scalp nevi in children and young adults typically exhibit a globular or reticular pattern with central hypopigmentation (eclipse nevus), scalp

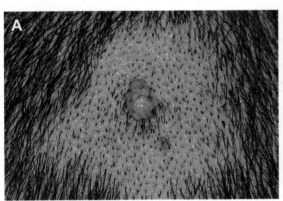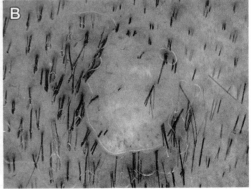

Fig. 5. (*A*) Clinical image of intradermal nevus: skin-colored papule, diameter 0.4 cm. (*B*) Dermoscopic image: unspecific pattern with comma-like vessels.

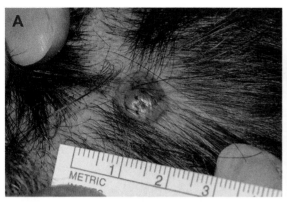

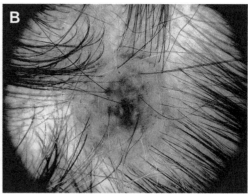

Fig. 6. (*A*) Clinical image of blue nevus: blue-gray papule, diameter 0.7 cm. (*B*) Dermoscopic image: homogenous blue-gray pattern with some white areas as sign of fibrosis. Note the irregular linear vessels.

nevi in older persons tend to be raised, papillomatous and hypopigmented or skin colored (intradermal nevus).

Blue nevi should be excised except when there is a history of an unchanged, stable lesion.

Atypical pigment network or pseudopigment network in association with regression areas is indicative for thin melanomas on the scalp.

A biopsy should be performed in lesions with prominent regression because differentiation of lichen planus–like keratosis, regressing seborrheic keratosis, and pigmented actinic keratosis from melanoma may be difficult.

Thick nodular melanomas are sometimes indistinguishable from blue nevi, pigmented basal cell carcinoma, pyogenic granuloma, and metastatic melanoma; thus, growing nodular lesions have to be excised without exception.

MUCOSAL LESIONS

Examination and evaluation of pigmented lesions located on the mucosa are considered problematic. First, especially in female patients, the lesion may be on a location difficult to examine; second, there are only a few studies describing the different dermoscopic patterns in this region. To avoid possible transmission of infections, the use of polyvinyl chloride food wrap covering the dermatoscope with the interposition of oil or alcohol both between the glass plate and the film and between the film and the skin is recommended.[13] In the author's opinion, the use and cleaning of the dermatoscope with isopropyl alcohol is sufficient to prevent nosocomial infection.[14]

Pigmented lesions on the mucocutaneous junction and mucous membrane include mucosal melanotic macule (mucosal melanosis), melanocytic nevus, malignant melanoma, and nonmelanocytic lesions, such as bowenoid papulosis. Estimates suggest that pigmented mucosal lesions are present in 10% to 12% of the general population and account for approximately 20% of vulvar disease.[15–17]

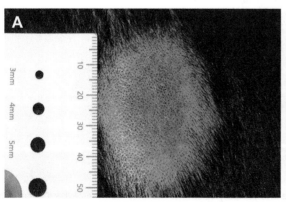

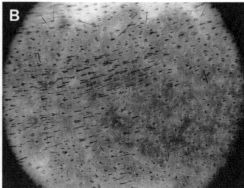

Fig. 7. (*A*) Clinical image of large blue nevus: blue-gray macule, diameter 3.5 cm × 1.5 cm. (*B*) Dermoscopic image of the central part of the lesions: homogenous blue pattern with subtle perifollicular hypopigmentation.

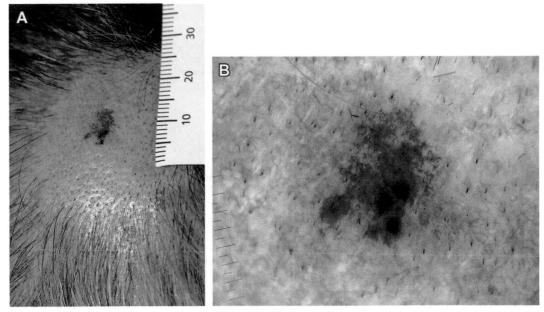

Fig. 8. (*A*) Clinical image of melanoma in situ in association with a lentigo actinica: brown macule with 3 black spots, diameter 1.5 cm × 0.5 cm. (*B*) Dermoscopic image: in the upper part, homogenous area representing the lentigo actinica; in lower part, 3 black blotches, which occlude asymmetrically the hair follicles. The latter is one of the early signs of melanoma in situ.

Mucosal Melanosis (Mucosal Melanotic Papule)

Mucosal melanosis is the most common pigmented mucosal lesion. It is defined as benign hyperpigmentation of basal keratinocytes. The number of melanocytes is normal or slightly increased, but they are not arranged in nests. Clinically mucosal melanosis presents as single or multiple brown macules. The diameter varies from 1 mm to 1 cm.

Mucosal melanosis can reveal different dermoscopy patterns. A general finding is the regularity of these mucosal lesions. They can display a homogenous, globular, or variant of reticular pattern (**Fig. 11**). Usually the border is regular.

The frequency of dermoscopic patterns differs in different studies. A study by Lin and colleagues[18] included 24 mucosal melanosis. The lesions presented a dotted-globular pattern (25%), a homogeneous pattern (25%), a fish scale–like pattern (18%), and a hyphal pattern (18%). In the author's opinion, the latter 2 are variants of a reticular pattern. The fish scale pattern was defined as multiple curves of semicircle, U shaped or V shaped, and arranged like scales of fish, whereas the

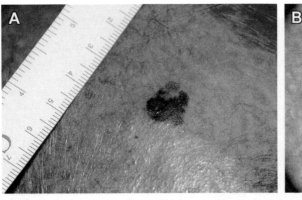
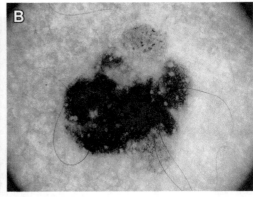

Fig. 9. (*A*) Clinical image of superficial spreading melanoma: polychromatic macule, diameter 1.1 × 0.8 cm. (*B*) Dermoscopic image: many of melanoma-specific criteria are visible; note the area of regression in the lower part of the lesions.

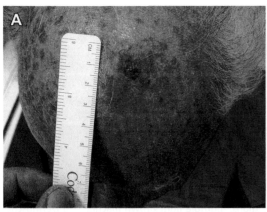
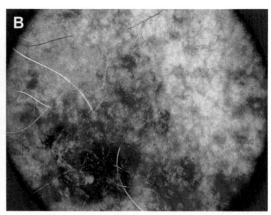

Fig. 10. (A) Clinical image of thick melanoma: blue-black nodule, diameter 1 cm, associated with multiple actinic lentigines. (B) Dermoscopic image: unspecific blue-red pattern, with striking shiny white streaks (chrysalis) in the nodular lesion.

hyphal pattern shows less regularly curved or flexed lines of different lengths, mimicking fungal hyphae. The other lesions displayed a homogenous, ringlike, or fingerprint-like pattern. Remarkably, none of the lesions revealed a multicomponent pattern (Fig. 12).

Based on dermoscopy, Mannone and colleagues[19] distinguished only 3 types of mucosal melanosis: structureless, parallel, and reticular types. The parallel pattern, characterized by regularly distributed pigmentation linearly arranged according to skin profile (furrows and reliefs), was predominant in clinically typical and small-in-diameter melanosis of the lip and penis. The second type was the structureless pattern, characterized by diffuse pigmentation ranging from light brown to dark brown. Structureless pattern was found in 10 of 11 clinically equivocal, large-in-diameter melanosis of the vulva (Fig. 13). The reticular pattern was less frequent in this case series.

A parallel pattern defined of linear and curved streaks, lines, or globules running parallel to the skin surface and the ringlike pattern characterized by multiple round to ovoid structures, with regular hyperpigmented well-defined borders, was found exclusively in benign melanocytic lesions in a monocentric study.[20] Ferrari and colleagues,[21] who described the ringlike pattern first, found it significantly more frequently in multifocal lesions than in single lesions of vulvar melanosis.

The structureless pattern was the predominant pattern, with presence in more than 50% of the histologically proved mucosal melanosis in the large retrospective study of the International Dermoscopy Society. All melanomas included in this study revealed zones of structureless pattern.[22]

To conclude, a regular parallel pattern formed by lines, dots, or globules and ringlike pattern are the main dermoscopic features of mucosal melanosis, indicating benignity. Frequently, mucosal melanosis displays a homogenous pattern, which is also found in mucosal melanoma. If, in large lesions with a homogenous pattern, more than

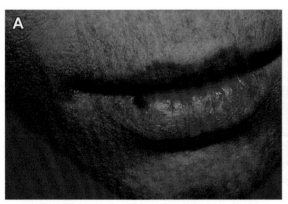
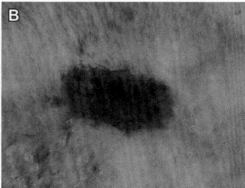

Fig. 11. (A) Clinical image of mucosal melanosis: brown macule on the lip. (B) Dermoscopic image: lines arranged in parallel order or circles form a regular pattern.

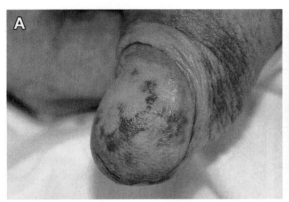

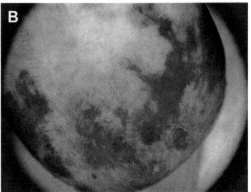

Fig. 12. (*A*) Clinical image of multifocal melanosis of the glans: multiple light brown macules. (*B*) Dermoscopic image: parallel lines, circles, and homogeneous areas are visible.

1 color or gray-blue color is evident, biopsy is recommended.

Melanocytic Nevus

Vulvar nevi are uncommon; in a study of 301 new patients in a gynecology practice, the prevalence of melanocytic nevi on vulvar skin was only 2.3%.[23] Nevi of mucosal membrane tend to be associated with younger age compared with melanoma or melanosis. Clinically, nevi appear, in most cases, as single 5-mm to 9-mm flat, slightly elevated, or nodular brown to gray lesions.

There are not many reports focused on the dermoscopic patterns of nevi of the mucosal membranes. Ferrari and colleagues,[24] investigating 37 cases of vulvar nevi, found the most common pattern was globular/cobblestone pattern or mixed pattern. The latter pattern was composed of parallel lines and a homogeneous brown-gray pigmentation or globules. This dermoscopic finding was correlated strongly to the histopathologic diagnosis of atypical melanocytic nevi of the genital type. Other studies revealed a different frequency of dermoscopic patterns, with homogeneous and globular pattern the most common features in their series of 8 and 16 melanocytic nevi, respectively.[20,22] All described blue nevi displaying the typical homogenous blue pattern.

In general, common melanocytic nevi on the mucosal membranes are brown to gray symmetric lesions with a globular or homogeneous pattern (**Fig. 14**).

Melanoma of Mucosal Membranes

Mucosal melanoma accounts for approximately 1.3% to 1.4% of all melanomas. Compared with cutaneous melanoma, the mean age of detection of mucosal melanomas is 10 years later. There is no evidence for racial predilection of mucosal melanoma. Mucosal melanomas account for 1.3% of melanomas in whites, whereas 11.8% of all melanomas in blacks are mucosal. Mucosal melanoma has a poorer prognosis than cutaneous melanoma. More than the half of patients develop advanced disease.[25]

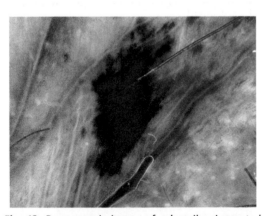

Fig. 13. Dermoscopic image of a heavily pigmented genital mucosal melanosis displaying a structureless (homogeneous) pattern.

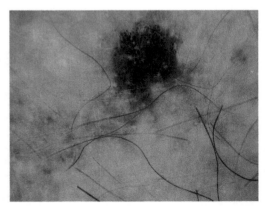

Fig. 14. Dermoscopic image of a genital nevus with a regular globular pattern.

Clinically, early mucosal melanomas present brown-black macules with shades of gray. The diameter is larger than 1 cm and multifocal growth is possible.

Advanced mucosal melanomas present as black or dark brown nodules combined frequently with the macular part at the basis of a tumor (see **Fig. 14**). In cases of amelanotic melanoma, red is the dominant color.

Dermoscopy of thin melanomas typically shows a multicolored and multicomponent pattern (**Figs. 15** and **16**). The multicomponent pattern consists of blue-white veil, irregular black dots, atypical network or streaks, and atypical (dotted and linear-irregular) vessels. Ferrari and colleagues[24] also found, in 4 of 5 vulvar melanomas, a reticular depigmentation, defined as delicate, white, crossing lines resembling a white network, and speculated that this might be an additional criterion for the diagnosis of melanoma.

In a study by Ronger-Savle and colleagues,[20] the investigators propose a scoring algorithm for vulvar pigmented lesions, which has sensitivity and specificity values of 100% and 94%, respectively. Different clinical and dermoscopic variables are included in this algorithm. Two points are given for a clinically palpable (raised or papular) lesion, for lesions showing dermoscopically a multicomponent pattern or for each of the following criteria: blue-whitish veil, white veil, irregular globules, peppering. Unilateral and unifocal, irregular pattern, more than 3 colors, and irregular vessels count each for 1 point. A total score greater than or equal to 4 is defined as a threshold for the diagnosis of melanoma.

Blum and colleagues developed 2 other algorithms for management of mucosal lesions. In the first algorithm the presence of blue, gray, or white color and the presence of a structureless zone, even if present in only parts of the lesion is suspicious. With regard to the diagnosis of melanoma, this algorithm had a sensitivity of 100% and a specificity of 82.2%. In the second model, they used only colors. Every lesion that contained blue, gray, or white color was regarded as suspicious, irrespective of the pattern. The sensitivity for melanoma of this model was 100% and the specificity was 64.3%.

Conclusion: Mucosal Lesions

Diameter larger than 1 cm, gray color, and the presence of structureless areas are highly suggestive for mucosal melanoma.

Only 1 color and regular dermoscopic structures are the main criteria of mucosal melanosis.

LESIONS ON THE MILK LINE

In the group of melanocytic nevi in special locations, there are also nevi located on the milk line and in flexural locations, such as axilla, inguinal region, popliteal, and antecubal fossa. These nevi show similar histopathologic features as nevi on the genitalia. Sometimes these nevi are difficult to differentiate histologically from melanoma and are diagnosed as superficial atypical melanocytic proliferation of uncertain significance (SAMPUS) or with a substantial dermal tumorigenic component—melanocytic tumor of uncertain malignant potential (MELTUMP).[15]

Clinically, these nevi are usually larger than 6 mm and display an irregular border. There are only a few case reports describing the dermoscopic features. In the personal experience of the author, the main dermoscopic finding is a prominent pigment network consisting of partly curved lines. Sometimes the lines form a parallel pattern similar to the parallel pattern of an acral nevus (**Fig. 17**). Sometimes large globules can be found in the center of these lesions histologically

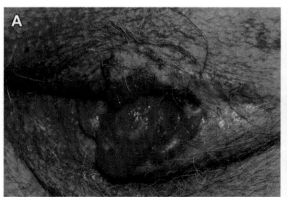 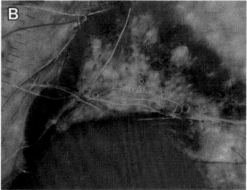

Fig. 15. (*A*) Clinical image of genital melanoma. The lesion consists of 2 parts the amelanotic nodular part and a pigmented macule at one site. (*B*) Dermoscopic image: the pigmented part shows homogenous gray-white areas and at the periphery irregular globules. Polymorphous vessels are visible in the red nodular part.

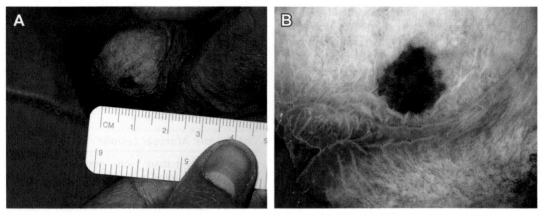

Fig. 16. (*A*) Clinical image of genital melanoma in situ: brown-black macule, diameter 0.6 cm. (*B*) Dermoscopic image: structureless (homogeneous) pattern with multiple colors; gray is the predominant color.

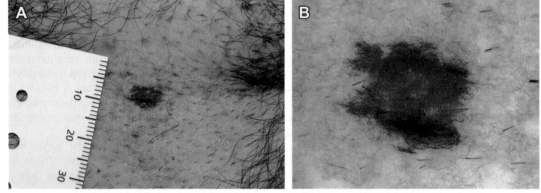

Fig. 17. (*A*) Clinical image of milk-line nevus: brown-red macule with a papule in the center, diameter 0.6 cm. (*B*) Dermoscopic image: pigment net with lines in a parallel pattern at the border of the lesion; in the center amelanotic part with comma vessels.

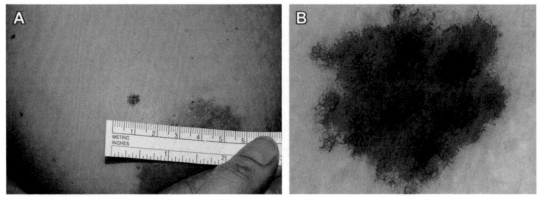

Fig. 18. (*A*) Clinical image of milk-line nevus: brown macule with an irregular border, diameter 0.6 cm. (*B*) Dermoscopic image: prominent pigment net with curved lines in some areas; note the large globules in some of the holes of the pigment net.

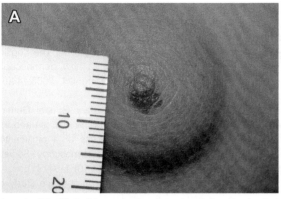
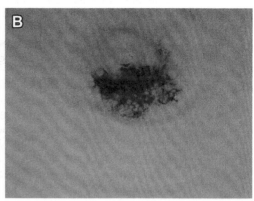

Fig. 19. (*A*) Clinical image of melanosis of the nipple: light brown patch maculebrown-black macule, diameter 0.4 cm. (*B*) Dermoscopic image: faint brown reticular pigmentation confined to the normal texture of skin of the areola.

corresponding to a large nest of melanocytes (**Fig. 18**). In the flexural lesions, a tiny white veil can be observed, probably due to the maceration of epidermis in these regions.

In a study investigating the correlation of anatomic location and the dermoscopic criteria of acquired nevi in patients with atypical nevus syndrome, Gamo and colleagues[26] found significantly more nevi with homogenous or homogenous-globular pattern in the neck, axilla, shoulders, and pectoral area than in other locations. Comma vessels were also more frequent on the neck, axillary area, and shoulders.

Nevi of the nipple display an unspecific pattern. Assessment of the dermoscopic criteria is difficult because of the brown background of the areola. In a case report of Kolm and colleagues,[27] an irregular brown to gray-blue pigmentation of the lobules of the nipple forming an irregular cobblestone pattern was present. Additionally, at the periphery of some lobules, the lesion displayed brown streaks and few irregular dark brown dots. Pastar and colleagues,[28] in their case report of a nevus of the nipple, described a globular pattern with the presence of focally light brown globules and irregular black globules in its center. Histology revealed a congenital nevus.

Reports of melanoma located on the breast are rare. Blum and Maltagliati-Holzner[29] reported 1 case of melanoma in situ, which was growing during pregnancy and developed an atypical pigment net.

Pigmented morbus Paget mammary disease can mimic melanoma clinically and dermoscopically. The major features described were irregular black dots and blue-gray structures and atypical reticular pigmentation.[30,31]

Another differential diagnosis is benign melanosis of the nipple (**Fig. 19**). Blum and colleagues[32] found

a cobblestone pattern representing the texture of the normal skin of the areola. Additionally, slightly narrow parallel lines were present at the periphery of the lesion. All 3 melanoses of the areola in the series of Mannone and colleagues[19] displayed a regular reticular pattern.

Conclusion: Melanocytic Lesions on Milk Line and Flexural Locations

Nevi located on the milk line and in flexural locations, such as axilla, inguinal region, popliteal, and antecubal fossa, can display specific dermoscopic patterns. Prominent pigment net, sometimes with bizarre lines, and large globules are characteristic. These nevi can mimic melanoma clinically and histopathologically.

REFERENCES

1. Stanganelli I, Argenziano G, Sera F, et al. Dermoscopy of scalp tumours: a multi-centre study conducted by the international dermoscopy society. J Eur Acad Dermatol Venereol 2012;26(8):953–63.

2. Chiu CS, Lin CY, Kuo TT, et al. Malignant cutaneous tumors of the scalp: a study of demographic characteristics and histologic distributions of 398 Taiwanese patients. J Am Acad Dermatol 2007; 56:448–52.

3. Lachiewicz AM, Berwick M, Wiggins CL, et al. Survival differences between patients with scalp or neck melanoma and those with melanoma of other sites in the Surveillance, Epidemiology, and End Results (SEER) program. Arch Dermatol 2008;144: 515–21.

4. Fabrizi G, Pagliarello C, Parente P, et al. Atypical nevi of the scalp in adolescents. J Cutan Pathol 2007;34:365–9.

5. Aguilera P, Puig S, Guilabert A, et al. Prevalence study of nevi in children from Barcelona:

dermoscopy, constitutional and environmental factors. Dermatology 2009;218:203–14.

6. Tcheung WJ, Bellet JS, Prose NS, et al. Clinical and dermoscopic features of 88 scalp nevi in 39 children. Br J Dermatol 2011;165:137–43.

7. Kessides MC, Puttgen KB, Cohen BA. No biopsy needed for eclipse and cockade nevi found on the scalps of children. Arch Dermatol 2009;145:1334–6.

8. Ferrara G, Soyer HP, Malvehy J, et al. The many faces of blue nevus: a clinicopathologic study. J Cutan Pathol 2007;34:543–51.

9. Martin RC, Murali R, Scolyer RA, et al. So-called "malignant blue nevus": a clinicopathologic study of 23 patients. Cancer 2009;115(13):2949–55.

10. Zalaudek I, Leinweber B, Soyer HP, et al. Dermoscopic features of melanoma on the scalp. J Am Acad Dermatol 2004;51:S88–90.

11. Argenziano G, Longo C, Cameron A, et al. Blue-black rule: a simple dermoscopic clue to recognize pigmented nodular melanoma. Br J Dermatol 2011; 165(6):1251–5.

12. Zaballos P, Carulla M, Ozdemir F, et al. Dermoscopy of pyogenic granuloma: morphological study. Br J Dermatol 2010;163(6):1229–37.

13. Zampino MR, Borghi A, Corazza M, et al. A preliminary evaluation of polyvinyl chloride film use in dermoscopic analysis of mucosal areas. Arch Dermatol 2005;141(8):1044–5.

14. Hausermann P, Widmer A, Itin P. Dermatoscope as vector for transmissible diseases - no apparent risk of nosocomial infections in outpatients. Dermatology 2006;212(1):27–30.

15. Elder DE. Precursors to melanoma and their mimics: nevi of special sites. Mod Pathol 2006;19:S4–20.

16. Hosler GA, Moresi JM, Barrett TL. Naevi with site-related atypia: a review of melanocytic naevi with atypical histological features based on anatomic site. J Cutan Pathol 2008;35:889–98.

17. Olszewska M, Banka A, Gorska R, et al. Dermoscopy of pigmented oral lesions. J Dermatol Case Rep 2008;2(3):43–8.

18. Lin J, Koga H, Takata M, et al. Dermoscopy of pigmented lesions on mucocutaneous junction and mucous membrane. Br J Dermatol 2009;161(6): 1255–61.

19. Mannone F, De Giorgi V, Cattaneo A, et al. Dermoscopic features of mucosal melanosis. Dermatol Surg 2004;30(8):1118–23.

20. Ronger-Savle S, Julien V, Duru G, et al. Features of pigmented vulval lesions on dermoscopy. Br J Dermatol 2011;164(1):54–61.

21. Ferrari A, Buccini P, Covello R, et al. The ringlike pattern in vulvar melanosis: a new dermoscopic clue for diagnosis. Arch Dermatol 2008;144(8): 1030–4.

22. Blum A, Simionescu O, Argenziano G, et al. Dermoscopy of pigmented lesions of the mucosa and the mucocutaneous junction: results of a multicenter study by the International Dermoscopy Society (IDS). Arch Dermatol 2011;147(10):1181–7.

23. Rock B, Hood AF, Rock JA. Prospective study of vulvar nevi. J Am Acad Dermatol 1990;22:104–6.

24. Ferrari A, Zalaudek I, Argenziano G, et al. Dermoscopy of pigmented lesions of the vulva: a retrospective morphological study. Dermatology 2011; 222:157–66.

25. Seetharamu N, Ott PA, Pavlick AC. Mucosal melanomas: a case-based review of the literature. Oncologist 2010;15(7):772–81.

26. Gamo R, Malvehy J, Puig S, et al. Dermoscopic features of melanocytic nevi in seven different anatomical locations in patients with atypical nevi syndrome. Dermatol Surg 2013;39(6):864–71.

27. Kolm I, Kamarashev J, Kerl K, et al. Diagnostic pitfall: pigmented lesion of the nipple–correlation between dermoscopy, reflectance confocal microscopy and histopathology. Dermatology 2011; 222(1):1–4.

28. Pastar Z, Massone C, Ahlgrimm-Siess V, et al. Dermoscopy and in vivo reflectance confocal microscopy of a congenital nevus of the nipple. Dermatology 2010;221(2):127–30.

29. Blum A, Maltagliati-Holzner P. Monitoring a melanocytic tumor. When is excision indicated? Hautarzt 2011;62(10):774–7.

30. Yanagishita T, Tamada Y, Tanaka M, et al. Pigmented mammary Paget disease mimicking melanoma on dermatoscopy. J Am Acad Dermatol 2011;64(6): 114–6.

31. Hida T, Yoneta A, Nishizaka T, et al. Pigmented mammary Paget's disease mimicking melanoma: report of three cases. Eur J Dermatol 2012;22(1): 121–4.

32. Blum A, Metzler G, Caroli U. Melanosis of the areola in dermoscopy. J Am Acad Dermatol 2004;51(4): 664–5.

Blue Lesions

Caterina Longo, MD, PhD[a],*, Alon Scope, MD[b,c],
Aimilios Lallas, MD[a], Iris Zalaudek, MD[a],
Elvira Moscarella, MD[a], Stefano Gardini, MD[a],
Giuseppe Argenziano, MD[a], Giovanni Pellacani, MD[d]

KEYWORDS

- Blue color • Melanoma • Blue nevi • Spitz/Reed nevi • Nonmelanocytic lesions
- Exogenous pigmentation

KEY POINTS

- Blue color can be found in a wide range of malignant and benign melanocytic and nonmelanocytic lesions as well as in lesions that result from penetration of exogenous materials.
- Careful patient examination and lesion assessment by integrating dermoscopy in clinical practice is useful to discriminate between different diagnostic entities that display blue color.
- As a fundamental rule, all blue nodular lesions that do not fulfill clear-cut clinical and dermoscopic criteria for a specific benign lesion with high confidence should be excised to avoid the risk of delaying or missing the diagnosis of a nodular melanoma.

INTRODUCTION

Colors that are seen under dermoscopic examination of skin lesions emanate from the presence of different chromophores in the epidermis and dermis, including melanin, hemoglobin, and collagen. The colors depend on the anatomic level of skin at which these chromophores are located.[1] Blue color in lesions that are not vascular in origin is mostly related to a dermal localization of melanin, arranged as either extracellular melanin granules or located within cells arranged as solitary units (eg, melanophages) or as clusters of cells (eg, melanocytic nests in a nevus or aggregates of basaloid neoplastic cells in basal cell carcinoma).[2] Thus, blue color can be found under dermoscopy in a wide range of melanocytic and nonmelanocytic lesions. Of these, lesions that show diffuse bluish pigmentation on dermoscopy can be particularly challenging to diagnose with specificity. The assessment of colors under dermoscopy is influenced by the type of dermatoscope that is being used for the analysis: polarized light dermoscopy (PD) versus nonpolarized light dermoscopy (NPD).[3] More specifically, under PD, blue colors appear darker and different shades of brown and blue seem to be highlighted compared with NPD. In particular, peppering and blue-white structures (BWSs) are seen better with NPD. The reason for these differences, simplistically stated, is that PD allows for better visualization of light coming from deeper layers of the dermis than NPD, because the polarized filters of PD block light that is backscattered from more superficial layers (eg, epidermis and dermal-epidermal junction). This difference, however, between PD and NPD does not seem to affect the overall lesion pattern and the diagnostic accuracy.

The authors have no conflict of interest to declare.
Funding Sources: Study supported in part by the Italian Ministry of Health (RF-2010-2316524).
[a] Skin Cancer Unit, Arcispedale Santa Maria Nuova-IRCCS, Viale Risorgimento 80, Reggio Emilia 42100, Italy;
[b] Department of Dermatology, Sheba Medical Center, Sackler School of Medicine, Tel Aviv University, Tel Aviv 52621, Israel; [c] Dermatology Service, Memorial Sloan-Kettering Cancer Center, New York, NY 10065, USA; [d] Dermatology Unit, University of Modena and Reggio Emilia, Modena 41121, Italy
* Corresponding author.
E-mail address: longo.caterina@gmail.com

derm.theclinics.com

This article reviews the diagnoses that appear predominantly blue in color under dermoscopy and the management rules for the various blue lesions in clinical practice.

MELANOCYTIC LESIONS
Blue Nevi

Blue melanocytic nevi represent the prototypical melanocytic neoplasm that is typified by a predominantly blue color under dermoscopy. The authors acknowledge that what is referred to clinically and dermoscopically as blue nevus actually represents various subtypes of melanocytic nevi that have in common a predominantly dermal proliferation of pigmented melanocytes on histopathology. Dermoscopically, blue nevi show a structureless, uniform steel-blue coloration (**Fig. 1**) that corresponds on histopathology to the presence of heavily pigmented melanocytes in the reticular dermis. Blue nevi are typically devoid of other dermoscopic criteria, such as pigment network, although multiple colors (blue, black, and brown)[4] can be observed in a small percentage of lesions. Recently, Di Cesare and colleagues[5] confirmed that the prototypical dermoscopic feature of blue nevi is homogeneous bluish to steel-blue pigmentation. This feature was significantly more frequent in blue nevi compared with melanomas and pigmented basal cell carcinomas, with a specificity of 99% and 96.8%, respectively, and a sensitivity of 48.4%.[5]

The clinical and dermoscopic diagnosis of blue nevus is usually straightforward and relies on the dermoscopic observation of diffuse, homogeneous bluish to steel-blue pigmentation in absence of specific melanoma criteria, and, importantly, on the clinical history of a long-standing, stable lesion. When lesion history is not available and, particularly in adult patients, when the lesion at hand is new or changing, a biopsy should be strongly considered to rule out the diagnosis of melanoma or melanoma metastasis.

Spitz/Reed Nevi

Dermoscopically, pigmented Spitz/Reed nevi (PSRN) often display a starburst pattern typified by multiple peripheral streaks or peripherally located pigmented globules, whereas the center of the lesion usually shows a homogeneous pattern ranging in color from blue-gray to brown-black.[6–13]

Clinically, PSRN presents as a flat or papular lesion that often arises on the face, limbs, and buttocks of children or young adults. Patient age is an important factor in determining whether a lesion with bluish color clinically and a starburst pattern dermoscopically is managed as a PSRN or melanoma; at times, melanoma can be completely indistinguishable from PSRN, clinically and dermoscopically. Furthermore, under confocal microscopy, PSRN often shows the presence of cytologic atypia, pagetoid spread, and architectural disorder, confocal features that overlap with those seen in melanoma; thus, confocal microscopy cannot always reliably differentiate between PSRN and melanoma.[13]

The difficulty clinicians may face in discriminating PSRN from melanoma is also encountered in the histopathologic analysis of so-called spitzoid lesions, and discordant diagnoses (of melanoma vs PSRN) are not infrequent when multiple pathologists review the slides of a given spitzoid neoplasm. Thus, prompt excision of any pigmented lesion that shows spitzoid features on clinical and dermoscopic examination should be performed in adults, including young adults after puberty, to avoid missing melanoma. Finally, new molecular analysis techniques may potentially enhance the diagnostic discrimination between PSRN and melanoma in the future.

Melanoma

The presence of blue color is a common dermoscopic finding in melanoma. In melanoma, blue color is often admixed with white; thus, these

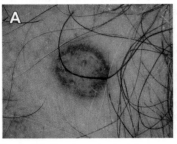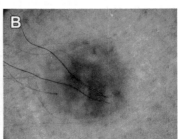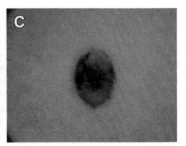

Fig. 1. (*A*) The stereotypical dermoscopic pattern of a blue nevus showing a steel-blue homogeneous pigmentation. (*B*) Blue nevus with polychromatic dermoscopic pattern (*blue-white and brown color*). (*C*) Blue nevus with brown and blue shades.

dermoscopic structures have been named BWSs. BWSs are often classified according to the clinical palpability of the area showing the blue color (eg, flat, palpable, and purely nodular melanoma). Foci of BWSs that are clinically flat often signify the presence of regression on histopathology, whereas palpable or nodular BWSs often signify melanomas in which the proliferation of neoplastic cells is present in the dermis (ie, invasive melanoma). A blue color that is associated with black color (BB rule; discussed later) typically occurs in nodular melanomas that lack, or have a limited, junctional component.

Regression (Flat Blue-white Structures)

Dermoscopically observed regression (flat BWSs) mostly appears as white scarlike depigmentation that is usually whiter in color than the surrounding skin, admixed with granularity or peppering (speckled multiple blue-gray granules within the hypopigmented areas).[14,15] On histopathology, regression shows fibrosis and a bandlike infiltrate of melanophages in the superficial dermis as well as a thin epidermis with effacement of the rete ridges.

Flat BWSs that show a combination of white scarlike areas and blue granularity are a dermoscopic finding that should raise suspicion for melanoma undergoing regression. Although the presence of flat BWSs can also be seen in nevi, the majority of these nevi usually reveal only blue color (ie, granularity) without white; moreover, the blue structure is most often centrally located in more than half of such nevi, whereas an irregular distribution (combination of a central and peripheral location) is most frequently found in melanomas.[16,17] The extent of BWSs within the lesion is also important, in that the more widespread the BWS, the greater the suspicion for melanoma. Zalaudek and colleagues[16] demonstrated that melanocytic lesions with BWSs covering more than 50% of the lesion area had a 44% probability of being histopathologically equivocal (ie, showing discordance between pathologists on the diagnosis of nevus vs melanoma), whereas lesions with BWSs covering less than 50% of the lesion area had a 91% probability of being diagnosed unequivocally as a nevus on histopathology. In summary, the presence of flat BWSs that includes both white and blue colors, that is, irregular in distribution or that involves more than 50% of the lesion, should prompt a clinician to excise the lesion to rule out melanoma.

The evaluation of lesions showing flat BWSs, however, also has to be considered in the context of a patient's other nevi.[18] Older patients with multiple nevi may have more than 1 lesion showing blue color as a result of an involution phenomenon.[19] In contrast, a solitary lesion with blue color should always raise suspicion for melanoma.

When regression structures are extensive and advanced in the lesion, and other dermoscopic criteria are scant or absent, it could be difficult to determine whether the lesion at hand is melanocytic (ie, a fully regressed melanoma) or nonmelanocytic (ie, a seborrheic keratosis undergoing regression, termed, lichen planus–like keratosis).[20–23] In this scenario, confocal microscopy may support the clinical decision making process because it can enable the detection of subtle remnants of the melanocytic proliferation; for example, confocal observation of a proliferation of single atypical melanocytes or even aggregates of cells interspersed within a florid inflammatory infiltrate, is suggestive of the diagnosis of melanoma (Fig. 2).[20,24–26] Lichen planus, however, like keratosis typically shows on confocal imaging the presence of cordlike structures or bulbous projections admixed with a variable amount of melanophages. The detection of a remnant melanocytic proliferation on confocal examination, however, is not always reliable; thus, biopsy should be strongly considered in cases that lack additional clear-cut dermoscopic or confocal criteria for the diagnosis of seborrheic keratosis. This approach has led to better management of fully regressed melanomas; if left to their own devices, these melanomas can eventually disappear completely, potentially leading to the occurrence of melanoma metastases with an unknown primary tumor.[27]

A peculiar morphology of dermoscopically observed regression, occurring preferentially in melanoma in situ, has been recently described. This early melanoma can display regression that appears reticula in distribution, seen as a coarse blue-gray net, with thick gray-blue lines (reticular blue areas) with large holes that correspond to pink-colored regression areas (Fig. 3).[28] The fading of the pigment network or of other dermoscopic structures results in areas of structureless light brown pigmentation.[29] This reticular-type of regression can be found in so-called slow-growing melanomas that are characterized dermoscopically by the simultaneous presence of network and regression.[30]

Blue-white Veil (Palpable Blue-white Structures)

Blue-white veil is a dermoscopic structure defined as an irregular, indistinct, confluent blue pigmentation with an overlying white, ground-glass haze (Fig. 4).[14] On histopathology, the blue-white veil

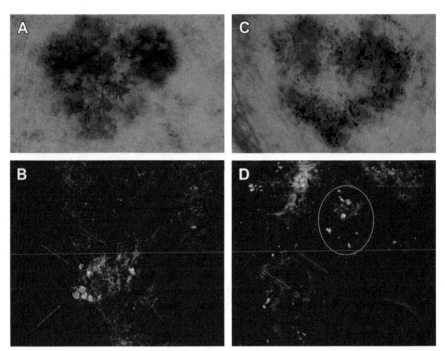

Fig. 2. (*A*) Melanoma undergoing regression, characterized by the presence of bluish gray granularity, fragmented pigmented network, and tan to dark brown background. (*B*) Confocal microscopy reveals the presence of small aggregates of atypical melanocytes (*red arrows*) that support the melanocytic nature of the lesion. (*C*) Lichen planus–like keratosis characterized by coarse bluish granularity and small brown dots. (*D*) Confocal microscopy shows the presence of melanophages (*blue circle*) and bulbous projections (*red arrows*) that represent the hallmark of lichen planus–like keratosis diagnosis.

seen on dermoscopy corresponds to an acanthotic epidermis with focal hypergranulosis and compact orthokeratosis overlying sheets of heavily pigmented neoplastic atypical melanocytes in the upper dermis. Among melanocytic neoplasms, blue-white veil is mostly seen in melanomas and PSRN. The presence of blue-white veil is associated with foci in the lesion that are clinically palpable, and thus, in the context of melanoma, blue-white veil signifies invasive melanomas. Additional dermoscopic criteria may be observed in the lesion, such as atypical network and vascular

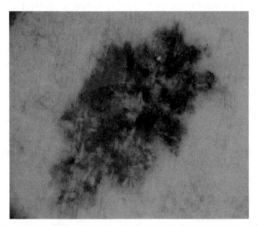

Fig. 3. Melanoma in situ showing the presence of regression that appears reticular in distribution, seen as a coarse blue-gray network with thick lines (termed, *reticular blue areas*) and large pink-colored holes that correspond to regression areas.

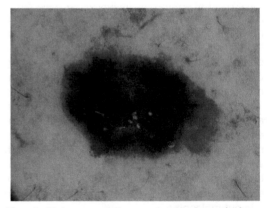

Fig. 4. Melanoma 0.7 mm in Breslow thickness revealing the presence of a blue-white veil that appears as an irregular, indistinct, confluent blue pigmentation with an overlying white, ground-glass haze.

pattern, and taken together with the blue-white veil, these criteria usually point to the correct dermoscopic diagnosis of melanoma.

Blue-black Color (BB Rule)

Nodular melanoma is a fast-growing malignant neoplasm[31] that often lacks classical dermoscopic criteria, such as atypical network, peripheral streaks, and regression that are usually found in superficial spreading melanoma. To complicate matters, the small initial size of this cancer and its occurrence de novo as a lesion that has not arisen from a preexisting nevus render this melanoma more difficult for patients to recognize. Recently, a simple rule has been described to aid in the detection of pigmented nodular melanoma. It consists of the simultaneous combination of blue and black colors (BB rule) in a given lesion (**Fig. 5**).[32] The presence of the BB rule combined with 1 or more of the standard dermoscopic criteria for the diagnosis of melanoma resulted in 91.9% specificity and 90.6% positive predictive value for melanoma diagnosis.

As exception to the BB rule, black-colored structures can also be seen under dermoscopy in seborrheic keratoses as comedo-like openings and in hemangiomas as dark lacunae. Historical and clinical details, however, as well as other dermoscopic features usually allow a ready differentiation of these benign lesions from nodular melanoma.

Confocal microscopy suggests that the black color in nodular melanoma results not only from an abundant and diffuse presence of melanin in the epidermis but also from a dense dermal proliferation of sheets of pigmented atypical melanocytes under a thinned epidermis. The authors'

confocal study also highlighted that dermoscopically observed black color may herald in some cases an incipient ulceration or a preulcerative state in nodular melanoma.[33]

Metastasis

Pigmented melanoma metastasis may show a variety of dermoscopic global patterns, such as a homogeneous blue color or saccular pattern and often demonstrate the presence of brown, blue, and black colors.[32–34] An additional clue, the presence of peripheral stellate telangiectasias has been recently described (**Fig. 6**).[35] The diagnosis of cutaneous melanoma metastasis is usually suspected based on a previous history of primary invasive melanoma. New lesions, located in proximity to the surgical scar of the primary melanoma (satellite metastases) or at a more distant location, that do not show convincing dermoscopic criteria of nevi or other benign diagnoses, should be promptly excised in suspicion of melanoma metastasis. In addition, the use of echography may help to differentiate blue nevi from a blue-colored melanoma metastasis, because blue nevi are generally dish-shaped and have a homogeneous echo whereas melanoma metastases are potato-shaped and show an inhomogeneous echo.[36]

NONMELANOCYTIC LESIONS

Seborrheic keratosis can show the presence of blue color, more commonly displaying a fuzzy grayish color with a bluish shade; these colors are related to the presence of melanin-laden melanophages in the superficial dermis (blue) and an acanthotic epidermis (gray). The presence of additional dermoscopic features, however, such as comedo-like openings, milia-like structures, and regular hairpin vessels, point to the correct diagnosis of seborrheic keratosis in most cases. A bluish coloration can be observed in seborrheic keratoses located on the hairline of the forehead or on the scalp of elderly women who dye their hair; the color is bright blue, and the dye saturates the fissures of the lesion as well as the comedo-like openings that appear as well-demarcated roundish to oval bluish structures with a darker outline (**Fig. 7**).

Hemangioma is another benign nonmelanocytic lesion that can present as a blue-colored papule. In hemangioma, the blue color is usually visualized as reddish purple to blue multiple, well-demarcated lacunae (**Fig. 8**).[14] The clear-cut demarcation of the lacunae helps in distinguishing the lesion from melanoma or melanoma metastasis.

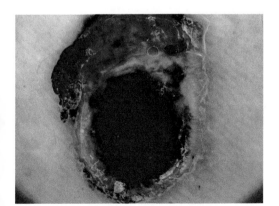

Fig. 5. Nodular melanoma characterized by the simultaneous presence of blue and black color (BB rule). Perilesional erythema is also visible at the right side of the tumor.

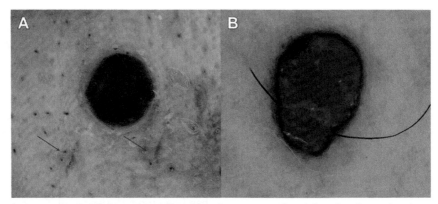

Fig. 6. New dermoscopic criteria for melanoma metastasis: presence of peripheral stellate telangiectasias (*arrows*) (*A*) and presence of blue and black colors (*B*).

Dermatofibroma in its classical appearance is characterized by a central white scarlike area surrounded by a delicate peripheral network.[37–39] A variant of dermatofibroma, the hemosiderotic type, may display a homogeneous bluish pigmentation (**Fig. 9**). This dermoscopic pattern, however, can be found in a variety of tumors and a diagnosis of malignancy is difficult to rule out. Furthermore, in blue nodular lesions that lack a specific dermoscopic pattern, the strategy of conservative monitoring is strongly discouraged because of the possibility of delaying the diagnosis of nodular melanoma; because nodular melanoma is typically a fast-growing and aggressive cancer, delay in diagnosis may adversely affect the prognosis a patient.

In pigmented basal cell carcinoma, blue color can be found under dermoscopy as large blue to gray ovoid nests and as blue-gray globules and dots.[14] Large blue to gray ovoid nests are well-circumscribed, confluent or near-confluent pigmented oval or elongated areas, larger than globules, that are not intimately connected to a central large pigmented blotch (**Fig. 10**). Multiple in-focus blue-gray dots describe small, pigmented dots that appear sharply in focus under dermoscopy, in contrast to the fuzzy appearance of the specks and dots in granularity seen in regression structures. Both blue-gray ovoid nests and globules represent aggregates of basaloid neoplastic cells in the dermis—when the aggregates are large, they are seen as large ovoid nests under dermoscopy, and when the aggregates are smaller, they appear as globules on dermoscopy. Conversely, blue-gray dots correspond histopathologically to dermal melanophages. These dermoscopic criteria, along with additional dermoscopic features, such as the presence of arborizing vessels or ulcerations, represent reliable and robust diagnostic parameters for basal cell carcinoma.

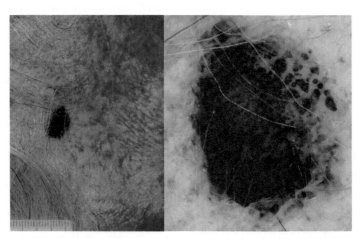

Fig. 7. Seborrheic keratosis located on the hairline of a woman who has dyed hair (*right*). The color of the dye is bright blue and saturates the fissures of the lesion. In particular, the comedo-like openings appear as well demarcated roundish to oval structures with a darker outline (*left*).

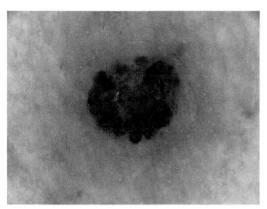

Fig. 8. Hemangioma characterized by the presence of multiple, fairly well demarcated reddish to purple-blue lacunae, separated by blue-white septae. A blackish, thrombosed lacuna is also visible in the inferior part of the lesion.

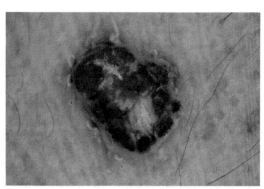

Fig. 10. This basal cell carcinoma shows a predominantly dark blue color that emanates from the presence of heavily pigmented large blue ovoid nests. A few telangiectasias are also visible at the periphery of the lesion but are obscured by the heavy pigmentation.

As a complementary tool, confocal microscopy can be used in cases of heavily pigmented basal cell carcinoma whereby dermoscopic criteria are sometimes obscured by the abundant pigmentation and the diagnosis of melanoma cannot be excluded with certainty.[40,41] In these cases, the recognition of bright tumor islands on confocal examination permits a rapid diagnosis of basal cell carcinoma.

Kaposi sarcoma is characterized under polarized dermoscopy by a bluish-reddish coloration, a scaly surface, small brown globules, and, most distinctively, a multicolored pattern that has been described as a rainbow pattern.[42,43] Although Kaposi sarcoma can appear as a blue-colored papule or nodule, the blue color is often associated with a reddish hue. In addition, on clinical examination, the presence of multiple lesions lends additional support for the diagnosis of Kaposi sarcoma.

Among malignant vascular neoplasms, the dermoscopic aspects of angiosarcoma have been recently described. Angiosarcoma often exhibits a patchy, structureless pattern, ranging in color from variable shades of red (light and dark) to purple or bluish colors (Fig. 11).[44] Dermoscopy can raise further suspicion of angiosarcoma, because dermoscopic criteria that are specific for benign vascular proliferations, such as the presence of discrete lacunae, are absent. This is particularly evident in cases where the clinical scenario is also suspicious for angiosarcoma, typically an enlarging violaceous plaque or nodule preferentially located on the scalp of an elderly man. The final confirmation of diagnosis of angiosarcoma rests on the histopathological examination. Further

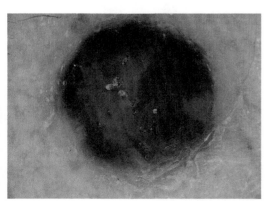

Fig. 9. This dermatofibroma, hemosiderotic variant displays a diffuse homogeneous bluish pigmentation. There is absence of any distinctive dermoscopic criteria for the diagnosis of dermatofibroma.

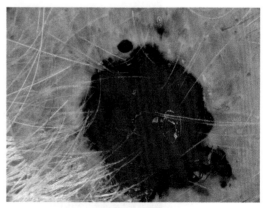

Fig. 11. Sporadic angiosarcoma of the scalp presenting as an ulcerated nodule with a central homogeneous blackish area, surrounded by a white-to-blue/purple structureless rim.

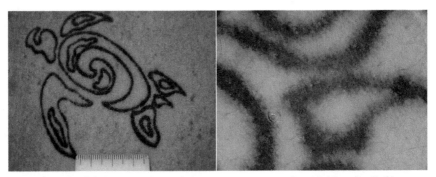

Fig. 12. Cosmetic tattoo (*right*) that reveals on dermoscopy a structureless bluish color (*left*).

study of the dermoscopic criteria of early angiosarcoma in large case series may elucidate the significance of dermoscopy in the diagnosis of this malignant neoplasm.

EXOGENOUS BLUE PIGMENTATION

The presence of any kind of exogenous dermal pigmentation, such as ink tattoo, radiation tattoo, amalgam tattoo, and traumatic penetration of pigmented materials, may be perceived as blue coloration on dermoscopy. In these cases of exogenous pigmentation, the color is usually associated with a structureless pattern, and, in case of cosmetic tattoo, the color is arranged in a pattern that forms a drawing (**Fig. 12**). India ink tattooing, a black pigment made of carbons, is used for radiation field positioning. The ink particles are taken up by macrophages and fibroblasts in the dermis and subcutis. The deeper location of India ink in the dermis causes a bluish appearance by a similar physical mechanism as seen with dermal melanin—the so-called Tyndall effect of the light scattering effect of blue pigmentation in the dermis.[45] In women undergoing radiotherapy for breast cancer, radiation tattoos are preferentially located around the chest areas (**Fig. 13**), and, similarly, in men treated with radiotherapy for prostate cancer, radiation tattoos are located around the pelvic area; dermoscopically, these tattoos are almost indistinguishable from blue nevi.

Amalgam tattoos are common, oral pigmented lesions that clinically present as isolated, blue, gray, or black macules and patches that occur most often on the gingivae and can also be seen on the buccal and alveolar mucosae, the palate, or the tongue (**Fig. 14**). They are due to a deposition of a mixture of silver, tin, mercury, copper, and zinc, which compose an amalgam filling, into the oral soft tissues. As a peculiar finding, amalgam tattoos can resemble a blue nevus or vascular lesion but occur in the context of a patient

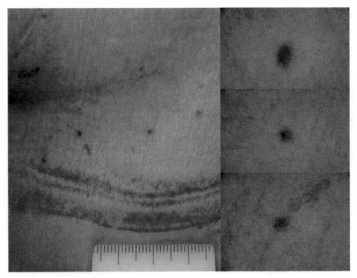

Fig. 13. Radiation tattoo in a woman with breast cancer. Dermoscopically, the lesions, as seen on the right panel, are indistinguishable from blue nevi.

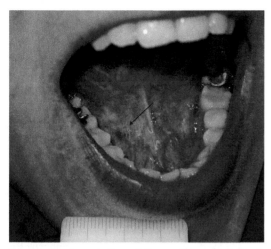

Fig. 14. Amalgam tattoo of the oral mucosa (*arrow*).

that has an adjacent dental filling. In cases of clinical doubt or when a mucosal melanoma has to be ruled out, radiography can be performed in search of a radiopaque signal, along with a small incisional punch biopsy.[46,47]

A traumatic injection of any kind of external dark-colored material, such as penetration of tar particles from abrasion against the road surface in a motorcycle accident, can give rise to blue coloration; under dermoscopy, this blue coloration is usually seen as scattered bluish granules.

SUMMARY

In the realm of lesions that predominantly show a blue color, the correct diagnostic evaluation always relies on the integration of data, including a patient's age, lesion history (duration of onset and rate of growth), palpability, and dermoscopic features. As a fundamental rule, all blue nodular lesions that do not fulfill clear-cut clinical and dermoscopic criteria for a specific benign lesion with high confidence should be excised to avoid the risk of delaying or missing the diagnosis of a nodular melanoma.

REFERENCES

1. Yadav S, Vossaert KA, Kopf AW, et al. Histopathologic correlates of structures seen on dermoscopy (epiluminescence microscopy). Am J Dermatopathol 1993;15:297–305.

2. Soyer HP, Kenet RO, Wolf IH, et al. Clinicopathologic correlation of pigmented skin lesions using dermoscopy. Eur J Dermatol 2000;10:22–8.

3. Benvenuto-Andrade C, Dusza SW, Agero AL, et al. Differences between polarized light dermoscopy and immersion contact dermoscopy for the evaluation of skin lesions. Arch Dermatol 2007; 143(3):329–38.

4. Ferrara G, Soyer HP, Malvehy J, et al. The many faces of blue nevus: a clinicopathologic study. J Cutan Pathol 2007;34:543–51.

5. Di Cesare A, Sera F, Gulia A, et al. The spectrum of dermatoscopic patterns in blue nevi. J Am Acad Dermatol 2012;67(2):199–205.

6. Argenziano G, Scalvenzi M, Staibano S, et al. Dermatoscopic pitfalls in differentiating pigmented Spitz naevi from cutaneous melanomas. Br J Dermatol 1999;141(5):788–93.

7. Argenziano G, Soyer HP, Ferrara G, et al. Superficial black network: an additional dermoscopic clue for the diagnosis of pigmented spindle and/or epithelioid cell nevus. Dermatology 2001;203(4): 333–5.

8. Marchell R, Marghoob AA, Braun RP, et al. Dermoscopy of pigmented Spitz and Reed nevi: the starburst pattern. Arch Dermatol 2005; 141(8):1060.

9. Ferrara G, Argenziano G, Soyer HP, et al. The spectrum of Spitz nevi: a clinicopathologic study of 83 cases. Arch Dermatol 2005;141(11):1381–7.

10. Argenziano G, Zalaudek I, Ferrara G, et al. Involution: the natural evolution of pigmented Spitz and Reed nevi? Arch Dermatol 2007;143(4):549–51.

11. Nino M, Brunetti B, Delfino S, et al. Spitz nevus: follow-up study of 8 cases of childhood starburst type and proposal for management. Dermatology 2009;218(1):48–51.

12. Pellacani G, Longo C, Ferrara G, et al. Spitz nevi: In vivo confocal microscopic features, dermatoscopic aspects, histopathologic correlates, and diagnostic significance. J Am Acad Dermatol 2009;60(2):236–47.

13. Pellacani G, Guitera P, Longo C, et al. The impact of in vivo reflectance confocal microscopy for the diagnostic accuracy of melanoma and equivocal melanocytic lesions. J Invest Dermatol 2007 Dec; 127(12):2759–65.

14. Argenziano G, Soyer HP, Chimenti S, et al. Dermoscopy of pig- mented skin lesions. Results of a consensus meeting via the internet. J Am Acad Dermatol 2003;48:679–93.

15. Massi D, De Giorgi V, Carli P, et al. Diagnostic significance of the blue hue in dermoscopy of melanocytic lesions: a dermo- scopic-pathologic study. Am J Dermatopathol 2001;23:463–9.

16. Zalaudek I, Argenziano G, Ferrara G, et al. Clinically equivocal melanocytic skin lesions with features of regression: a dermoscopic-pathological study. Br J Dermatol 2004;150(1):64–71.

17. Ferrara G, Argenziano G, Soyer HP, et al. Dermoscopic and histopathologic diagnosis of equivocal melanocytic skin lesions: an interdisciplinary study on 107 cases. Cancer 2002;95:1094–100.

18. Argenziano G, Catricalà C, Ardigo M, et al. Dermoscopy of patients with multiple nevi: Improved management recommendations using a comparative diagnostic approach. Arch Dermatol 2011;147(1):46–9.

19. Zalaudek I, Docimo G, Argenziano G. Using dermoscopic criteria and patient-related factors for the management of pigmented melanocytic nevi. Arch Dermatol 2009;145(7):816–26.

20. Pellacani G, Bassoli S, Longo C, et al. Diving into the blue: in vivo microscopic characterization of the dermoscopic blue hue. J Am Acad Dermatol 2007;57(1):96–104.

21. Braun RP, Gaide O, Oliviero M, et al. The significance of multiple blue-grey dots (granularity) for the dermoscopic diagnosis of melanoma. Br J Dermatol 2007;157(5):907.

22. Pastar Z, Lipozencić J, Rados J, et al. Regressing seborrheic keratosis- clinically and dermoscopically mimicking a regressing melanoma. Acta Dermatovenerol Croat 2007;15(1):24–6.

23. Zaballos P, Martí E, Cuéllar F, et al. Dermoscopy of lichenoid regressing seborrheic keratosis. Arch Dermatol 2006;142(3):410.

24. Moscarella E, Zalaudek I, Pellacani G, et al. Lichenoid keratosis-like melanomas. J Am Acad Dermatol 2011;65(3):e85–7.

25. Bassoli S, Rabinovitz HS, Pellacani G, et al. Reflectance confocal microscopy criteria of lichen planus-like keratosis. J Eur Acad Dermatol Venereol 2012;26(5):578–90.

26. Longo C, Casari A, Pellacani G. Superficial spreading melanoma. In: Hofmann-Wellenhof R, Pellacani G, Malvehy J, et al, editors. Reflectance confocal microscopy for skin disease. 1st edition. Berlin, Heidel-berg (Germany): Springer-Verlag; 2012. p. 151–78.

27. Bories N, Dalle S, Debarbieux S, et al. Dermoscopy of fully regressive cutaneous melanoma. Br J Dermatol 2008;158(6):1224–9.

28. Seidenari S, Ferrari C, Borsari S, et al. Reticular grey-blue areas of regression as a dermoscopic marker of melanoma in situ. Br J Dermatol 2010;163(2):302–9.

29. Annessi G, Bono R, Sampogna F, et al. Sensitivity, specificity, and diagnostic accuracy of three dermoscopic algorithmic methods in the diagnosis of doubtful melanocytic lesions: the importance of light brown structureless areas in differentiating atypical melanocytic nevi from thin melanomas. J Am Acad Dermatol 2007;56(5):759–67.

30. Argenziano G, Kittler H, Ferrara G, et al. Slow-growing melanoma: a dermoscopy follow-up study. Br J Dermatol 2010;162(2):267–73.

31. Liu W, Dowling JP, Murray WK, et al. Rate of growth in melanomas: characteristics and associations of rapidly growing melanomas. Arch Dermatol 2006;142(12):1551–8.

32. Argenziano G, Longo C, Cameron A, et al. Blue-black rule: a simple dermoscopic clue to recognize pigmented nodular melanoma. Br J Dermatol 2011;165(6):1251–5.

33. Longo C, Farnetani F, Moscarella E, et al. Can noninvasive imaging tools potentially predict the risk of ulceration in invasive melanomas showing blue and black colors? Melanoma Res 2013;23(2):125–31.

34. Bono R, Giampetruzzi AR, Concolino F, et al. Dermoscopic patterns of cutaneous melanoma metastases. Melanoma Res 2004;14(5):367–73.

35. Julian Y, Argenziano G, Moscarella E, et al. Peripheral stellate telangiectasias: a clinical-dermoscopic clue for diagnosing cutaneous melanoma metastases. J Dermatol Case Rep 2012;6(4):102–4.

36. Samimi M, Perrinaud A, Naouri M, et al. High-resolution ultrasonography assists the differential diagnosis of blue naevi and cutaneous metastases of melanoma. Br J Dermatol 2010;163(3):550–6.

37. Ozdemir F, Kilinc I, Akalin T. Homogeneous blue pigmentation in dermatofibroma simulating a blue naevus. J Eur Acad Dermatol Venereol 2006;20(6):733–4.

38. Kilinc Karaarslan I, Gencoglan G, Akalin T, et al. Different dermoscopic faces of dermatofibromas. J Am Acad Dermatol 2007;57(3):401–6.

39. Zaballos P, Puig S, Llambrich A, et al. Dermoscopy of dermatofibromas: a prospective morphological study of 412 cases. Arch Dermatol 2008;144(1):75–83.

40. Casari A, Pellacani G, Seidenari S, et al. Pigmented nodular basal cell carcinomas in differential diagnosis with nodular melanomas: confocal microscopy as a reliable tool for in vivo histologic diagnosis. J Skin Cancer 2011;2011:406859.

41. Longo C, Farnetani F, Ciardo S, et al. Is confocal microscopy a valuable tool in diagnosing nodular lesions? A study on 140 cases. Br J Dermatol 2013;169(1):58–67. http://dx.doi.org/10.1111/bjd.12259.

42. Hu SC, Ke CL, Lee CH, et al. Dermoscopy of Kaposi's sarcoma: areas exhibiting the multicoloured 'rainbow pattern'. J Eur Acad Dermatol Venereol 2009;23(10):1128–32.

43. Cheng ST, Ke CL, Lee CH, et al. Rainbow pattern in Kaposi's sarcoma under polarized dermoscopy: a dermoscopic pathological study. Br J Dermatol 2009;160(4):801–9.

44. Zalaudek I, Gomez-Moyano E, Landi C, et al. Clinical, dermoscopic and histopathological features of spontaneous scalp or face and radiotherapy-induced angiosarcoma. Australas J Dermatol 2012 Sep 4. http://dx.doi.org/10.1111/j.1440-0960.2012.00943.x. [Epub ahead of print].

45. Scope A, Benvenuto-Andrade C, Agero AL, et al. Non-melanocytic lesions defying the two-step dermoscopy algorithm. Dermatol Surg 2006;32(11):1398–406.

46. Tsiklakis K, Patsakas A. Differential diagnosis of bluish and pigmented lesions of the oral mucosa. Hell Stomatol Chron 1989;33(2):113–20 [in Greek, Modern].

47. Grazzini M, Rossari S, Gori A, et al. Pigmented lesions in the oral mucosa: the ugly but good. QJM 2012;105(5):483.

Pink Lesions

Jason Giacomel, MBBS[a],*, Iris Zalaudek, MD[b,c]

KEYWORDS

- Pink lesions • Non-pigmented skin tumors • Amelanotic/hypomelanotic melanoma
- Actinic keratosis • Basal cell carcinoma • Squamous cell carcinoma • Dermoscopy
- Dermatoscopy

KEY POINTS

- Dermoscopy is a valuable tool for the diagnosis of pink or nonpigmented skin lesions. Patient history and clinical examination, however, remain fundamental in helping to reach a correct diagnosis for a given lesion and represent the first step in deciding whether a particular lesion is tumoral (and possibly malignant) or whether it is part of an inflammatory or infectious process.
- Pink lesions lack pigment or are only partially pigmented. Therefore, the dermoscopic diagnosis of a given pink lesion relies on evaluation of the blood vessel types and patterns observed within it as well as on additional dermoscopic criteria, such as ulceration or scale. A 3-step algorithm has been formulated to assist in this regard.
- Benign pink lesions are typified dermoscopically by symmetry of color and pattern. Vessels seen on dermoscopy are usually of a single (or predominant) morphology and occur in a fairly regular pattern.
- Malignant pink tumors typically have a history of incessant growth. They often present on dermoscopy with an atypical or polymorphous vascular pattern (defined as having 2 or more vessel morphologies), with the vessels arranged irregularly. Additional clues for malignancy can also frequently be detected by dermoscopy.
- Dermoscopy has the potential to improve the detection of malignant pink tumors while reducing the number of excisions of benign pink lesions, for the ultimate benefit of patients.

INTRODUCTION

Pink, or nonpigmented, cutaneous lesions are a large heterogeneous group comprising both tumoral and inflammatory and infectious conditions. Pink tumoral (ie, neoplastic) lesions are the focus of this article. Nonpigmented skin tumors can present as macules, plaques, papules, or nodules and may be benign or malignant (**Table 1**). Although clinical evaluation is fundamental for the diagnosis and subsequent management of these conditions, a naked eye diagnosis in many cases is inconclusive and dermoscopy has become a valuable ancillary diagnostic tool.

Pigmented structures within skin tumors provide important clues to improve the diagnosis of these lesions. Pink lesions lack or have scarce pigmentation, so in these cases the morphology and patterns of their blood vessels become essential in helping clinicians formulate a diagnosis (or differential diagnoses) and management plan.[1–4] The definitions and morphology of these various vessels are provided in **Table 2**. **Table 3** details

The authors declare no conflict of interest.

[a] Skin Spectrum Medical Services, 400 Canning Highway, Como, Perth, Western Australia 6152, Australia;
[b] Department of Dermatology, Medical University of Graz, Auenbruggerplatz 8, Graz 8036, Styria, Austria;
[c] Dermatology and Skin Cancer Unit, Arcispedale Santa Maria Nuova IRCCS, Viale Risorgimento 80, Reggio Emilia, Province of Reggio Emilia 42100, Italy
* Corresponding author.
E-mail address: jasongiacomel@gmail.com

Dermatol Clin 31 (2013) 649–678
http://dx.doi.org/10.1016/j.det.2013.06.005

derm.theclinics.com

Table 1
Examples of benign and malignant nonpigmented (pink) skin tumors, for which dermoscopic features have been described

	Benign	Malignant
Melanocytic	Compound and dermal nevi Red Clark nevi Spitz nevi	Primary AHM, including eczema-like melanoma CMMs
Nonmelanocytic	SH SK CCA Acantholytic dyskeratoma Angioma PG Dermatofibroma Benign adnexal lesions	BCC AKs SCCIS (Bowen disease) Invasive SCC Keratoacanthoma AS MCC Malignant adnexal lesions

some important architectural or distribution patterns of vessels seen in pink tumors.

As shown in **Table 4**, a 3-step algorithm can be used to help diagnose pink tumors.[3] Initially, patient history and the overall clinical presentation of the lesion (or lesions) should be assessed to determine whether the latter is part of an inflammatory or infectious disease (such as psoriasis, lichen planus, scabies, or molluscum contagiosum) or whether it is tumoral. Once it is decided that the lesion (or lesions) is tumoral, the first step of the algorithm can be performed. In this step, the morphology of the vessels within the tumor is assessed. The second step involves noting the architectural pattern or distribution (arrangement) of the vessels within the lesion. The third step is to observe any additional dermoscopic features, such as remnants of pigmentation, scale, or ulceration. After performing these 3 steps, a diagnosis (or differential diagnoses) is formulated and an appropriate management plan organized.

INSTRUMENTATION AND TECHNIQUE OF DERMOSCOPY

Regarding dermoscopic instrumentation, various handheld devices are available, which use either nonpolarized (eg, Heine Delta 20) or polarized light (eg, DermLite II Pro HR, DermLite III, or DermLite FOTO). Each modality has its strengths and limitations. For example, red color (eg, of erythema or vessels) and whitish streaks are enhanced visually with polarized instruments, whereas the white of milia cysts and blue and gray hues (eg, peppering seen in regression) are visualized better with nonpolarized light dermoscopy.[5]

Generally, tumoral vessels are visualized well with noncontact polarized dermoscopy. A scaly surface atop a lesion may, however, obstruct the

view of underlying vessels and make diagnosis difficult. In these situations, applying a fluid (eg, alcohol or immersion oil) onto the surface of the tumor helps reduce surface reflection from the scale, improving the visualization of underlying vascular features.[3] Conversely, if the presence of surface scale is being assessed (eg, in cases of actinic keratosis [AK] or squamous cell carcinoma in situ [SCCIS]), dry dermoscopy without immersion fluid should be performed (using either a polarized or nonpolarized instrument).

Immersion fluids are routinely used in polarized or nonpolarized contact dermoscopy. In contact dermoscopy, care must be taken to exert minimal downward pressure on the tumoral surface. Excessive pressure can diminish or completely conceal vascular features and lead to difficulty with dermoscopic diagnosis. Immersion fluids (eg, oil) can be used in this context, but ultrasound gel is of higher viscosity and generally achieves superior results, that is, it permits good optical contact between the surface of the tumor and the glass plate of the dermatoscope even when the latter is applied lightly to the tumoral surface.[3,6]

BENIGN PINK (NONPIGMENTED) LESIONS
Dermal Nevi

Summary

On dermoscopy, dermal nevi display a fairly regular arrangement of comma vessels. Remnants of pigmentation and hair may additionally be seen.

Dermal nevi are commonly occurring, benign melanocytic tumors that mostly develop in

Table 2
Definitions of the various morphologic types of vascular structures, as seen by dermoscopy

Vascular Morphology	Description
Dotted	Red-colored dots that are usually arranged fairly closely Highly specific for melanocytic lesions (if not surrounded by white haloes)
Comma	Vessels that are broad, curved, slightly unfocused, and may be scarcely branching; stereotypically present in dermal nevi
Glomerular	Tortuous vessels, frequently arranged in clusters and resembling the glomerular apparatus of the kidney; classically seen in Bowen disease
Crown	Barely branching vessels located around the periphery of the lesion; characteristic for SH
Hairpin	Vascular loops resembling a hairpin, which may be twisted in morphology; typically surrounded by a whitish halo when occurring in keratinizing tumors, such as invasive SCC and KA
Linear irregular	Linear vessels, which are usually irregular in width and shape
Milky-red globules	Unfocused (ie, not well-demarcated), milky red-colored circular or ovoid structures May contain vessels (eg, linear irregular or corkscrew); classically seen in invasive melanoma
Corkscrew	Helical vessels twisted along a central axis and resembling a corkscrew; can occur in both primary (ie, nodular or desmoplastic) melanoma and CMMs
Polymorphous (atypical) vascular pattern	A combination of 2 or more different types of vascular structures; a frequent combination is dotted and linear irregular vessels; classical pattern indicative of malignancy (eg, invasive SCC or melanoma)

(continued on next page)

Table 2
(continued)

Vascular Morphology	Description
Arborizing	Classical arborizing telangiectasias resemble tree branches in morphology. Stem vessels of large diameter branch irregularly into finer capillaries The vessels are bright red in color and sharply focused. Stereotypically seen in nBCC or nodulocystic BCC.
Short fine arborizing	A variation on the theme of arborizing vessels. These vessels are fine, red, focused, linear, and barely branching. They are irregularly shaped and generally finer and shorter than classical arborizing telangiectasias. Typical of sBCC.
Lacunes	Well-demarcated, red to red-purple–colored vascular structures, visible in hemangioma
Reddish pseudonetwork	A pattern on facial skin comprising erythema located between keratotic (and targetoid) hair follicles. These features form a peculiar strawberry-like pattern and are typically seen in facial AKs. Fine, linear-wavy vessels may also surround the follicles in some facial AK.
Red homogeneous color	In PG, usually associated with intersecting white rail lines. A yellowish collarette may also be seen (pictured). Pink-red homogeneous color can also be seen in BCC, where it may be associated with ulceration/s, whitish streaks and arborizing (or microarborizing) vessels.

adulthood. They can be categorized into 2 main subtypes, which differ clinically and dermoscopically: Miescher nevi (on the face) and Unna nevi (located particularly on the trunk, extremities, and neck). Clinically, both Miescher and Unna nevi are usually long-standing lesions without a history of recent change. Miescher nevi, however, are smooth and dome-shaped, with a semifirm consistency (which may at times mimic nodular basal cell carcinoma [nBCC]). Conversely, Unna nevi are soft and papillomatous.[7]

Both types of dermal nevi are characterized dermoscopically by coarse comma-shaped vessels, which are pinkish in color and slightly blurred. Comma vessels have a positive predictive value (PPV) for dermal nevi of 94%[8] and are a significant negative predictor for amelanotic/hypomelanotic melanoma (AHM).[9] The vessels of Miescher nevi are basically comma-shaped but can be somewhat variable in morphology (ie, varying in size and shape and frequently elongated) (**Fig. 1**A). These vessels differ from the sharply focused, bright red arborizing telangiectasias of nBCC, which at times may be mistaken clinically for dermal nevus on the face. Like Miescher nevi, the comma vessels of Unna nevi are pinkish and slightly unfocused, but they differ in having a more classically comma shape, with less variation in size or shape (see **Fig. 1**B).

Additional dermoscopic features of Miescher nevi include structureless tan-brown remnants of pigmentation and/or remnants of a pigmented pseudonetwork. Conversely, Unna nevi often display exophytic papillary structures, keratin-filled crypts, residual brown globules, and hairs.[3]

Nonpigmented (Red) Clark Nevi

Summary

Nonpigmented or red Clark nevi show a combination of dotted and comma vessels in a fairly regular arrangement, occurring on a pinkish-tan background. Comparison with other clinically similar lesions in patients should be performed to ensure comparable dermoscopic features of these nevi.

Table 3
Common vascular patterns in nonpigmented (pink) skin tumors, as seen dermoscopically

Vascular Pattern	Definition
Regular	Vessels that are arranged fairly regularly throughout lesion (eg, the arrangement of hairpin vessels in SK, comma vessels in dermal nevi, and dot vessels in Spitz nevus or thin AHM)
Irregular	Vessels distributed irregularly throughout tumor; for example, polymorphous vessels in invasive SCC or melanoma (pictured) or the irregular distribution of arborizing telangiectasias in BCC
Clustered	Pattern wherein vessels are arranged in clustered groups, classically referring to glomerular vessels in Bowen disease
Stringlike (or reticular)	Vessels arranged in lines, which may crisscross to form a peculiar reticular pattern; usually refers to the distribution of dotted and/or tortuous (ie, coiled or glomerular) vessels in CCA, but this pattern may also be seen in LCA
Radial	Vessels are distributed around the periphery of the tumor; stereotypical example, radial arrangement of hairpin vessels in KA (surrounding a central keratin mass)
Strawberry	A pattern seen in facial AK, comprising a reddish pseudonetwork around hair follicles; fine, linear-wavy vessels may also surround the follicles; hair follicle openings often filled with yellowish keratotic plugs and surrounded by a white halo

Nonpigmented or red Clark (atypical) nevi usually present as pink to pinkish-tan lesions of diameter greater than 5 mm in fair-skinned white patients (ie, skin phototype I or II). Red nevi are often multiple but may present as solitary lesions (ie, with or without the presence of other, pigmented nevi).[10] Red nevi may present as macules, papules, or maculopapular tumors and can be difficult at times to distinguish clinically from AHM, particularly when presenting as ugly duckling lesions. Such ugly duckling lesions include solitary or relatively large red nevi.

On dermoscopy, red Clark nevi typically show dotted and comma vessels, arranged fairly regularly throughout the lesions and occurring on a pinkish-tan background (**Fig. 2**). The tan background may have a reticular or homogeneous appearance. These features generally contrast with nonpigmented Spitz nevi, which are usually solitary and fast growing and typically display a more dense arrangement of dot vessels on a pink-to-red background. In addition, reticular depigmentation, whitish striae, and remnants of pigmentation (eg, black dots, brown globules, and blue color) may additionally be seen in Spitz nevi. Dermoscopic examination of red nevi is also helpful in differentiating these tumors from AHM. Like Spitz nevi, AHM can present as solitary, fast-growing lesions and can exhibit a fairly dense arrangement of dot vessels on a pink-to-red background. In AHM, reticular depigmentation, whitish striae, remnants of pigmentation (eg, black dots, brown globules, blue color, and other melanoma-specific features), atypical

Table 4
Three-step algorithm for the diagnosis of nonpigmented (pink) skin tumors

1st Step: Vessel Morpholoy	2nd Step: Vessel Arrangement	3rd Step: Additional Features	Diagnosis	Management
Arborizing (branching)	Large-stem vessels, branching over lesion irregularly	Blue-gray ovoid nests and/or globules	nBCC or nodulocystic BCC	Biopsy
	Fine microarborizing vessels, scattered irregularly	Multiple erosions; brown-gray leaflike and/or spoke-wheel areas, hublike pigmentation	sBCC	Biopsy
Comma	Regular	Residual brown globules (or pseudonetwork on face), hairs	Congenital melanocytic nevus, compound or dermal nevus	No action
Dotted + comma	Regular	Pinkish-tan background pigmentation	Red Clark nevus	Follow up if similar to other nevi. Excise if solitary lesion.
Dotted	Regular	Reticular depigmentation; whitish striae; remnants of pigmentation (eg, brown globules, black dots, blue color)	Spitz nevus or thin AHM	Excision
Dotted	Stringlike (or reticular)	White halo or whitish background	CCA (or LCA)	No action
Dotted + glomerular	Clustered	Surface scale, white halo around vessels.	Bowen disease (SCCIS)	Biopsy
Dotted	Usually regular (central position)	Central whitish patch; delicate peripheral pigment network	DF	No action
Hairpin	Regular	Milia-like cysts; crypts; white halo around vessels	SK	No action
	Radial or irregular (±polymorphous vessels)	White haloes and/or whitish background; central scale or keratin mass; ulceration/blood crusts; targetoid follicles; whitish pearls	SCC or KA	Excision

Linear irregular	Irregular	Red homogeneous areas; pigment remnants (including blue-black color); ±hairpin vessels	Nodular AHM (or PG)	Excision
Linear irregular + dotted	Irregular	Red homogeneous areas; intersecting white rail lines; white collarette; ulceration	PG (or nodular AHM)	Excision
	Central or irregular	Whitish striae; remnants of pink to brown-gray pigmentation	Thin or intermediate-thickness AHM	Excision
Linear irregular + hairpin, corkscrew or arborizing	Central or irregular	Multiple colors; milky red globules or areas	Thick AHM or melanoma metastases	Excision
Red homogeneous areas	Throughout lesion	Intersecting white rail lines; white collarette; ulceration; ±linear irregular, dotted, hairpin vessels.	PG (or nodular AHM)	Excision
Crown	Radial	Central white to yellow lobular structures; ostia	SH	No action
Reddish pseudonetwork (face)	Confluent erythema located around hair follicles	Surface scale; targetoid follicles; linear-wavy vessels around follicles	AK	Topical therapy
Well-demarcated reddish lacunes	Regular	Whitish septae between lacunes	Angioma	No action

vessels (eg, hairpin and linear irregular vessels) and ulceration may be additional clues for the diagnosis.

In patients presenting with multiple red Clark nevi, dermoscopic comparison of all the lesions should be performed to ensure comparable dermoscopic features of these nevi. To avoid missing a possible AHM, dermoscopic ugly duckling red Clark nevi–like tumors (ie, dermoscopically unlike the other red nevi on a given patient), solitary red tumors, lesions with a history of recent change, or lesions showing melanoma specific criteria should be excised.[3]

Spitz Nevi

Summary

On dermoscopy, flat nonpigmented Spitz nevi display regularly distributed dotted vessels on a pink to red background. Other features include reticular depigmentation, whitish striae, and pigment remnants.

Nonpigmented atypical or nodular Spitz tumors often show a polymorphous vascular pattern on dermoscopy.

Nonpigmented or hypopigmented Spitz lesions can closely mimic melanoma clinically and dermoscopically.

Spitz lesions were originally described in 1948 as juvenile melanomas by the pathologist, Sophie Spitz.[11] Spitz believed that these lesions were childhood melanomas with a largely innocuous course (ie, rarely metastasizing, unlike adult melanomas).[12] Of Spitz' original 13 cases, at least 1 proved to be an actual malignancy (as evidenced by metastases and death), with the remainder having a benign biologic course.

Spitz lesions nowadays are generally considered benign entities (ie, nevi) that can mimic malignant melanoma both clinically and histopathologically. Recently, however, some investigators have challenged this mainstream view and echoed Spitz' original conclusions, hypothesizing that Spitz tumors may actually be a low-grade cutaneous malignancy with a high tendency to self-limitation and involution.[13]

Spitz nevi classically present as fast-growing, smooth, dome-shaped papules or nodules. They are frequently pink or reddish in color but also commonly pigmented. They occur more commonly in children, especially on facial sites.[14] As discussed previously, Spitz nevi assume significance because they are at times difficult to distinguish from melanoma on clinical grounds. In this setting,

dermoscopy can be of assistance to clarify the diagnosis or at least raise a red flag for excision.

In flat nonpigmented Spitz nevi, dermoscopy stereotypically reveals dotted vessels that appear fairly closely aligned in a regular arrangement. The vessels lack whitish haloes and typically occur on a pink to red (milky red) background (**Fig. 3**A). Dot vessels lacking white haloes are highly predictive for melanocytic skin tumors (PPV of 90%) and are particularly prevalent in Spitz nevi.[8] Other dermoscopic features of flat Spitz nevi include reticular depigmentation (or negative network), a white network-like structure formed by intersecting white lines that surround the abovementioned dot vessels.[15] White striae (chrysalis structures) can also be seen in some lesions and consist of shiny white orthogonal lines visible under polarized light dermoscopy.[16] In Spitz nevi having pigment remnants, black dots, brown globules, bluish areas, and regions of pigmented network or streaks (ie, a residual starburst pattern) may also be apparent.[15]

Nonpigmented atypical and nodular Spitz tumors typically display a polymorphous vascular pattern, with linear irregular vessels, coiled vessels, and/or milky red or pink globules.[3] If partially pigmented, pigment remnants, such as homogeneous bluish areas and brown globules, may be visualized (see **Fig. 3**B).

Because AHM, Spitz nevi, and atypical Spitz tumors can show similar dermoscopic features, excision should be performed for all nonpigmented spitzoid-looking lesions in adult patients. In children (ie, up to the age of 12 years), a more conservative approach is currently used when dealing with nonpigmented Spitz lesions exhibiting a stereotypical appearance.[3,17] Contrarily, excision should be performed for large (>1 cm), nodular, rapidly changing, ulcerated, or otherwise atypical Spitz tumors appearing in childhood.

Sebaceous Hyperplasia

Summary

Sebaceous hyperplasia (SH) is typified dermoscopically by crown vessels around the periphery of the lesion, with a white polylobular center.

SH is a benign, nonpigmented neoplasm frequently presenting as multiple papules on the forehead, nose, and cheeks of middle-aged to elderly patients. Lesions are smooth, have a yellowish hue, and may have a central dell visible to the naked eye.[18] Although a diagnosis is reliably made in many instances on clinical grounds alone, SH

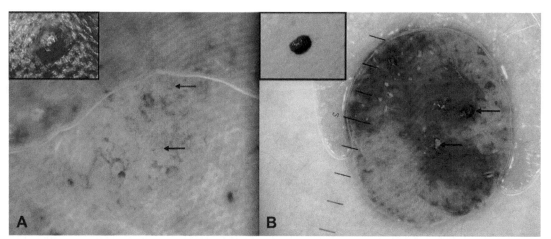

Fig. 1. (*A*) Clinical (*inset*) and dermoscopic views of a long-standing dermal (Miescher) nevus on the upper cutaneous lip of a 61-year-old woman. Clinically, the lesion had a diameter of 4 mm, was semifirm, smooth, and dome-shaped. On polarized contact dermoscopy, slightly blurred, pinkish comma-shaped vessels can be discerned (*arrows*), along with remnants of a tan pseudonetwork. Although Miescher nevi on the face may clinically mimic nBCC, dermoscopy usually facilitates a ready differentiation between the sharply focused, bright red arborizing vessels of BCC and the slightly blurred, pinkish comma vessels of dermal nevi. (*B*) Clinical (*inset*) and dermoscopic images of a long-standing dermal (Unna) nevus, located on the abdomen of a 42-year-old woman. Clinically, the lesion was soft and papillomatous. Nonpolarized contact dermoscopy exhibits exophytic papillary structures, keratin-filled crypts (*arrows*), and a fairly regular arrangement of comma vessels. A fairly homogeneous, tan-colored background was also apparent. The patient requested removal of the lesion due to it catching on clothing. Histopathologic examination revealed a dermal nevus.

may at times be difficult to distinguish from other conditions, such as basal cell carcinoma (BCC).

Dermoscopy aids in the correct identification of SH by revealing crown (wreathlike) vessels, seen as pinkish, elongated, slightly blurred, and scarcely branching telangiectasias that surround the tumor (ie, in a radial arrangement). These vessels do not usually cross over the central parts of the lesion. The latter is in contrast to the arborizing telangiectasias of nBCC, which are typically bright red in color, sharply focused, and often pass over the center of the lesion. Multiple white to yellow, aggregated, homogeneous globular areas are also characteristically seen, which correspond histopathologically to the enlarged sebaceous lobules of SH. Moreover, a small centrally located yellowish crater (or craters) may be present on dermoscopy, which correlates with the dilated ostium (or ostia) of the infundibulum of the sebaceous glands (**Fig. 4A**).[4,6,19–22]

Seborrheic Keratosis

Summary

Nonpigmented seborrheic keratoses (SKs) display regularly distributed hairpin vessels, surrounded by a white halo. In addition, multiple milia cysts and crypts are often seen.

SKs are common benign acanthomas that commonly present as rough, well-demarcated, skin-colored to brown to black papules and plaques in adult patients. They are particularly prevalent on the trunk, face, and extremities and stereotypically have a stuck-on appearance. When nonpigmented, SK may clinically resemble other lesions, such as verruca, squamous cell carcinoma (SCC), or even AHM.[23]

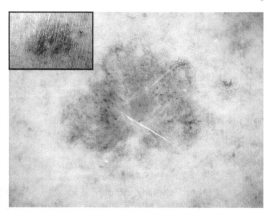

Fig. 2. Red Clark nevus. Clinical view of an 8 × 6 mm soft, smooth, pinkish plaque on the back of a 43-year-old Australian man with skin phototype I/II and a history of BCC (*inset*). The tumor was one of many similar pink lesions on the trunk. Polarized noncontact dermoscopy reveals dotted and comma vessels in a fairly regular arrangement, occurring on a pinkish-tan background.

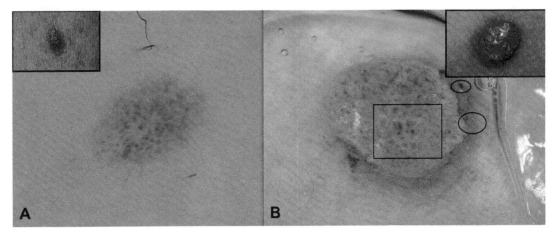

Fig. 3. (A) Clinical (*inset*) and dermoscopic images of a 4 × 3 mm pinkish plaque, located on the dorsum of the foot of a 21-year-old woman. Polarized contact dermoscopy reveals whitish reticular depigmentation (negative network), dotted and coiled vessels. The vessels lack white haloes and are fairly closely and regularly arranged. Tan pigmentation is seen peripherally. Histopathologic examination confirmed the diagnosis of Spitz nevus. (B) Clinical (*inset*) and dermoscopic photographs of a 1-cm pinkish, verrucous nodule, located on the knee of a 4-year-old boy. Polarized contact dermoscopy demonstrates whitish surface scale, exophytic papillary structures, and a polymorphous vascular pattern. The latter comprises a combination of dotted, coiled, hairpin, linear irregular, and a few branching vessels. The vessels lack whitish haloes and occur on a pinkish-white background. Numerous milky pink globules (*rectangle*) and a few brown dots and globules (*ovals*) are also present. Histopathologic examination confirmed the diagnosis of Spitz nevus.

Dermoscopy assists in improving the accuracy of diagnosis of nonpigmented SK by revealing hairpin vessels (capillary loops) of fairly monomorphous morphology, arranged in a regular pattern. Hairpin vessels may occur in several different types of skin tumors but, when surrounded by white haloes, are suggestive of keratinizing lesions. Furthermore, hairpin vessels are particularly characteristic of SK, having a PPV for SK of 70%, compared with only approximately 13% for (invasive) SCC.[8] In further contrast to SK, hairpin vessels in invasive SCC are usually elongated and irregular in morphology and occur in an irregular distribution.[4]

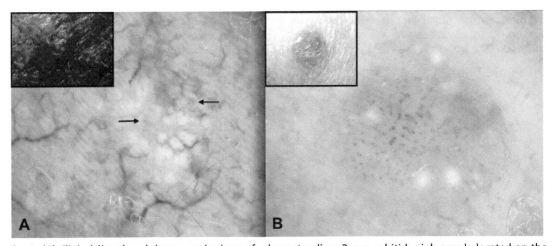

Fig. 4. (A) Clinical (*inset*) and dermoscopic views of a long-standing, 3-mm, whitish-pink papule located on the forehead of a 79-year-old man with skin phototype II. Polarized contact dermoscopy highlights the aggregated whitish globular structures, yellowish ostia (ie, openings of the infundibula) (*arrows*), and crown vessels at the periphery. The latter are scarcely branching and pass toward the center of the lesion but do not cross over it. The crown vessels of SH contrast with arborizing vessels of nBCC, which are bright red, sharply focused, and often course over the central parts of the tumor. (B) Clinical (*inset*) and dermoscopic views of a 4–5 mm, slightly raised, lightly pigmented plaque, located on the back of a 77-year-old woman (with skin phototype I/II). Nonpolarized contact dermoscopy supports the diagnosis of SK by revealing multiple large whitish milia cysts and a fairly regular arrangement of fine hairpin vessels.

Additional dermoscopic features of SK include a well-demarcated edge, a brainlike appearance with gyri and sulci (ridges and fissures), multiple whitish milia cysts, and pseudocomedone openings (crypts) (see **Fig. 4**B).[24]

Irritated or traumatized SK may at times pose a diagnostic and management dilemma, because they can clinically simulate malignant conditions, such as melanoma or SCC. This is especially the case if a history of recent trauma is not recalled by a patient. On dermoscopy, the hairpin vessels may be enlarged or elongated and appear somewhat irregular in morphology. Signs of recent trauma, namely blood crusts and/or erythema (inflammation), are also typically seen. Such features can make a dermoscopic diagnosis challenging. Remnant areas showing specific features of SK (ie, well-demarcated edge, multiple large milia cysts, crypts, fissures and ridges), however, may be present, which suggest the correct diagnosis of traumatized SK. Close clinical follow-up typically reveals that the features of trauma subside within a few weeks. In doubtful cases, however, where a diagnosis of malignancy cannot be ruled out, biopsy at the outset is recommended.

Benign pink lichenoid keratosis (LK) is considered a variant of SK and presents as a scaly or smooth, pinkish macule, plaque, or papule that may be pruritic. The lesion is especially prevalent on the trunk and extremities of middle-aged to elderly patients and can clinically mimic several lesions, such as psoriasis, AK, SCCIS, BCC, and even amelanotic melanoma (AM). Dermoscopically, surface scale may be highlighted and dotted or coiled and/or telangiectatic vessels may be seen, the vessels typically arranged in a fairly regular pattern (**Fig. 5**). In lesions with pigment remnants, tan-gray blotches may be present. Because the dermoscopic features of pink LK can overlap with nonpigmented malignant tumors, however, such as early SCCIS, BCC, or AHM, biopsy is recommended.

Clear Cell Acanthoma (and Large Cell Acanthoma)

Summary

Clear cell acanthoma (CCA) reveals dotted and/or coiled vessels in a stringlike arrangement. A scaly surface and collarette may also be seen. Stringlike vessels may also occur in large cell acanthoma (LCA).

CCA, also called Degos or pale cell acanthoma, is an uncommon benign epithelial tumor that usually presents clinically as a solitary, pink to red plaque,

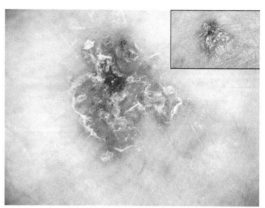

Fig. 5. Clinical (inset) and dermoscopic images of a scaly, reddish macule located on the thigh of a 63-year-old woman, who had a history of psoriasis. The lesion had been pruritic. On polarized noncontact dermoscopy, diffuse whitish scale is seen in conjunction with a fairly regular array of dotted and coiled vessels. The dermoscopic differential diagnoses included psoriasis, pink LK, and early SCCIS. Histopathologic examination confirmed the diagnosis of benign LK.

papule, or nodule in middle-aged or elderly patients. Additionally, a scaly surface is sometimes present and a scaly collarette may be visible around the edge of the lesion. Many other benign and malignant nonpigmented skin lesions may resemble CCA clinically, including SK, BCC, SCC, and AM.[23,25,26]

Dermoscopy assists in the identification of CCA by showing a striking pattern of dot and/or coiled vessels arranged in a linear, stringlike distribution (**Fig. 6**A). At times, these linear patterns may assume a reticular arrangement. In addition, a whitish scaly surface may be highlighted by dry dermoscopy (ie, without immersion fluid) as well as a translucent to whitish peripheral scaly collarette.[20,27–29] In contrast to the dot vessels seen in melanocytic lesions (including melanoma), the vessels in CCA are surrounded by whitish haloes or occur on a whitish background, as is customary for keratinizing tumors. Furthermore, the stringlike pattern of CCA contrasts with the typically regular arrangement of dot vessels in melanocytic skin lesions. In thicker variants of CCA, the vessels may appear coiled (or even glomerular), but they essentially retain their typical stringlike arrangement.[4]

LCA is another rare, benign acanthoma that can at times present as a (scaly) pink papule or plaque on the trunk or extremities of middle-aged to elderly patients. Differential diagnoses may include SK, SCCIS (Bowen disease), BCC, and AM.[30] Although considered highly specific for CCA, it is the experience of the authors that a

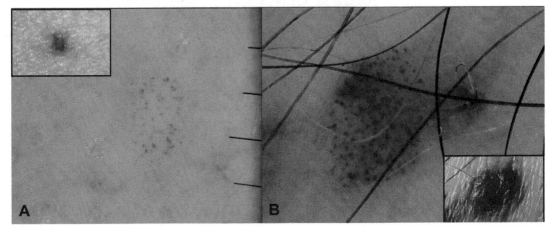

Fig. 6. (*A*) Clinical (*inset*) and dermoscopic images of a 2–3 mm smooth, solitary pink papule, located on the chest of a 57-year-old Australian man. Nonpolarized contact dermoscopy revealed a string of pearls vascular pattern (ie, dotted and coiled vessels arranged in a linear fashion) on a whitish background. Histopathologic examination confirmed the diagnosis of CCA. (*B*) Clinical (*inset*) and dermoscopic photographs of a 4-mm pink papule situated on the right lower back of a 61-year-old man. Polarized contact dermoscopy disclosed dotted and coiled vessels in linear arrays, reminiscent of CCA. The lesion was biopsied and histopathologic examination revealed a LCA. (Note: an incidental focus of acute suppurative folliculitis is present at the right side of the dermoscopic image.)

stringlike (or reticular) arrangement of dotted and coiled vessels may also be seen in LCA (see **Fig. 6B**). Further studies on the dermoscopic features of LCA, however, are needed.

Acantholytic Dyskeratotic Acanthoma (Acantholytic Dyskeratoma)

Summary

Brown colored, scaly, starlike shapes can occur in acantholytic dyskeratoma, surrounded by a white to pink to tan background. Very fine and regular vessels may also be visible.

Acantholytic dyskeratotic acanthoma (acantholytic dyskeratoma) is a benign lesion typically presenting as a smooth to scaly-topped papular, pinkish tumor on the trunk of middle-aged to elderly patients. The lesion usually presents as a solitary tumor less than 1 cm in diameter and clinical differential diagnoses may include SK, verruca, nevus, BCC, AK, SCCIS, and invasive SCC.[31]

On dermoscopy, acantholytic dyskeratoma may reveal tan to darker brown–colored, starlike (stellate) shapes consisting of surface scale and/or superficial indentations (microfissures). These features are hardly visible with the unaided eye. Tan-brown areas can appear in some lesions as broken-up and branching lines and/or discrete rounded areas. Similar brown stellate

shapes can be seen in papules of transient acantholytic dermatosis (Grover disease), another condition displaying acantholytic dyskeratosis on histopathology.[32,33]

In addition, the tan-brown superficial scaly star-like areas typically have whitish edges and occur on a white to pink to tan background (**Fig. 7**). Very faint and fine dotted hairpin and linear vessels may also be visible, having a regular morphology and whitish haloes, the latter feature typically seen in keratinizing tumors.[6] The tan-brownish keratotic areas of acantholytic dyskeratoma may at times be relatively large and round or oval in shape, reminiscent dermoscopically of the central yellowish-brown keratotic plugs or (giant) pseudocomedones seen in Darier disease.[34]

Angioma

Summary

Angiomas are characterized dermoscopically by multiple well-demarcated reddish or reddish-purple lacunae.

Angiomas (hemangiomas or cherry angiomas) are benign vascular lesions that usually present clinically as soft, pink, red, purple, or reddish-black papules or nodules on the trunk and extremities of adult patients. Although the clinical diagnosis is usually straightforward, at times angioma may mimic other lesions, such as AM.[35]

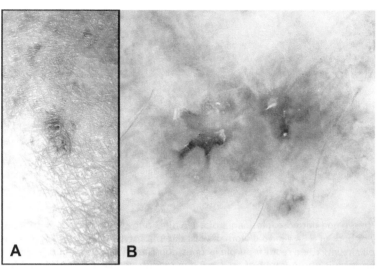

Fig. 7. (*A*) Clinical photograph of a solitary 4–5 mm pink papule on the back of a 73-year-old Australian man with chronically sun-damaged skin (skin phototype I/II). (*B*) On noncontact polarized light dermoscopy, tan-colored starlike shapes and rounded areas are seen. The tan-colored areas appear scaly, have whitish edges, and occur on a pinkish-tan background. Histopathologic examination revealed features of acantholytic dyskeratosis. The clinical, dermoscopic and histopathologic findings were consistent with the diagnosis of acantholytic dyskeratotic acanthoma. (*From* Giacomel J, Zalaudek I, Argenziano G. Dermatoscopy of Grover's disease and solitary acantholytic dyskeratoma shows a brown, star-like pattern. Australas J Dermatol 2012;53:315–6. In reproducing this figure the author acknowledges the Australasian Journal of Dermatology, the Australasian College of Dermatologists and Blackwell Publishing.)

On dermoscopy, angiomas reveal multiple well-circumscribed red, reddish-blue/purple, or reddish-black lacunes (**Fig. 8**A). On histopathology, these reddish lacunes correspond to dilated vessels in the upper dermis. Thrombosed angiomas contain thrombus within the vessels of the lesion and are suggested dermoscopically by a reddish-black color.[36,37]

Pyogenic Granuloma

Summary

Red homogeneous areas surrounded by a white collarette and intersected by white lines are suggestive of pyogenic granuloma (PG), but an important differential diagnosis is nodular AHM.

PG (lobular hemangioma) characteristically presents as a fast-growing, reddish, or reddish-black papule or nodule and as such can clinically mimic nodular amelanotic or hypomelanotic melanoma (ie, both are elevated, firm, and growing [EFG-positive] lesions; discussed later).[4,35,38,39]

In a 2006 study of 13 cases of PG, Zaballos and colleagues[38] found that reddish homogeneous areas (92%), a white collarette (85%), white rail lines that intersect the lesion (31%), and ulceration (46%) were the most frequent dermoscopic signs of PG (see **Fig. 8**B). They

concluded, however, that no single criterion allows exclusion of nodular AHM with a high degree of confidence.

In a later work, Zaballos and colleagues[39] examined 122 histopathologically proved cases of PG and found the dermoscopic pattern comprising reddish homogeneous areas, white collarette, and white rail lines showed the highest sensitivity (22.1%) and a specificity of 100% for the diagnosis of PGs. The investigators again concluded that although dermoscopy is useful for assisting in the diagnosis of PG, histopathologic confirmation is recommended for all cases, to exclude the possibility of nodular AHM (**Fig. 9**). This was especially the case if vessels were visible within the lesion dermoscopically.[39]

Dermatofibroma

Summary

Dermatofibroma (DF) classically exhibits a delicate peripheral pigment network on dermoscopy, which surrounds a central whitish, scarlike area. In addition, dotted vessels are typically seen within the central area.

DFs (histiocytomas) are common, benign fibrous skin lesions that may arise at a site of minor injury,

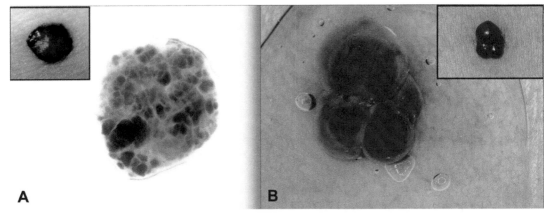

Fig. 8. (*A*) Clinical (*inset*) and dermoscopic images of a 4–5 mm, long-standing, smooth, soft, reddish-black papule located on the lower back of a 74-year-old woman with skin phototype II. Polarized contact dermoscopy reveals multiple, small, well-circumscribed reddish-purple lacunes, consistent with the diagnosis of hemangioma. (*B*) Clinical (*inset*) and dermoscopic photographs of an 8 × 6 mm reddish nodule, located on the chest of a 21-year-old woman. A botryoid (grapelike) appearance is apparent clinically. Nonpolarized contact dermoscopy demonstrates a few large, fairly homogeneous reddish areas, separated by whitish rail lines. Histopathologic examination confirmed the diagnosis of PG (lobular hemangioma).

such as an insect bite. Clinically, DFs commonly present as partially pigmented lesions, with the diagnosis suggested by firmness on palpation (being button hard) and a positive dimpling sign. On occasion, however, DFs may be difficult to distinguish from other lesions, such as a melanocytic nevus or even melanoma.[40,41]

Dermoscopy assists in the diagnosis of DF by typically revealing a delicate peripheral pigment network surrounding a central whitish, scarlike area. Sometimes the peripheral network is incomplete, making the diagnosis somewhat challenging. Dotted vessels are frequently seen within the central scarlike area of DF (**Fig. 10**).[42] The scarlike areas generally have a pinkish hue when viewed using noncontact polarized light dermoscopy (or polarized dermoscopy using a faceplate but with minimal downward pressure applied to the surface of the lesion).[43] Although these characteristics describe the stereotypical dermoscopic features of DF, there are cases where the dermoscopic diagnosis is unclear. In such situations, there may be a mismatch between clinical and dermoscopic characteristics and biopsy is recommended.[40,41]

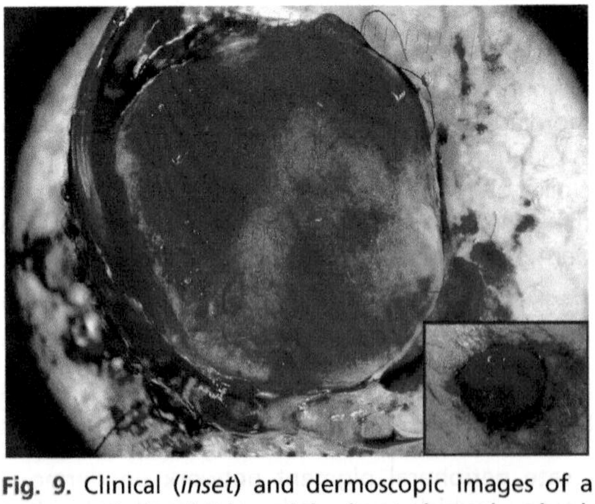

MALIGNANT PINK (NONPIGMENTED) SKIN LESIONS
Amelanotic and Hypomelanotic Melanoma

Summary

Amelanotic and hypomelanotic melanoma frequently displays dot vessels or atypical vessels (eg, a combination of dot and irregular vessels) on a pinkish background, with or without remnants of pigmentation.

Fig. 9. Clinical (*inset*) and dermoscopic images of a 2-cm, eroded reddish nodule, located on the cheek of an 80-year-old man. Polarized contact dermoscopy reveals abundant linear irregular vessels (of variable caliber and length) and arborizing vessels on a milky pink to red background. Histopathologic examination confirmed the diagnosis of invasive (nodular) melanoma (Breslow thickness 4 mm).

Nonpigmented (pink) melanoma can be divided into 2 main groups, AM and hypopigmented melanoma. True AM lacks pigmentation macroscopically and on dermoscopy. In this subtype, dot vessels or an atypical vascular pattern (especially dotted plus linear irregular vessels), a milky pink-red background color, whitish streaks, and ulceration are key features to search for

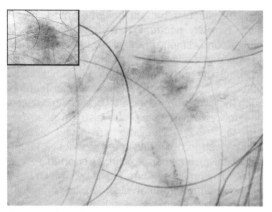

Fig. 10. Clinical view of a 5–6 mm flat, solitary, pinkish-tan lesion located on the calf of a 60-year-old man with skin phototype I and a history of hypomelanotic melanoma (*inset*). It was button hard on palpation and had a positive dimpling sign. Polarized contact dermoscopy reveals remnants of a delicate peripheral pigment network surrounding a central whitish, scarlike area. In addition, dot vessels are visible centrally. The diagnosis of dermatofibroma was confirmed by histopathologic evaluation.

dermoscopically.[3,9,44] Hypopigmented melanoma can be further divided into the 2 following subtypes: partially pigmented melanoma, generally defined as those melanomas having pigmentation (eg, residual pigment network or bluish areas) in up to 25% to 30% of the surface area of the tumor (**Fig. 11A**), and light-colored melanoma,

which has a light tan/brown pigmentation visible throughout the lesion, usually imparting a pinkish-tan background hue dermoscopically.[3,45]

Although historical and clinical information is important in helping to make the correct diagnosis of AHM, such information is often incomplete. Moreover, AHM is a great clinical masquerader of other lesions, such as BCC, SK, PG, and pink melanocytic nevi.[46] Important clinical clues for AHM include any pink lesion that has a history of progressive growth, including any EFG-positive tumor.[47,48] Although not specific for melanoma, the EFG rule has a potentially high sensitivity for the detection of aggressive malignancies, including Merkel cell carcinoma (MCC) and invasive SCC.[49] Despite these clinical clues, a naked eye diagnosis of AHM is frequently challenging. In this context, dermoscopy may provide additional information that can raise a red flag for clinically nonsuspicious AHM, which prompts biopsy or excision.

On dermoscopy, AHM frequently displays dot vessels or atypical vessels (eg, a combination of dot and linear irregular vessels) on a pinkish (milky pink) or pinkish-tan background, with or without remnants of pigmentation. The latter includes tan-brown homogeneous areas, multiple blue-gray dots, irregular brown dots or globules, regions of residual (atypical/broadened) pigment network, and homogeneous bluish or blue-white areas.[9,44]

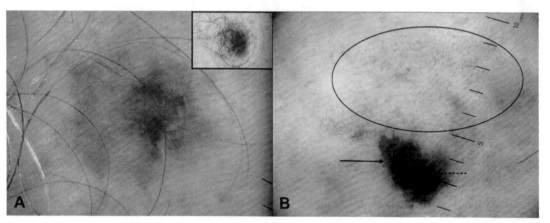

Fig. 11. (*A*) Clinical view of a solitary, slightly raised, pinkish-tan lesion on the thigh of a 60-year-old man with skin phototype I (*inset*). On polarized, contact dermoscopy, the predominant vascular feature is dot vessels without white haloes, suggesting a probable melanocytic lesion. A few hairpin vessels are also present. In addition, whitish striae are visible and there is homogeneous tan pigmentation with residual areas of pigment network. Histopathologic evaluation of the excised specimen revealed an invasive melanoma (Breslow thickness 0.6 mm), arising in association with a dysplastic compound nevus. (*B*) Nonpolarized, contact dermoscopic image of a thin, invasive hypomelanotic melanoma. The lesion presented as a solitary, flat pinkish tumor on the lower leg of a 76-year-old man with skin phototype II. Numerous dotted and coiled vessels are seen in the upper part of the lesion (*oval*). In addition, remnants of an atypical (broadened) pigment network can be seen at the inferior aspect of the lesion (*solid arrow*), adjacent to an area of homogeneous brown pigmentation (*dotted arrow*). Histopathologic examination of the excised specimen revealed an invasive melanoma (Breslow thickness 0.5 mm).

Early cases of AHM (ie, Breslow thickness <1 mm) are flat or slightly raised clinically and tend to show dot vessels, often arranged in a fairly regular pattern and not surrounded by whitish haloes.[3,8,9,45] As such, these lesions may closely simulate nonpigmented Spitz nevi on surface microscopy. In addition, pigment remnants may be present and on the lower leg, coiled vessels may be seen (see **Fig. 11B**).

In intermediate-thickness AHM (ie, 1–2 mm tumor thickness), the tumor may be raised clinically and frequently reveals dotted and linear irregular vessels on dermoscopy (**Fig. 12A**). The latter are typically devoid of white haloes and have been reported to have a PPV for melanoma of approximately 68%.[8] Hairpin vessels may also be seen. These vessel types usually occur in an irregular arrangement within the lesion. Additional dermoscopic features include pigment remnants (eg, irregular brown dots/globules, multiple blue-gray dots, and blue-white veil), whitish streaks (chrysalis structures), irregular depigmentation, and a milky pink-reddish background color.[9] As for thin tumors, the surface microscopy findings for intermediate-thickness AHM can overlap with Spitz nevus, and it is recommended that all such lesions be removed for histopathologic evaluation.[3]

In thick (ie, elevated/nodular and palpable) lesions with greater than 2-mm thickness, the atypical vascular pattern becomes more prominent, typically occurring on a milky pink to red background. Linear irregular and hairpin vessels are generally wider, longer, and more variable in morphology and are distributed in an irregular pattern within the tumor. Other vascular features, such as corkscrew vessels, branching vessels, and milky red globules, can also be seen (see **Fig. 9**).[3,9,45,50,51] The latter are round or ovoid and pinkish in color and are a distinctive feature of (invasive) melanoma, with a reported PPV of 78%.[8] They may be surrounded by whitish striae and contain a central atypical (eg, linear irregular or corkscrew) vessel or vessels.

Studies differ regarding their inclusion of melanoma with significant regression as a subtype of AHM. These tumors, however, can present clinically and dermoscopically as nonpigmented or partly pigmented lesions owing to extensive areas of whitish depigmentation. Other dermoscopic features, such as blue-gray dots (peppering), whitish streaks or bands (under polarized light), dotted vessels, and linear irregular vessels, may be present as further clues for the diagnosis of these tumors.[45,52,53]

Eczematous, or eczema-like, melanoma is a rare variant of AHM, which usually presents as a nonpigmented, scaly, ill-defined patch or plaque.[54,55] It can mimic several inflammatory or

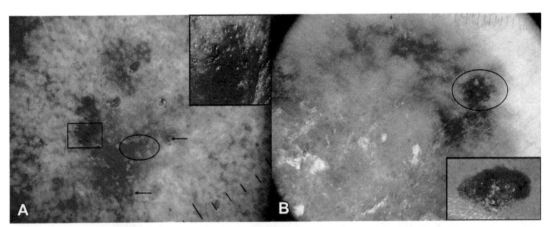

Fig. 12. (*A*) Clinical (*inset*) and dermoscopic photographs of an invasive hypomelanotic lentigo maligna melanoma located on the cheek of a 59-year-old man with skin phototype I/II. The lesion was mostly flat but was slightly raised in the eroded pinkish area located in the inferior part of the image. Polarized contact dermoscopy reveals a marked asymmetry of colors and structures. There are remnants of pigmentation (peripherally), surrounding a central pinkish-red homogeneous area. The pigmentation comprises asymmetric pigmented follicular openings (*arrows*) and brown rhomboidal structures (*rectangle*). In the central-inferior pinkish area dot vessels are present (*oval*) along with linear-irregular vessels in the vicinity of the ulcerated area. Whitish striae are also seen. Histopathologic evaluation of the excised specimen revealed an invasive melanoma (ie, level 4, Breslow thickness 1.5 mm). (*B*) Clinical (*inset*) and dermoscopic images of a 3.5 × 2.5 cm, flat, scaly, pink, and partly pigmented lesion located on the lower leg of a 59-year-old woman. Polarized contact dermoscopy shows whitish surface scale and prominent dotted and coiled vessels on a pink-to-tan background. Remnants of an atypical pigment network are also visible (*oval*). Histopathologic examination revealed an invasive melanoma (Breslow thickness 1.3 mm).

infective skin conditions, such as tinea corporis, psoriasis, nummular eczema, or verrucous lichen planus. As such, it may be unsuccessfully treated using a variety of topical therapies before a correct diagnosis is finally made. Dermoscopy may assist, however, in an earlier diagnosis by revealing remnant pigmentation (eg, residual brown, gray, and/or bluish pigmentation) in conjunction with dotted vessels or an atypical vascular pattern. The latter may include combinations of dotted, coiled (or glomerular), linear irregular, and/or corkscrew vessels (see **Fig. 12B**).[51,55]

Cutaneous melanoma metastases (CMMs) typically present as multiple firm papules or nodules arising in patients with a known past history of invasive melanoma. CMMs may be pigmented or nonpigmented and the latter may arise from both pigmented and nonpigmented primary melanomas. Relevant clinical differential diagnoses for nonpigmented CMMs include hemangiomas, primary malignancies, or cutaneous metastases from other tumors.[56]

Dermoscopy may prove useful for the diagnosis of CMM, in particular, early lesions or those with a nonspecific clinical appearance. As is the case for thin primary AHM, thinner nonpigmented CMM exhibit predominantly dotted vessels on dermoscopy. In thicker lesions, however, the vessels are generally larger and more irregular in morphology and pattern. Such vascular morphologies include corkscrew, linear irregular, hairpin, branching and/or tortuous (ie, glomerular-like) vessels, reddish lacunae-like (or saccular) areas, and/or milky red globules/areas. Lacunae-like structures or sacculi can resemble the lacunae of angiomas (see **Fig. 8A**), being reddish in color and round or ovoid in shape, but differ in being not well demarcated. Whitish striae, perilesional erythema, and peripheral stellate telangiectasias may also be visualized in some CMMs.[57–59]

Nodular BCC

Summary

Dermoscopically, nBCC shows striking, bright red and focused arborizing vessels, which envelope the pinkish lesion. Ulceration and an erythematous blush may also be present. If pigmented, blue-gray globules, blue-gray ovoid nests, and spoke-wheel and leaflike areas may be visible.

nBCC is a common subtype of BCC, frequently occurring on the head and neck region.[60] Nonpigmented nBCC typically presents clinically as a smooth, semitranslucent pinkish papule or nodule. Ulceration and arborizing telangiectasias may be visible to the naked eye. Clinical differential diagnoses may include both benign and malignant tumors, such as dermal nevus (especially on the face), SH, epidermoid cyst, SCC, and AHM.[61]

On dermoscopy, nonpigmented nBCC is characterized by its hallmark arborizing telangiectasias, which usually arise as large, bright red, stem vessels dividing into finer, sharply focused ramifications over the surface of the lesion. The vessels typically occur on a fairly homogeneous white-to-pinkish background and white streaks may also be present (**Fig. 13A**). Orange-red, reddish-brown, or reddish-black ulceration and an erythematous blush (under noncontact polarized dermoscopy) may also be seen in some lesions.[62] In partly pigmented nBCC, discrete tan-brown to gray to bluish areas of pigmentation may occur. These latter areas particularly include blue-gray globules and blue-gray ovoid nests, but spoke-wheel and leaflike areas may also be found.[63]

nBCC can assume a peculiar appearance on the lower leg in that classical arborizing telangiectases may occasionally be absent. Instead, hairpin and/or coiled vessels are often visible in nBCC at this special site, which may be associated with an homogeneous whitish-pink background, ulceration, whitish striae, and pigmentation patterns, such as blue-gray globules or ovoid nests.

Superficial BCC

Summary

On dermoscopy, superficial BCC (sBCC) generally shows fine, scarcely branching, microarborizing vessels and multiple erosions or ulcerations occurring on a whitish-pink to red homogeneous background. If pigmented, blue-gray globules and spoke-wheel, leaflike, and hublike pigmentation may additionally be seen.

Nonpigmented sBCC is another common subtype of BCC that presents clinically as a flat erythematous macule or patch, often located on the trunk and limbs.[60] Clues to the clinical diagnosis may include a slightly raised outer edge and shiny surface, which are often visible with tangential lighting. Further hints include the presence of multiple small ulcerations or blood crusts on the surface of the lesion. Nonetheless, the clinical diagnosis may at times be challenging and differential diagnoses may include SCCIS (Bowen disease), AK, pink LK, tinea corporis, or inflammatory lesions, such as discoid eczema or psoriasis.

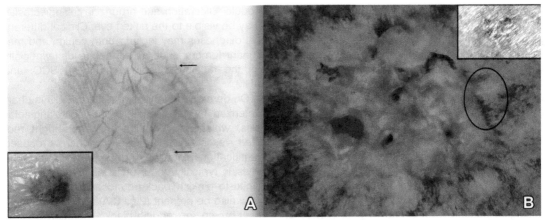

Fig. 13. (*A*) Clinical (*inset*) and dermoscopic photographs of a smooth, shiny pink papule located on the upper arm of a 78-year-old woman with skin phototype I/II and a history of BCC. Polarized noncontact dermoscopy reveals red, focused arborizing telangiectasias on a fairly homogeneous white-to-pinkish background. A few whitish streaks are also visible (*arrows*). Histopathologic examination confirmed the diagnosis of nBCC. (*B*) Clinical (*inset*) and dermoscopic views of a 6-mm pinkish macule located on the back of a 53-year-old Australian man with skin phototype II. Polarized contact dermoscopy demonstrates multiple ulcerations/erosions or blood crusts, short fine telangiectasias, and a fairly homogeneous white-to-pink-to-red background with whitish striae. Tan-colored leaflike areas are also visible at the periphery of the lesion (*oval*). Histopathologic examination confirmed the diagnosis of sBCC.

Dermoscopy is useful for improving the accuracy of diagnosis of sBCC by revealing the essential features of fine, barely branching microarborizing vessels, multiple orange-red to reddish-black erosions or ulcerations, and a whitish-pink to red structureless background.[64–66] Shiny whitish streaks (chrysalis or crystalline structures) can also be seen under polarized light dermoscopy.[16,67] When containing pigment, sBCC may display blue-gray globules or smaller blue-gray ovoid nests as well as spoke-wheel and leaflike areas (see **Fig. 13B**). Hublike areas are a more recently described feature[4] and comprise a brown circular pigmented area with a lighter tan halo (ie, forming a concentric pattern) (**Fig. 14A**). In the authors' view, hublike areas are a possible precursor to spoke-wheel and leaflike areas and blue-gray ovoid nests.

A signature BCC pattern has recently been postulated by Zalaudek and colleagues.[68] In detail, they found that multiple sBCCs in the same patient and same anatomic area revealed similar dermoscopic (including pigmentation) patterns.

Similar to nBCC, the lower leg may be considered a special site for sBCC in that typical microarborizing telangiectases may be absent. Instead, hairpin and/or coiled vessels are frequently seen in sBCC on the lower limbs, which may be associated with a homogeneous whitish-pink background, erosions or ulcerations, whitish striae, and pigmentation patterns (discussed previously).

Infiltrative BCC

Summary

On dermoscopy, infiltrative BCC can exhibit finely arborized, scattered telangiectasias. The latter occurs on a whitish background that has poorly defined borders.

Infiltrative BCC—the term used in this article also includes morphoeic or sclerosing BCC—is the least common of the 3 main subtypes of BCC but generally the most aggressive. This variant can be challenging to diagnose with the naked eye, tending to present clinically as a whitish, scar-like plaque with ill-defined edges.[61]

The dermoscopic features of infiltrative BCC have barely been described, but it is the authors' experience that this variant often demonstrates finely arborized, scattered telangiectasias, which appear to show fewer ramifications than the classic arborizing telangiectasias of nBCC. In the authors' view, the vessels typically occur on a whitish background that has poorly defined borders (see **Fig. 14B**). In contrast, nBCC usually shows arborizing vessels that envelope a fairly well defined, translucent pinkish tumor.[4] Mixed nodular and infiltrative BCC can show a combination of these features.

Pyne and colleagues[69] studied a group of aggressive BCC subtypes (that included infiltrating BCC, micronodular BCC, and BCC with squamous

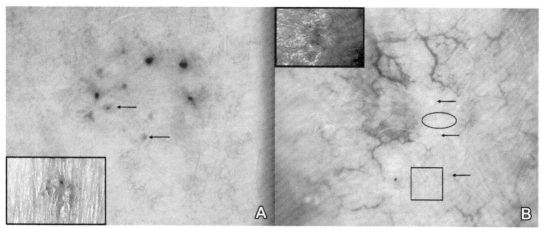

Fig. 14. (*A*) Clinical (*inset*) and dermoscopic photographs of a 3–4 mm, smooth pink macule situated on the back of a 56-year-old woman with skin phototype II. Speckling of pigmentation is seen in the clinical image. Polarized contact dermoscopy demonstrates short fine telangiectasias, a fairly homogeneous pinkish background (the pinkish hue is difficult to appreciate due to the downward pressure of the faceplate on the lesion), leaflike areas, and hublike pigmentation (*arrows*). The latter is a possible precursor to leaflike and spoke-wheel pigmentation. Histologic evaluation reported an sBCC. (*B*) Clinical (*inset*) and dermoscopic pictures of a whitish lesion on the dorsum of the nose of a 72-year-old woman with skin phototype II and a history of BCC. The lesion had a central depression with slightly elevated, smooth edges. Polarized contact dermoscopy reveals a poorly defined lesion with fine arborizing vessels in a scattered distribution (*arrows*). Whitish streaks (*square*) and structureless areas (*oval*) are also visible. Histopathologic examination reported a morphoeic BCC.

differentiation) and found less pink color in these tumors compared with less aggressive subtypes (ie, sBCC or nBCC). Furthermore, they reported that vessels were more likely to occupy a peripheral location in aggressive BCC rather than a central site.

Fibroepithelial BCC

Summary

Dermoscopically, fibroepithelioma of Pinkus (FEP) shows shiny whitish streaks and finely arborizing vessels. Ulcerations, dot vessels, and milia cysts are also present in some lesions. Pigmented cases may display blue-gray dots and areas of structureless gray to brown pigmentation.

FEP was originally described by Hermann Pinkus in 1953 as a "premalignant fibroepithelial tumor"[70] but is now considered an uncommon subtype of BCC (fibroepithelial BCC). It usually presents clinically as a solitary, elevated, flesh-colored, or erythematous tumor that may be pedunculated. It occasionally displays the features of gray to brown pigmentation or ulceration and may sometimes present as multiple lesions. Pinkus tumor commonly occurs in middle-aged and elderly individuals and has a predilection for the lumbosacral region. Furthermore, FEP clinically mimics several benign skin lesions, including dermal nevus, acrochordon (skin tag), and SK, making it a challenge to diagnose with the naked eye.[70–72]

FEP is characterized histopathologically by multiple thin branching and anastomosing cords of atypical basaloid cells extending downwards from the epidermis into the dermis, embedded in a fibrovascular stroma.[73]

Dermoscopy assists in the diagnosis of FEP by revealing shiny whitish streaks (striae) or septal lines (seen under polarized light) and fine arborizing vessels (**Fig. 15A**).[74] The latter are typically smaller in caliber and have fewer ramifications than the classical treelike arborizing vessels of nBCC. The finely arborized vessels of FEP differ from the comma vessels found in dermal nevi, the fine linear or elongated vessels of acrochordons, and the regular hairpin vessels of SKs.[8] Orange-red to brown erosions or ulcerations are visible in some lesions. Dotted vessels and milia cysts can also be seen in some cases of FEP. These latter features may be found in other lesions, such as melanocytic tumors and SKs, respectively.[3,4,8] The constellation of dermoscopic findings in FEP should alert clinicians, however, to the possibility of this diagnosis and the need for biopsy. If pigmented, FEP may exhibit irregularly distributed, structureless areas of gray to brown pigmentation as well as blue-gray dots.[74]

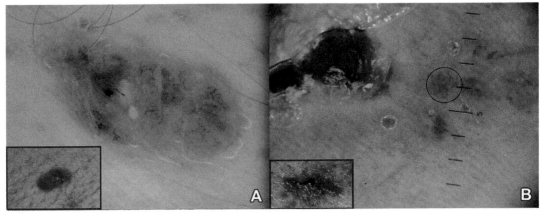

Fig. 15. (*A*) Clinical (*inset*) and dermoscopic images of a 13 × 6 mm smooth pinkish-tan plaque located in the axilla of a 75-year-old woman. Clinically, the tumor resembles a dermal nevus. Polarized contact dermoscopy raised suspicion, however, for FEP by revealing fine, focused arborizing vessels, whitish striae, large white milia cysts, brown-gray homogeneous pigmentation, blue-gray dots, and a few dotted vessels. Histopathologic examination confirmed the diagnosis of Pinkus tumor. (*B*) Clinical image of a 22 × 12 mm scaly, reddish plaque on the lower leg of an 82-year-old man with skin phototype II (*inset*). Nonpolarized, contact dermoscopy shows overlapping features of BCC and invasive SCC. SCC-like features include whitish surface scale, a keratin mass with orange-to-black hemorrhagic pigmentation and blood spots, whitish homogeneous areas (particularly adjacent to the keratin mass), and multiple dotted, hairpin, and linear-irregular vessels. BCC-related criteria include an ill-defined blue-gray blotch, and slightly unfocused arborizing telangiectasias (*circle*). Histopathologic examination confirmed the diagnosis of BSC.

Infundibulocystic BCC

Summary

Infundibulocystic BCC is a rare BCC variant that frequently shows arborizing vessels, fine elongated vessels, blue-gray ovoid nests, and blue-gray globules on dermoscopic examination.

Infundibulocystic BCC was first described as a histopathologic entity by Walsh and Ackerman in 1990[75] and is particularly common in nevoid BCC (Gorlin) syndrome. This rare variant of BCC often presents as a small smooth (shiny) papule or pedunculated lesion, which resembles a benign nevus or skin tag, respectively.[76,77] Patients with Gorlin syndrome may present with numerous lesions and favored sites include the face, neck, trunk, and extremities.

There is a scarcity of reports concerning the dermoscopic features of infundibulocystic BCC. Feito-Rodríguez and colleagues[78] described the dermoscopic features of 11 acrochordon-like BCCs in a 7-year-old child with Gorlin syndrome. Ten of the 11 lesions studied were subsequently diagnosed histopathologically as infundibulocystic BCC. Dermoscopic findings in these latter lesions most commonly disclosed arborizing vessels, fine elongated vessels, blue-gray ovoid nests, single blue-gray globules, and/or multiple blue-gray globules. No maple leaflike areas, spoke-wheel–like areas, or ulceration was observed. These dermoscopic features seem useful in differentiating infundibulocystic BCC from lesions which may mimic it clinically, such as melanocytic nevi and acrochordons.

Basosquamous Carcinoma

Summary

Basosquamous carcinoma (BSC) displays dermoscopic features reminiscent of both BCC and invasive SCC. BCC-like features include unfocused arborizing vessels, ulceration, and blue-gray blotches. SCC-related criteria include surface scale, white structureless areas, targetoid follicles, keratin masses, and blood spots within keratin masses.

BSC, also called metatypical carcinoma, was first described by MacCormac in 1910.[79] It is generally considered an uncommon variant of BCC, having clinical and histologic features of both BCC and SCC.[80,81] Histopathologically, BSC is composed of areas of both classical BCC and SCC, with a transition zone linking the two.[82] It must be differentiated on histopathology from a collision lesion comprising BCC and SCC and from a keratotic subtype of BCC.[81–83] It is a rare skin malignancy, estimated to represent less than 0.5% of all BCCs.[81] BSC commonly occurs on the head and neck region and has been reported to be more prevalent in elderly men.[81,84]

Clinically, the tumor may have a history of rapid and aggressive local growth and exhibit surface scale, a rust-red coloration, and ulceration.[80,81,84–86] The macroscopic appearance is generally regarded as nonspecific, however, because BSC can mimic several benign and malignant skin lesions, such as verruca (viral wart), hyperkeratotic or bowenoid AK, less-aggressive subtypes of BCC, invasive SCC, SCCIS, and AHM.

BSC has a potential for aggressive biologic behavior, marked by local tissue destruction in addition to possible local recurrence and even lymph node and distant metastasis.[84–86] The rate of distant metastasis of BSC has been reported to be higher than for either BCC or SCC alone.[81] The nonspecific clinical appearance of BSC and its propensity for local and distant spread underlines the need for early diagnosis and excision, to avoid significant morbidity and even mortality.

The dermoscopic features of BSC have recently been studied by Giacomel and colleagues.[87] In an assessment of 22 BSCs, overlapping dermoscopic features of BCC and invasive SCC were seen, mirroring its peculiar histopathology. BCC-like features included unfocused arborizing vessels (preferentially located at the periphery of the tumors), ulceration or blood crusts, and blue-gray blotches. The blue-gray blotches seen in BSC were slightly ill defined, in contrast to the more well-demarcated appearance of this criterion in less-aggressive subtypes of BCC (in particular, nBCC). Multiple brown dots and leaflike areas were also visualized. SCC-related criteria included surface scale, white structureless areas, targetoid follicles (white circles), keratin masses, and reddish to reddish-black blood spots within the latter keratin masses. Dotted, hairpin, and linear irregular vessels were also noted, typically with whitish haloes (see **Fig. 15**B). In all but 1 BSC at least 1 of the BCC-like criteria was detected in addition to 1 of the features related to invasive SCC.[4,63,88,89] Further studies are required, however, to investigate the sensitivity and specificity of these dermoscopic criteria in differentiating BSC from other benign and malignant skin tumors.

Actinic Keratosis

Summary

On dermoscopy, facial nonpigmented AKs typically reveal a strawberry pattern, comprising an erythematous pseudonetwork surrounding keratotic hair follicles. In addition, whitish-yellow surface scale is commonly present.

Actinic (or solar) keratoses (AKs) are neoplastic skin lesions within the biologic continuum of SCC. They may be considered an early form of superficial SCC that if left untreated may progress to full-thickness SCCIS or invasive SCC.[90,91] Although the risk of progression of an individual AK to invasive SCC is unclear, estimates vary between 0.1% and 10%.[92] Furthermore, patients with numerous (ie, >10) AKs are estimated to have a cumulative probability of 14% of developing invasive SCC within 5 years.[92,93] Early diagnosis and treatment of AK are, therefore, recommended.[91]

AKs are a marker of chronic sun exposure. As such, they are most commonly seen in middle-aged to elderly individuals with fair skin phototypes (in particular, I and II), who have evidence of chronically sun-damaged skin (ie, dermatoheliosis and/or solar lentigines). AKs are usually nonpigmented and present as multiple scaly erythematous macules, papules, or small plaques on the chronically sun-exposed surfaces of the dorsa of the hands, forearms, face, bald scalp, and lower legs.[94] Although traditionally diagnosed by clinical appearance alone, nonpigmented AKs may at times be clinically difficult to distinguish from several benign and malignant skin lesions, such as small plaques of SCCIS, invasive SCC, sBCC, SK, verruca, and discoid eczema.[64,95]

On dermoscopy, facial nonpigmented AKs typically reveal whitish-yellow surface scale and a strawberry pattern, the latter consisting of an erythematous (pink to red colored) pseudonetwork surrounding hair follicles. The hair follicle openings are surrounded by a white halo and filled with a yellowish keratotic plug, forming a peculiar targetoid appearance. In addition, fine, linear-wavy vessels are often seen surrounding the hair follicles (**Fig. 16**A).[96] Furthermore, small coiled vessels are occasionally visible in AK on the face. These small coiled vessels should be distinguished from the glomerular vessels (GVs) typical of SCCIS. Although coiled vessels are usually located around hair follicle openings, GVs are generally more convoluted, larger in size, and classically distributed in clusters.[96]

Dermoscopy is also useful in assessing clearance of facial AK after the use of topical treatments, such as imiquimod. In detail, clearance of AK is assessed by disappearance of the various dermoscopic features of AK. The latter involves particularly surface scale and keratotic plugs but also includes disappearance of signs of neovascularization, such as the reddish pseudonetwork and linear wavy vessels. In this way, dermoscopy may have superior sensitivity in detecting treatment failure compared with naked eye examination alone.[97] Further studies on a large number of AKs are required, however, to investigate this latter point.

AK on nonfacial sites typically lack this strawberry pattern but dermoscopically frequently display surface scale on an erythematous background, along with dot vessels. Whitish haloes may be seen around these dot vessels, as is typical of keratinizing lesions.[6] In particularly hyperkeratotic AK, the underlying vascular structures may be obscured, which may make diagnosis by dermoscopy difficult.

Squamous Cell Carcinoma In Situ (Bowen Disease or Intraepidermal Carcinoma)

Summary

The dermoscopy of SCCIS is characterized by surface scales and clustered groups of dotted and glomerular vessels.

Clinically, SCCIS classically presents as a gradually enlarging, fairly well demarcated, scaly, pink to reddish macule or plaque. It may clinically resemble several conditions, including psoriasis, eczema, verruca, AK, BCC, and eczematous AM.[51,98] Uncommonly, SCCIS may present as a pigmented lesion and mimic several conditions, such as pigmented AK, BCC, SK, (junctional) nevus, and melanoma.[95,98]

Dermoscopy is useful in helping to diagnose SCCIS accurately because nonpigmented variants typically display islands of whitish surface scale with intervening clusters of glomerular (ie, highly convoluted) and/or dotted vessels (see **Fig. 16**B). Zalaudek and colleagues[95] reported GVs in 100% of nonpigmented SCCIS studied in their initial series. A whitish halo is usually seen around these vessels, as is customary for keratinizing lesions.[6,95] In pigmented SCCIS, GV may be difficult to discern but were still visible in approximately 80% of the cases studied by Zalaudek and colleagues.[95] Regarding pigment patterns, homogeneous tan/brown areas and tan/brown globules may be visible in pigmented SCCIS.

GVs may also be seen on skin of the lower leg in patients with chronic venous stasis.[99] GVs may also occur in other types of lesions (eg, AKs and BCCs) in these patients on this anatomic location. The distribution of GVs in these instances, however, is more homogeneous, rather than clustered, and other lesion-specific features may be present (eg, arborizing vessels and/or blue-gray globules in BCC). On the face, nonpigmented SCCIS may present with peripherally located and clustered

GV or dot vessels surrounding central white to yellow scale, with or without small erosions (blood crusts).[88]

Invasive Squamous Cell Carcinoma

Summary

Dermoscopy of invasive SCC typically reveals surface scale, ulceration, and an atypical vascular pattern. The vessels have white haloes and occur over a whitish background.

Like AK, invasive SCC typically occurs in chronically sun-damaged individuals with fair skin phototypes (ie, I and II). The majority of invasive SCCs are thought to arise from superficial SCC (ie, AK and SCCIS).[91] As such, invasive SCCs are usually seen in patients with numerous AKs. Invasive SCC usually enlarges quickly, over a period of weeks or months. Initially, early invasive SCC presents as a scaly, reddish papule or ill-defined plaque that may mimic other lesions, such as verruca vulgaris, inflamed or irritated SK, hyperkeratotic AK, or SCCIS. Less scaly tumors may simulate BCC or AHM. If left untreated, SCC typically becomes a firm, ulcerated, often tender and indurated nodule or nodule/plaque.[98,100]

On dermoscopy, invasive SCC usually exhibits white to yellow surface scale, keratin (which may contain blood spots), ulceration, and/or orange-reddish blood crusts. A polymorphous or atypical vascular pattern is stereotypically present, with the vessels surrounded by whitish haloes and occurring on a white background.[6,8,98] Dotted, linear irregular, and/or hairpin vessels are often visible in invasive SCC. The latter 2 vessel types are usually elongated and irregular in shape and distribution (**Fig. 17**A).[4,88,98] Another feature that can be visualized in invasive SCC as well as keratoacanthoma is whitish hyperkeratotic follicles, often with central yellowish keratinous plugs (ie, targetoid follicles, also termed white circles). White rounded areas (keratin pearls) have also been reported in keratoacanthoma and well-differentiated invasive SCC.[88,89,101]

On the face, invasive SCC can usually be differentiated dermoscopically from AK and SCCIS, enhancing diagnostic accuracy over clinical examination alone. In detail, facial AK classically shows surface scale and a strawberry pattern, whereas SCCIS exhibits scale and clusters of dotted and/or glomerular vessels (often located peripherally).[88,96] Small superficial erosions or ulcerations may also be seen in SCCIS on the face.[88]

Keratoacanthoma

Summary

Keratoacanthoma is characterized by peripheral hairpin vessels or a polymorphous vascular pattern, arranged radially on a whitish background. A central yellowish plug of keratin or scale is typically present, often with blood crusts.

Keratoacanthoma (KA), a somewhat peculiar self-healing skin tumor, is considered a variant of SCC because of its close histopathologic resemblance to well-differentiated invasive SCC.[102] KA typically arises on the sun-damaged skin of fair-skinned, middle-aged to elderly patients. It usually presents clinically as a fast-growing, nonpigmented, firm, and exophytic tumor. It grows quickly over a period of weeks before stabilizing in size and then finally may undergo spontaneous involution. On macroscopic examination, KA appears as a dome-shaped papule or nodule, with smooth rolled edges, surrounding a central mass of keratin (keratin plug). Although usually solitary, multiple lesions may occur as part of Muir-Torre syndrome, after BRAF inhibitor (eg, vemurafenib) therapy for metastatic melanoma, or as a Grzybowski, Ferguson Smith, or Witten-Zak–type presentation.[103–109]

On dermoscopy, KA typically displays a central whitish-yellow to brown mass of keratin, which may contain blood spots. This mass of keratin is usually surrounded by a smooth rolled edge, housing elongated and radially arranged hairpin vessels. Other vessel types may also be present, such as dotted, coiled, and linear irregular vessels (ie, forming a polymorphous vascular pattern). The vessels typically have white haloes, as is customary for keratinizing tumors (see **Fig. 17B**).[4,6,8,20,98] As discussed previously, hyperkeratotic targetoid follicles and keratin pearls may be seen in KA and well-differentiated SCC.[88,89,101]

In KA, the peripheral arrangement of hairpin vessels around a central keratin mass is helpful in differentiating the condition from skin tumors, which may simulate it clinically. The latter includes SKs, in which hairpin vessels occur in a regular distribution throughout the tumor as well as other lesions, such as hyperkeratotic AK, BCC, and AHM.

Angiosarcoma

Summary

Classical nodular angiosarcoma (AS) often reveals red to bluish-purple areas interspersed with whitish lines. Flatter parts of classical AS show structureless red to bluish-purple areas, intermingled with yellowish globular structures. Radiation-associated AS shows homogeneous whitish-pink areas, with increased color intensity at the periphery. An atypical vascular pattern may also be seen in some lesions.

AS (hemangiosarcoma) is a rare and aggressive vascular malignancy that typically has a poor prognostic outcome.[110–112] The tumor usually presents as an enlarging, diffuse, red to purple patch or plaque that may in time become nodular. AS has 3 main clinical variants. The first and commonest subtype is idiopathic (sporadic or classical) AS, which mainly occurs on the scalp and face of elderly patients. The second variant is lymphedema-associated AS and the third subtype is postradiation AS.[113] Although the clinical diagnosis of AS may be suspected in many instances, AS may at times simulate other lesions, such as AHM, hemorrhage (bruising), other vascular tumors, rosacea, or cutaneous infections, such as cellulitis and erysipelas. Confusion with benign entities may result in a delayed diagnosis with a potentially adverse prognostic outcome.[112]

To date, there have been only a few reports published on the dermoscopic characteristics of AS. Oiso and colleagues[114] reported dermoscopic features found in a case of classical AS of the scalp of an 86-year-old Japanese man. Findings included a color gradation within the lesions, from pink to red to purple. Furthermore, the reddish areas displayed an atypical vascular pattern, which included dotted, linear irregular, and glomerular-like vessels.

de Giorgi and colleagues[115] examined 2 cases of cutaneous AS arising in 2 women who had a history of breast carcinoma and subsequent radiotherapy. On dermoscopic examination of the ringlike lesions, they found central white to skin-colored areas surrounded by a more intensely colored pink to purple peripheral zone.

In a larger series, Zalaudek and colleagues[112] reported on the dermoscopic features seen in 11 cases of AS, seen in 11 patients (ie, 6 men and 2 women with spontaneous AS and 3 women with radiation-associated AS). In the spontaneous

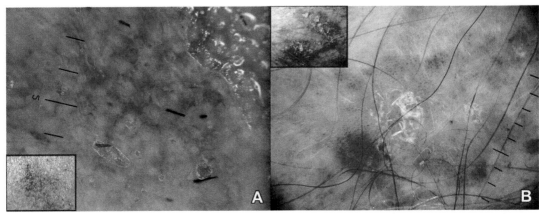

Fig. 16. (A) Macroscopic view of an 8-mm scaly, erythematous macule on the cheek of a 74-year-old man with skin phototype II (*inset*). Nonpolarized contact dermoscopy discloses a strawberry appearance, comprising a blurred, reddish pseudonetwork located between hyperkeratotic (and targetoid) hair follicles. Whitish surface scale and fine focused (linear wavy) vessels are also seen, the latter surrounding the follicles. Histopathologic examination confirmed the diagnosis of AK. (B) Clinical image of a 12-mm scaly, reddish plaque on the lower leg of a 64-year-old Australian man with skin phototype I and a history of chronic sun exposure (*inset*). The lesion had been present for some years and was enlarging gradually. Polarized, contact dermoscopy shows clusters of dotted and tortuous (ie, coiled and glomerular) vessels and whitish surface scale. Histopathologic evaluation confirmed the diagnosis of SCCIS.

(classical) AS group, structureless red to bluish-purple areas were seen in flatter tumors or parts of tumors, which were intermingled with yellowish globular structures. The latter corresponded histopathologically to the openings of the pilosebaceous units. In the cases of classical AS having a nodular component (ie, 3 patients), deep purple areas were visualized, with intersecting whitish lines (**Fig. 18**A). Regarding the radiation-associated AS tumors, structureless whitish-pink

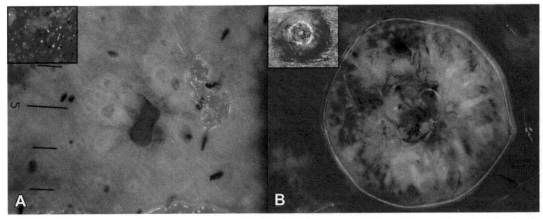

Fig. 17. (A) Clinical image of a scaly, nonpigmented, nontender, slightly indurated papule on the cheek of a 77-year-old Australian man with skin phototype II (*inset*). The lesion had been enlarging over the preceding few weeks. On nonpolarized, contact dermoscopy there is central ulceration, peripherally located hyperkeratotic follicles (with a targetoid appearance), and a polymorphous vascular pattern. The latter appears on a whitish background and comprises a combination of dotted, hairpin and linear-irregular vessels. Histopathologic examination confirmed well-differentiated invasive SCC, extending into the mid-dermis. (B) Clinical (*inset*) and dermoscopic photographs of a 6-mm nodule on the back of a 50-year-old Australian man with skin phototype I/II. The lesion had appeared a few weeks previously and grown quickly. Polarized contact dermoscopy shows numerous peripheral hairpin vessels arranged radially on a whitish background (ie, in the smooth rolled edge of the lesion). Dotted and linear-irregular vessels are also present, making this a polymorphous vascular pattern. The vessels surround a central yellowish mass of keratin with blood spots. The clinicodermoscopic suspicion of keratoacanthoma was confirmed histopathologically.

areas were reported, which seemed to correlate with dermal fibrosis or sclerosis histopathologically. The latter dermoscopic feature was associated with purple globules or with increased color intensity (strengthening of color) at the periphery of the lesion. This observation was similar to the findings of de Giorgi and colleagues[115] in their cases of radiation-associated AS.

Merkel Cell Carcinoma

Summary

MCC is a rare and aggressive malignant skin tumor that usually presents clinically as a smooth pink or red nodule. On surface microscopy, linear irregular vessels or an atypical vascular pattern is frequently seen, occurring on a pinkish background. Ulceration may also be visualized.

MCC, also called neuroendocrine carcinoma, was first described by Toker in 1972 as "trabecular carcinoma of the skin."[116] Primary MCC is a rare and highly aggressive malignancy, usually found on the sun-exposed areas of elderly patients. MCC typically presents as a fast-growing, firm, nontender, reddish (often cherry red) nodule that may at times show ulceration.[49,117] The correct diagnosis is often delayed and clinical differential diagnoses include benign cysts, acneiform lesions, and vascular lesions (including PG) as well as malignancies, such as AHM, invasive SCC, and cutaneous metastasis.[118] Similar to other fast-growing, aggressive skin tumors, such as nodular melanoma and invasive SCC, MCC can, therefore, present as a clinically worrisome EFG-positive skin lesion.[47,48]

Although most patients (70%–80%) present with localized disease, 9% to 26% have regional (lymph node) involvement at the time of diagnosis and 1% to 4% distant metastases.[117] Dermoscopy may potentially help clinicians recognize and excise MCC at the earliest possible stage, when the prognosis may be more favorable.

There have been a few reports on the dermoscopic findings of MCC. In 1 case study, an 83-year-old man with chronically sun-damaged skin presented with a reddish, nodular MCC on the forehead.[49] Dermoscopy revealed linear irregular vessels on a pinkish-red background.

Other recent reports cite linear irregular vessels or a polymorphous vascular pattern (ie, arborizing vessels, dotted vessels, glomerular vessels, linear irregular vessels, and/or milky red globules), whitish streaks and patches, and milky pink or milky red structureless areas as prominent dermoscopic features of MCC (see **Fig. 18B**).[119–121] Furthermore, although the sample size was small, Dalle and colleagues[120] reported that plaque-like MCC showed dotted or glomerular vessels on dermoscopy, without elongated vessels. Conversely, nodular lesions (excluding the special location of the leg) contained elongated vessels, namely linear irregular and/or arborizing vessels (with or without dot vessels).

Accordingly, any reddish, EFG-positive tumor that exhibits linear irregular vessels or a polymorphous vascular pattern on a pinkish-red background should raise the possibility of an aggressive malignant skin tumor (including NM or MCC) and prompt excision.

OTHER UNCOMMON BENIGN AND MALIGNANT PINK (NONPIGMENTED) LESIONS
Pink Adnexal Lesions

Summary

Benign adnexal lesions may clinically and dermoscopically resemble malignant pink tumors, such as BCC and melanoma.

Sgambato and colleagues[122] have reported 3 types of benign adnexal lesions that simulated BCC clinically and on dermoscopy, namely angiohistiocytoma, hydradenoma, and intraepidermal poroma. On dermoscopy, arborizing vessels suggestive of BCC were visible in all these lesions, with the angiohisticytoma also displaying peripheral tan-colored, leaflike pigmentation. The latter feature has been previously reported as 100% specific for pigmented BCC.[63] Moreover, Cabo and colleagues[123] recently documented a case of solitary cylindroma that mimicked BCC on surface microscopy by revealing arborizing telangiectasias, a pinkish background color, bluish globules, and surface ulceration. Furthermore, a recent study by Zaballos and colleagues[124] reported the presence of BCC-like arborizing vessels in apocrine hydrocystoma. In their series of 22 nonpigmented and pigmented lesions, arborizing vessels were seen in 68% of tumors and frequently occurred on a skin-colored to yellowish, translucent background (**Fig. 19**). The benign adnexal tumors listed above can, therefore, closely resemble BCC both clinically and dermoscopically, and biopsy is recommended.[4]

It is noteworthy that nonpigmented eccrine poroma may display a polymorphous vascular

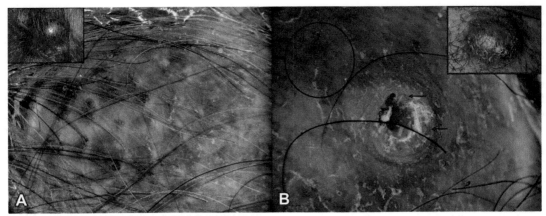

Fig. 18. (*A*) Clinical (*inset*) and dermoscopic images of a 30 × 25 mm smooth red to bluish-purple plaque located on the scalp of an 80-year-old man. Polarized contact dermoscopy of the flatter reddish area revealed whitish-pink areas containing atypical (dotted and linear irregular) vessels. Dermoscopic examination of the raised bluish, nodular part of the lesion showed structureless bluish-purple areas interspersed with whitish bands. Histopathologic examination confirmed the diagnosis of AS. (*B*) Clinical (*inset*) and dermoscopic images of a 2.5-cm, smooth pinkish nodule located on the lower leg of a 54-year-old man. Polarized contact dermoscopy of the 4-mm raised, focally ulcerated area reveals whitish surface scale, an area of red to reddish-black ulceration, and linear irregular vessels (*arrows*). In addition, dotted vessels (*oval*) are visible in the upper part of the dermoscopic image, thus forming an atypical vascular pattern. Furthermore, a fairly homogeneous pinkish background is apparent in the tumor. Histopathologic examination confirmed the diagnosis of MCC.

pattern on dermoscopy. Constituent vascular features include dotted, linear irregular, hairpin, and glomerular vessels as well as structures reminiscent of milky-red globules. White-to-pink meshlike bands are sometimes present, often surrounding glomerular vessels and milky red areas. These dermoscopic features may mimic malignant nonpigmented tumors, such as AM, and biopsy is indicated.[125–128] A polymorphous vascular pattern has also been reported for nonpigmented eccrine

porocarcinoma (malignant eccrine poroma) and biopsy is similarly required.[129–131]

SUMMARY

Dermoscopy can improve the accuracy of diagnosis and thus help facilitate appropriate management decisions for a range of nonpigmented or pink skin lesions. These include benign and malignant as well as melanocytic and nonmelanocytic tumors.

A combined approach for arriving at a diagnosis is advocated, which integrates historical and clinical information with the dermoscopic appearance of the skin lesion or lesions. In this way, the removal of malignant pink skin tumors can be maximized and the biopsy of benign lesions reduced, for the ultimate benefit of patients.

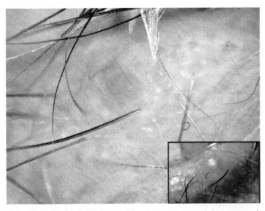

Fig. 19. Clinical image of a 2-mm nonpigmented, cystic lesion located on the palpebral border of the lower eyelid of a 63-year-old man (*inset*). Dermoscopic examination shows finely branched and linear vessels on a homogeneous skin-colored to pink background. Histopathologic examination revealed apocrine hidrocystoma.

REFERENCES

1. Kittler H, Pehamberger H, Wolff K, et al. Diagnostic accuracy of dermoscopy. Lancet Oncol 2002;3:159–65.
2. Rosendahl C, Tschandl P, Cameron A, et al. Diagnostic accuracy of dermatoscopy for melanocytic and nonmelanocytic pigmented lesions. J Am Acad Dermatol 2011;64:1068–73.
3. Zalaudek I, Kreusch J, Giacomel J, et al. How to diagnose nonpigmented skin tumors: a review of vascular structures seen with dermoscopy. Part I. Melanocytic skin tumors. J Am Acad Dermatol 2010;63:361–74.

4. Zalaudek I, Kreusch J, Giacomel J, et al. How to diagnose nonpigmented skin tumors: a review of vascular structures seen with dermoscopy: part II. Nonmelanocytic skin tumors. J Am Acad Dermatol 2010;63:377–86.

5. Pan Y, Gareau DS, Scope A, et al. Polarized and nonpolarized dermoscopy: the explanation for the observed differences. Arch Dermatol 2008;144:828–9.

6. Kreusch JF. Vascular patterns in skin tumors. Clin Dermatol 2002;20:248–54.

7. Argenziano G, Soyer HP, De Giorgio V, et al. Interactive atlas of dermoscopy. Milan (Italy): Edra Medical Publishing & New Media; 2000. Available at: www.dermoscopy.org. Accessed January 28, 2013.

8. Argenziano G, Zalaudek I, Corona R, et al. Vascular structures in skin tumors. A dermoscopy study. Arch Dermatol 2004;140:1485–9.

9. Menzies SW, Kreusch J, Byth K, et al. Dermoscopic evaluation of amelanotic and hypomelanotic melanoma. Arch Dermatol 2008;144:1120–7.

10. Zalaudek I, Leinweber B, Johr R. Nevi with particular pigmentation: black, pink, and white nevus. In: Soyer HP, Argenziano G, Hofmann-Wellenhof R, et al, editors. Color atlas of melanocytic lesions of the skin. Berlin, Heidelberg (Germany): Springer Verlag; 2007. p. 142–6.

11. Spitz S. Melanomas of childhood. Am J Pathol 1948;24:591–609.

12. Ackerman AB, Elish D, Shami S. Spitz's nevus: reassessment critical, revision radical. New York: Ardor Scribendi; 2007. p. 30–42.

13. Zalaudek I, Bonifazi E, Ferrara G, et al. Keratoacanthomas and spitz tumors: are they both 'self-limiting' variants of malignant cutaneous neoplasms? Dermatology 2009;219:3–6.

14. Caputo R, Gelmetti C. Pediatric dermatology and dermatopathology: a concise atlas. London: Martin Dunitz; 2002. p. 8.

15. Ferrara G, Argenziano G, Soyer HP, et al. The spectrum of Spitz nevi: a clinicopathologic study of 83 cases. Arch Dermatol 2005;41:1381–7.

16. Marghoob AA, Cowell L, Kopf AW, et al. Observation of chrysalis structures with polarized dermoscopy. Arch Dermatol 2009;145:618.

17. Argenziano G, Scalvenzi M, Staibano S, et al. Dermatoscopic pitfalls in differentiating pigmented Spitz naevi from cutaneous melanomas. Br J Dermatol 1999;141:788–93.

18. Ackerman AB, Boer A. Histopathologic diagnosis of adnexal epithelial neoplasms: atlas and text. New York: Ardor Scribendi; 2008. p. 113–4.

19. Zaballos P, Ara M, Puig S, et al. Dermoscopy of sebaceous hyperplasia. Arch Dermatol 2005;141: 808.

20. Zalaudek I, Argenziano G, Di Stefani A, et al. Dermoscopy in general dermatology. Dermatology 2006;212:7–18.

21. Kim NH, Zell DS, Kolm I, et al. The dermoscopic differential diagnosis of yellow lobularlike structures. Arch Dermatol 2008;144:962.

22. Bryden AM, Dawe RS, Fleming C. Dermatoscopic features of benign sebaceous proliferation. Clin Exp Dermatol 2004;29:676–7.

23. Kempf W, Burg G. Tumors of the epidermis. In: Burg G, editor. Atlas of cancer of the skin. 1st edition. Philadelphia: Churchill Livingstone; 2000. p. 1–26.

24. Braun RP, Rabinovitz HS, Krischer J, et al. Dermoscopy of pigmented seborrheic keratosis: a morphological study. Arch Dermatol 2002;138:1556–60.

25. Lacarrubba F, De Pasquale R, Micali G. Videodermatoscopy improves the clinical diagnostic accuracy of multiple clear cell acanthoma. Eur J Dermatol 2003;13:596–8.

26. Blum A, Metzler G, Bauer J, et al. The dermatoscopic pattern of clear-cell acanthoma resembles psoriasis vulgaris. Dermatology 2001;203:50–2.

27. Bugatti L, Filosa G, Broganelli P, et al. Psoriasis-like dermoscopic pattern of clear cell acanthoma. J Eur Acad Dermatol Venereol 2003;17:452–5.

28. Zalaudek I, Hofmann-Wellenhof R, Argenziano G. Dermoscopy of clear-cell acanthoma differs from dermoscopy of psoriasis. Dermatology 2003;207: 428.

29. Akin FY, Ertam I, Ceylan C, et al. Clear cell acanthoma: new observations on dermatoscopy. Indian J Dermatol Venereol Leprol 2008;74:285–7.

30. Sánchez Yus E, del Rio E, Requena L. Large-cell acanthoma is a distinctive condition. Am J Dermatopathol 1992;14:140–7 [discussion: 148].

31. Ko CJ, Barr RJ, Subtil A, et al. Acantholytic dyskeratotic acanthoma: a variant of a benign keratosis. J Cutan Pathol 2008;35:298–301.

32. Giacomel J, Zalaudek I, Argenziano G. Dermatoscopy of Grover's disease and solitary acantholytic dyskeratoma shows a brown "star-like" pattern. Australas J Dermatol 2012;53:315–6.

33. Ackerman AB. Focal acantholytic dyskeratosis. Arch Dermatol 1972;106:702–6.

34. Vázquez-López F, Lopez-Escobar M, Maldonado-Seral C, et al. The handheld dermoscope improves the recognition of giant pseudocomedones in Darier's disease. J Am Acad Dermatol 2004;50: 454–5.

35. Puig S, Argenziano G, Zalaudek I, et al. Melanomas that failed dermoscopic detection: a combined clinicodermoscopic approach for not missing melanoma. Dermatol Surg 2007;33:1262–73.

36. Wolf IH. Dermoscopic diagnosis of vascular lesions. Clin Dermatol 2002;20:273–5.

37. Wang SQ, Katz B, Rabinovitz H, et al. Lessons on dermoscopy #7. Dermatol Surg 2000;26:891–2.

38. Zaballos P, Llambrich A, Cuellar F, et al. Dermoscopic findings in pyogenic granuloma. Br J Dermatol 2006;154:1108–11.

39. Zaballos P, Carulla M, Ozdemir F, et al. Dermoscopy of pyogenic granuloma: a morphological study. Br J Dermatol 2010;163:1229–37.

40. Blum A, Bauer J. Atypical dermatofibroma-like pattern of a melanoma on dermoscopy. Melanoma Res 2003;13:633–4.

41. Zalaudek I, Ferrara G, Di Stefani A, et al. Dermoscopy for challenging melanoma; how to raise the 'red flag' when melanoma clinically looks benign. Br J Dermatol 2005;153:200–2.

42. Ferrari A, Soyer HP, Peris K, et al. Central white scar-like patch: a dermatoscopic clue for the diagnosis of dermatofibroma. J Am Acad Dermatol 2000;43:1123–5.

43. Agero AL, Taliercio S, Dusza SW, et al. Conventional and polarized dermoscopy features of dermatofibroma. Arch Dermatol 2006;142:1431–7.

44. Zalaudek I, Argenziano G, Kerl H, et al. Amelanotic/hypomelanotic melanoma: is dermatoscopy useful for the diagnosis? J Dtsch Dermatol Ges 2003;1:369–73.

45. Pizzichetta MA, Talamini R, Stanganelli I, et al. Amelanotic/hypomelanotic melanoma: clinical and dermoscopic features. Br J Dermatol 2004;150:1117–24.

46. Kreusch J. Amelanotic melanoma. In: Soyer HP, Argenziano G, Hofmann-Wellenhof R, et al, editors. Color atlas of melanocytic lesions of the skin. Berlin, Heidelberg (Germany): Springer Verlag; 2007. p. 204–12.

47. Chamberlain AJ, Fritschi L, Kelly JW. Nodular melanoma: patients' perceptions of presenting features and implications for earlier detection. J Am Acad Dermatol 2003;48:694–701.

48. Kelly JW, Chamberlain AJ, Staples MP, et al. Nodular melanoma. No longer as simple as ABC. Aust Fam Physician 2003;32:706–9.

49. Rosendahl C, Cameron A, Zalaudek I. Risk of ablative therapy for "elevated firm growing" lesions: merkel cell carcinoma diagnosed after laser surgical therapy. Dermatol Surg 2009;35:1005–8.

50. Cavicchini S, Tourlaki A, Bottini S. Dermoscopic vascular patterns in nodular "pure" amelanotic melanoma. Arch Dermatol 2007;143:556.

51. Giacomel J, Zalaudek I, Ferrara G, et al. Dermoscopy patterns of eczemalike melanoma. Arch Dermatol 2007;143:1081–2.

52. Zalaudek I, Argenziano G, Ferrara G, et al. Clinically equivocal melanocytic skin lesions with features of regression: a dermoscopic-pathological study. Br J Dermatol 2004;150:64–71.

53. Bories N, Dalle S, Debarbieux S, et al. Dermoscopy of fully regressive cutaneous melanoma. Br J Dermatol 2008;158:1224–9.

54. Tschen JA, Fordice DB, Reddick M, et al. Amelanotic melanoma presenting as inflammatory plaques. J Am Acad Dermatol 1992;27:464–5.

55. Coras B, Hohenleutner S, Raff K, et al. The "red melanoma" - a rare form of amelanotic malignant melanoma. J Dtsch Dermatol Ges 2004;2:597–600.

56. Pizzichetta MA. Cutaneous metastatic melanoma. In: Soyer HP, Argenziano G, Hofmann-Wellenhof R, et al, editors. Color atlas of melanocytic lesions of the skin. Berlin, Heidelberg (Germany): Springer Verlag; 2007. p. 260–3.

57. Bono R, Giampetruzzi AR, Concolino F, et al. Dermoscopic patterns of cutaneous melanoma metastases. Melanoma Res 2004;14:367–73.

58. Jaimes N, Halpern JA, Puig S, et al. Dermoscopy: an aid to the detection of amelanotic cutaneous melanoma metastases. Dermatol Surg 2012;38:1437–44.

59. Julian Y, Argenziano G, Moscarella E, et al. Peripheral stellate telangiectasias: a clinical-dermoscopic clue for diagnosing cutaneous melanoma metastases. J Dermatol Case Rep 2012;6:102–4.

60. McCormack CJ, Kelly JW, Dorevitch AP. Differences in age and body site distribution of the histological subtype of basal cell carcinoma: a possible indicator of differing causes. Arch Dermatol 1997;133:593–6.

61. Cockerell CJ, Tran KT, Carucci J, et al. Basal cell carcinoma. In: Rigel DS, Robinson JK, Ross MI, et al, editors. Cancer of the skin. 2nd edition. Philadelphia: Elsevier Saunders; 2011. p. 99–123.

62. Liebman TN, Jaimes-Lopez N, Balagula Y, et al. Dermoscopic features of basal cell carcinomas: differences in appearance under non-polarized and polarized light. Dermatol Surg 2012;38:392–9.

63. Menzies SW, Westerhoff K, Rabinovitz H, et al. Surface microscopy of pigmented basal cell carcinoma. Arch Dermatol 2000;136:1012–6.

64. Giacomel J, Zalaudek I. Dermoscopy of superficial basal cell carcinoma. Dermatol Surg 2005;31:1710–3.

65. Felder S, Rabinovitz H, Oliviero M, et al. Dermoscopic differentiation of a superficial basal cell carcinoma and squamous cell carcinoma in situ. Dermatol Surg 2006;32:423–5.

66. Pan Y, Chamberlain AJ, Bailey M, et al. Dermatoscopy aids in the diagnosis of the solitary red scaly patch or plaque–features distinguishing superficial basal cell carcinoma, intraepidermal carcinoma, and psoriasis. J Am Acad Dermatol 2008;59:268–74.

67. Salerni G, Alonso C, Bussy RF. Crystalline structures as the only dermoscopic clue for the diagnosis of basal cell carcinoma. Arch Dermatol 2012;148:776.

68. Zalaudek I, Moscarella E, Longo C, et al. The "signature" pattern of multiple basal cell carcinomas. Arch Dermatol 2012;148:1106.

69. Pyne J, Sapkota D, Wong JC. Aggressive basal cell carcinoma: dermatoscopy vascular features as clues to the diagnosis. Dermatol Pract Concept

2012;2:3–11. Available at: www.derm101.com. Accessed February 28, 2013.

70. Pinkus H. Premalignant fibroepithelial tumors of skin. AMA Arch Derm Syphilol 1953;67:598–615.

71. Barr RJ, Herten RJ, Stone OJ. Multiple premalignant fibroepitheliomas of Pinkus: a case report and review of the literature. Cutis 1978;21:335–7.

72. Yaffee HS. Premalignant fibroepithelioma of Pinkus. Arch Dermatol 1964;89:768–9.

73. Elder D, Elenitsas R, Ragsdale BD. Tumors of the Epidermal Appendages. In: Elder D, Elenitsas R, Jaworsky C, et al, editors. Lever's Histopathology of the Skin. 8th edition. Philadelphia: Lippincott-Raven; 1997. p. 727–8.

74. Zalaudek I, Ferrara G, Broganelli P, et al. Dermoscopy patterns of fibroepithelioma of Pinkus. Arch Dermatol 2006;142:1318–22.

75. Walsh N, Ackerman AB. Infundibulocystic basal cell carcinoma: a newly described variant. Mod Pathol 1990;3:599–608.

76. Burgdorf WH. Cancer-associated genodermatoses. In: Burg G, editor. Atlas of cancer of the skin. Philadelphia: Churchill Livingstone; 2000. p. 200.

77. Kelly SC, Ermolovich T, Purcell SM. Non-syndromic segmental multiple infundibulocystic basal cell carcinomas in an adolescent female. Dermatol Surg 2006;32:1202–8.

78. Feito-Rodríguez M, Sendagorta-Cudós E, Moratinos-Martínez M, et al. Dermatoscopic characteristics of acrochordon-like basal cell carcinomas in Gorlin-Goltz syndrome. J Am Acad Dermatol 2009;60:857–61.

79. MacCormac H. The relation of rodent ulcer to squamous cell carcinoma of the skin. Arch Middx Hosp 1910;19:172–83.

80. Menaker GM, Chiu DS. Basal cell carcinoma. In: Sober AJ, Haluska FG, editors. Atlas of clinical oncology: skin cancer. Hamilton, Ontario (Canada): BC Decker; 2001. p. 65–7.

81. Bowman PH, Ratz JL, Knoepp TG, et al. Basosquamous Carcinoma. Dermatol Surg 2003;29:830–3.

82. Mitsuhashi T, Itoh T, Shimizu Y, et al. Squamous cell carcinoma of the skin: dual differentiations to rare basosquamous and spindle cell variants. J Cutan Pathol 2006;33:246–52.

83. Maloney ML. What is basosquamous carcinoma? Dermatol Surg 2000;26:505–6.

84. Costantino D, Lowe L, Brown DL. Basosquamous carcinoma – an under-recognized, high-risk cutaneous neoplasm: case study and review of the literature. J Plast Reconstr Aesthet Surg 2006;59: 424–8.

85. Farmer ER, Helwig EB. Metastatic basal cell carcinoma: a clinicopathologic study of 17 cases. Cancer 1980;46:748–57.

86. Sendur N, Karaman G, Dikicioglu E, et al. Cutaneous basosquamous carcinoma infiltrating cerebral tissue. J Eur Acad Dermatol Venereol 2004;18:334–6.

87. Giacomel J, Lallas A, Argenziano G, et al. Dermoscopy of basosquamous carcinoma. Br J Dermatol 2013;169(2):358–64.

88. Zalaudek I, Giacomel J, Schmid K, et al. Dermatoscopy of facial actinic keratosis, intraepidermal carcinoma, and invasive squamous cell carcinoma: a progression model. J Am Acad Dermatol 2012; 66:589–97.

89. Rosendahl C, Cameron A, Argenziano G, et al. Dermoscopy of squamous cell carcinoma and keratoacanthoma. Arch Dermatol 2012;148:1386–92.

90. Ackerman AB, Mones JM. Solar (actinic) keratosis is squamous cell carcinoma. Br J Dermatol 2006; 155:9–22.

91. Czarnecki D, Meehan CJ, Bruce F, et al. The majority of cutaneous squamous cell carcinomas arise in actinic keratoses. J Cutan Med Surg 2002;6:207–9.

92. Robinson JK. Squamous cell carcinoma. In: Sober AJ, Haluska FG, editors. Atlas of clinical oncology: skin cancer. Hamilton, Ontario (Canada): BC Decker Inc; 2001. p. 74–5.

93. Salasche SJ. Epidemiology of actinic keratoses and squamous cell carcinoma. J Am Acad Dermatol 2000;42:S4–7.

94. Moy RL. Clinical presentation of actinic keratoses and squamous cell carcinoma. J Am Acad Dermatol 2000;42:S8–10.

95. Zalaudek I, Argenziano G, Leinweber B, et al. Dermoscopy of Bowen's disease. Br J Dermatol 2004; 150:1112–6.

96. Zalaudek I, Giacomel J, Argenziano G, et al. Dermoscopy of facial non-pigmented actinic keratosis. Br J Dermatol 2006;155:951–6.

97. Kacar N, Sanli B, Zalaudek I, et al. Dermatoscopy for monitoring treatment of actinic keratosis with imiquimod. Clin Exp Dermatol 2012;37:567–9.

98. Zalaudek I, Giacomel JS, Leinweber B. Squamous cell carcinoma including actinic keratosis, Bowen's disease and keratoacanthoma and its pigmented variants. In: Soyer HP, Argenziano G, Hofmann-Wellenhof R, et al, editors. Color atlas of melanocytic lesions of the skin. Berlin, Heidelberg (Germany): Springer Verlag; 2007. p. 295–302.

99. Vazquez-Lopez F, Kreusch J, Marghoob AA. Dermoscopic semiology: further insights into vascular features by screening a large spectrum of nontumoral skin lesions. Br J Dermatol 2004;150:226–31.

100. Bhambri S, Dinehart S, Bhambri A. Squamous cell carcinoma. In: Rigel DS, Robinson JK, Ross MI, et al, editors. Cancer of the skin. 2nd edition. Philadelphia: Elsevier Saunders; 2011. p. 124–39.

101. Jaimes N, Zalaudek I, Braun RP, et al. Pearls of keratinizing tumors. Arch Dermatol 2012;148:976.

102. Beham A, Regauer S, Soyer HP, et al. Keratoacanthoma: a clinically distinct variant of well

differentiated squamous cell carcinoma. Adv Anat Pathol 1998;5:269–80.

103. Grzybowski M. A case of peculiar generalized epithelial tumours of the skin. Br J Dermatol Syph 1950;62:310–3.

104. Smith JF. Multiple primary, self-healing squamous epithelioma of the skin. Br J Dermatol Syph 1948; 60:315–9.

105. Witten VH, Zak FG. Multiple, primary, self-healing prickle-cell epithelioma of the skin. Cancer 1952; 5:539–50.

106. Ponti G, Ponz de Leon M. Muir–Torre syndrome. Lancet Oncol 2005;6:980–7.

107. Wee SA. Multiple eruptive keratoacanthomas, de novo. Dermatol Online J 2004;10(3):19.

108. Alloo A, Garibyan L, LeBoeuf N, et al. Photodynamic therapy for multiple eruptive keratoacanthomas associated with vemurafenib treatment for metastatic melanoma. Arch Dermatol 2012;148: 363–6.

109. Haas N, Schadendorf D, Henz BM, et al. Nine-year follow-up of a case of Grzybowski type multiple keratoacanthomas and failure to demonstrate human papillomavirus. Br J Dermatol 2002;147:793–6.

110. Morgan MB, Swann M, Somach S, et al. Cutaneous angiosarcoma: a case series with prognostic correlation. J Am Acad Dermatol 2004;50:867–74.

111. Wollina U, Hansel G, Schönlebe J, et al. Cutaneous angiosarcoma is a rare aggressive malignant vascular tumour of the skin. J Eur Acad Dermatol Venereol 2011;25:964–8.

112. Zalaudek I, Gomez-Moyano E, Landi C, et al. Clinical, dermoscopic and histopathological features of spontaneous scalp or face and radiotherapy-induced angiosarcoma. Australas J Dermatol 2013;54:201–7.

113. Krayenbuehl BH, Cockerell CJ, Franklin G, et al. Vascular neoplasms. In: Burg G, editor. Atlas of cancer of the skin. Philadelphia: Churchill Livingstone; 2000. p. 82.

114. Oiso N, Matsuda H, Kawada A. Various colour gradations as a dermatoscopic feature of cutaneous angiosarcoma of the scalp. Australas J Dermatol 2013;54:36–8.

115. de Giorgi V, Grazzini M, Rossari S, et al. Dermoscopy pattern of cutaneous angiosarcoma. Eur J Dermatol 2011;21:113–4.

116. Toker C. Trabecular carcinoma of the skin. Arch Dermatol 1972;105:107–10.

117. Pectasides D, Pectasides M, Economopoulos T. Merkel cell cancer of the skin. Ann Oncol 2006; 17:1489–95.

118. Iyer JG, Thibodeau R, Nghiem P. Merkel cell carcinoma. In: Rigel DS, Robinson JK, Ross MI, et al, editors. Cancer of the skin. 2nd edition. Philadelphia: Elsevier Saunders; 2011. p. 179–85.

119. Jalilian C, Chamberlain AJ, Haskett M, et al. Clinical and Dermoscopic Characteristics of Merkel Cell Carcinoma. Br J Dermatol 2013;169:294–7.

120. Dalle S, Parmentier L, Moscarella E, et al. Dermoscopy of merkel cell carcinoma. Dermatology 2012;224:140–4.

121. Harting MS, Ludgate MW, Fullen DR, et al. Dermatoscopic vascular patterns in cutaneous Merkel cell carcinoma. J Am Acad Dermatol 2012;66:923–7.

122. Sgambato A, Zalaudek I, Ferrara G, et al. Adnexal tumors: clinical and dermoscopic mimickers of basal cell carcinoma. Arch Dermatol 2008;144:426.

123. Cabo H, Pedrini F, Cohen Sabban E. Dermoscopy of cylindroma. Dermatol Res Pract 2010;2010. http://dx.doi.org/10.1155/2010/285392. pii:285392. Epub 2010 Aug 24.

124. Zaballos P, Banuls J, Medina C, et al. Dermoscopy of apocrine hidrocystomas: a morphological study. J Eur Acad Dermatol Venereol 2012. http://dx.doi.org/10.1111/jdv.12044. [Epub ahead of print].

125. Altamura D, Piccolo D, Lozzi GP, et al. Eccrine poroma in an unusual site: a clinical and dermoscopic simulator of amelanotic melanoma. J Am Acad Dermatol 2005;53:539–41.

126. Ferrari A, Buccini P, Silipo V, et al. Eccrine poroma: a clinical-dermoscopic study of seven cases. Acta Derm Venereol 2009;89:160–4.

127. Nicolino R, Zalaudek I, Ferrara G, et al. Dermoscopy of eccrine poroma. Dermatology 2007;215: 160–3.

128. Minagawa A, Koga H, Takahashi M, et al. Dermoscopic features of nonpigmented eccrine poromas in association with their histopathological features. Br J Dermatol 2010;163:1264–8.

129. Johr R, Saghari S, Nouri K. Eccrine porocarcinoma arising in a seborrheic keratosis evaluated with dermoscopy and treated with Mohs' technique. Int J Dermatol 2003;42:653–7.

130. Blum A, Metzler G, Bauer J. Polymorphous vascular patterns in dermoscopy as a sign of malignant skin tumors. A case of an amelanotic melanoma and a porocarcinoma. Dermatology 2005; 210:58–9.

131. Suzaki R, Shioda T, Konohana I, et al. Dermoscopic features of eccrine porocarcinoma arising from hidroacanthoma simplex. Dermatol Res Pract 2010;2010:192371. http://dx.doi.org/10.1155/2010/192371. Epub 2010 Oct 11.

Dermoscopy in General Dermatology

Aimilios Lallas, MD[a],*, Iris Zalaudek, MD[a,b],
Giuseppe Argenziano, MD[a], Caterina Longo, MD, PhD[a],
Elvira Moscarella, MD[a], Vito Di Lernia, MD[c],
Samer Al Jalbout, MD[d], Zoe Apalla, MD[e]

KEYWORDS

• Dermoscopy • Dermatoscopy • General dermatology • Inflammoscopy • Entomodermoscopy

KEY POINTS

• In addition to its traditional use for evaluation of skin tumors, dermoscopy is increasingly used in general dermatology.
• The new-generation hand-held dermatoscope, which does not require immersion fluid and contact with the skin, represents the optimal equipment for dermoscopic examination of inflammatory and infectious skin diseases.
• Vascular structures, color variegation, follicular abnormalities, and specific features are the main criteria to be considered when applying dermoscopy in general dermatology.
• Dermoscopy is a valuable tool that improves diagnostic accuracy in several clinical scenarios, such as the differential diagnosis of erythematosquamous skin diseases or the diagnosis of scabies.
• Dermoscopic findings should always be interpreted within the clinical context of the patient and integrated with all relevant information from history and macroscopic examination.

INTRODUCTION

The introduction of dermoscopy in dermatology revealed structures and features invisible to the naked eye, providing additional morphologic information during clinical examination of skin lesion. The technique has been applied to evaluation of melanocytic tumors, with research efforts focusing mainly on identification of dermoscopic characteristics of melanoma. With time, the value of dermoscopy in improving melanoma detection was established, and the technique gained global acceptance for assessment of pigmented skin tumors.[1,2] More recently, several investigators reported on dermoscopic patterns of nonpigmented tumors, as well as nonneoplastic dermatoses.[3] The latter were based on the observation that, apart from pigmentation structures formed by melanin deposition, dermoscopy may also reveal vascular alterations, color variegations, follicle disturbances, and other features invisible to the unaided eye. The dermatoscope is now equivalent to the dermatologist's stethoscope, providing a clinician experienced in the technique with

Funding Sources: The study was supported in part by the Italian Ministry of Health (RF-2010-2316524).
Conflict of Interest: None.
[a] Skin Cancer Unit, Arcispedale Santa Maria Nuova, IRCCS, Viale Risorgimento 80, Reggio Emilia 42100, Italy;
[b] Department of Dermatology, Medical University of Graz, Auenbruggerplatz 8, 8036 Graz, Austria; [c] Unit of Dermatology, Arcispedale Santa Maria Nuova, IRCCS, Viale Risorgimento 80, Reggio Emilia 42100, Italy;
[d] Department of Dermatology and Venereology, Medical University of Modena and Reggio Emilia, Viale Risorgimento 80, Reggio Emilia 42100, Italy; [e] State Clinic of Dermatology, Hospital of Skin and Venereal Diseases, 124 Delfon Street, Thessaloniki 54643, Greece
* Corresponding author.
E-mail address: emlallas@gmail.com

Dermatol Clin 31 (2013) 679–694
http://dx.doi.org/10.1016/j.det.2013.06.008
0733-8635/13/$ – see front matter © 2013 Elsevier Inc. All rights reserved.

additional information on the morphology of skin lesions or eruptions.[4,5]

In 2006, a review article summarized existing evidence on dermoscopy in general dermatology, suggesting a 5-step diagnostic algorithm when evaluating nonpigmented skin lesions.[4] Since then, numerous articles describing dermoscopic characteristics of inflammatory and infectious diseases have been published, enriching the available knowledge on the topic. Most of the published data on dermoscopy of nonneoplastic dermatoses come from reports of 1 or few cases and, accordingly, additional research is required to clarify the role of dermoscopy in clinical diagnosis. However, in several fields, such as psoriasis and its differential diagnosis, or diagnosis of scabies, dermoscopic criteria have been tested in appropriately designed diagnostic accuracy studies, providing evidence that the technique significantly improves the clinical diagnostic performance.[6,7]

This article provides an up-to-date summary of data on dermoscopy in general dermatology to assist clinicians to use and apply the available knowledge in everyday practice.

DERMOSCOPY IS AN INTEGRAL PART OF CLINICAL EXAMINATION

Clinical examination is the mainstay of diagnosis in inflammatory and infectious diseases, because it represents a synthesis of several components. The patient's personal and family history, history of the current eruption, macroscopic characteristics, and distribution of the lesion(s) are some of the parameters to be considered and combined during the diagnostic approach of a given patient. Dermoscopy provides additional morphologic information at a submacroscopic level, completing the puzzle of clinical examination. Dermoscopic findings should therefore be interpreted within the overall clinical context of the patient.

SELECTION OF THE OPTIMAL EQUIPMENT

Vascular structures represent the most important group of criteria during dermoscopic evaluation of inflammatory skin diseases. Therefore, selection of equipment that preserves vessels' morphology and enhances their optimal visualization is considered essential. Standard hand-held dermatoscopes require direct contact of the optical lens with the skin surface, which may result in alteration or even disappearance of the morphology of the underlying vascular structures. Although using ultrasound gel and applying minimal pressure was considered the optimal practice

in the past, this problem was radically resolved by the introduction of the second-generation hand-held dermatoscopes, using polarized light and not requiring contact with the skin.

To acquire a dermoscopic image, a camera attached to a new-generation dermatoscope is preferable, compared with photographic equipment requiring direct contact of the dermoscopic lens and the skin surface.

DERMOSCOPY OF INFLAMMATORY SKIN DISEASES (INFLAMMOSCOPY)

Dermoscopic patterns of several inflammatory skin diseases have been described to date. This article summarizes the dermoscopic criteria of each disease and discusses their value in enhancing clinical diagnosis.

PSORIASIS

First described a decade ago, the dermoscopic pattern of plaque psoriasis (PP) was recently further investigated concerning its reliability for differentiating the disease from other erythematosquamous dermatoses (Fig. 1).[6,8–12]

Dotted and coiled (or glomerular) vessels represent the commonest dermoscopic feature of PP, typically being present in every psoriatic plaque. Detection of any other morphologic type of vessel should raise doubts about the diagnosis of PP. The term red globules has also been used to describe the same dermoscopic feature.[8] Distinction between dots and globules is based on the diameter of the structure (dots are smaller; ie, diameter up to 0.1 mm), and it is important in dermoscopy of melanocytic tumors. In psoriasis, both terms may be used, because the roundish vascular structures

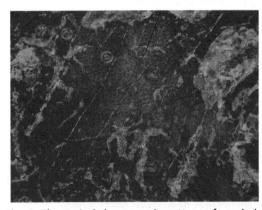

Fig. 1. The typical dermoscopic pattern of psoriasis, consisting of dotted vessels with a regular distribution within the lesion. White scales represent a common additional finding.

can be of various diameters, although they are usually of similar size within a given lesion. Under high magnifications (100–400×), the psoriatic vessels appear as dilated, elongated, and convoluted capillaries.[13] On histopathology, red dots correspond with the loops of vertically arranged vessels within the elongated dermal papillae.

Although red dots are the commonest criterion, their uniform or regular distribution within the lesion represents the dermoscopic hallmark of the disease, being particularly useful in differential diagnosis. As described later, dotted vessels may be detected in several inflammatory dermatoses. However, PP is characterized by a symmetric and homogenous arrangement of vessels all over the lesion, if not covered by thick superficial scales, which impede visualization of underlying vascular structures.[6] Even in the hyperkeratotic sites, scale removal reveals the characteristic vascular pattern of psoriasis, possibly together with tiny red blood drops, which can be characterized as the dermoscopic Auspitz sign.

Vázquez-López and colleagues[9] described a peculiar dermoscopic distribution of vessels in PP, the so-called red globular rings. This pattern was later shown to be a highly specific finding for the diagnosis of psoriasis, but nonsensitive.[6] Other types of vessel distribution are rare in PP.

Light red background color and white superficial scales represent two common additional dermoscopic criteria of PP. As shown by a recent diagnostic accuracy study, scale color is of particular value for differentiating PP among erythematosquamous dermatoses. Yellow scales were the strongest negative predictor of PP, suggesting the diagnosis of dermatitis.[6]

Limited data are available concerning the dermoscopic findings in other subtypes of the disease, such as scalp, inverse, or palmoplantar psoriasis.[14] However, in our experience, the dermoscopic pattern of the disease in specific body sites is similar to PP, with single variations in the amount of scaling, dependent on localization of lesions. In psoriatic balanitis and inverse psoriasis lesions that lack scaling, the typical vascular pattern of regularly distributed red dots is prominent under dermoscopic examination. In contrast, in scalp or palmoplantar psoriasis, the thick hyperkeratotic plaque surface does not allow visualization of the underlying vascular structures, which are highlighted after removal of the scales (**Fig. 2**).

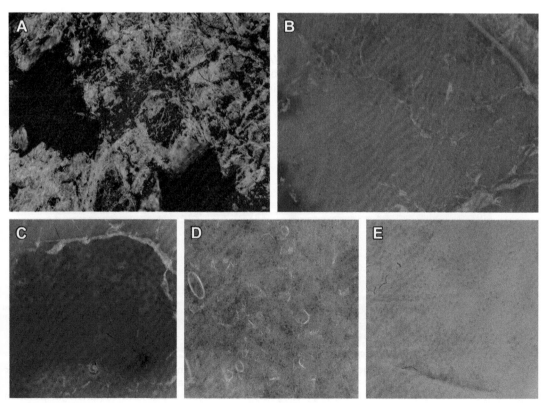

Fig. 2. Apart from variability in the degree of hyperkeratosis, the dermoscopic pattern of psoriasis is similar at specific sites, such as scalp (*A*), palms (*B*), gluteal region (*C*), face (*D*), and glans penis (*E*), comprising regularly distributed dotted vessels and white scales.

Beyond its well-documented value in differentiating psoriasis from other erythematosquamous inflammatory skin diseases, dermoscopy is now being used in monitoring patients under treatment with topical or systemic agents. **Fig. 3** shows the evolution of dermoscopic characteristics of psoriatic plaques in patients undergoing treatment with biologic agents. Apart from the assessment of treatment outcome, the additional morphologic information provided by dermoscopy might also be useful for early detection of disease recurrence, which would be highly relevant because the loss of drug effectiveness represents a major problem in the therapeutics of psoriasis.[15] Furthermore, the technique has been shown to detect steroid-induced skin atrophy at an early stage, by revealing characteristic linear vessels, before telangiectasias become clinically apparent.[16] In this context, application of dermoscopy in patients under long-term treatment with topical steroids is advisable.

DERMATITIS

Dermatitis encompasses several inflammatory entities with different causes and features and that share similar histopathologic characteristics. On dermoscopy, dermatitis usually shows red dots in a patchy distribution and fine, diffuse, yellowish scales.[6] No difference exists between the morphology of vessels of dermatitis and those of psoriasis. However, unlike psoriasis, the vessel distribution within dermatitis is not homogenous and symmetric (regular). Instead, the vessels are usually aggregated or clustered in some sites of a lesion and undetectable in others, forming an overall asymmetric, patchy pattern (**Fig. 4**).[6]

Superficial scaling is commonly detected in dermatitis lesions, and the fineness of the scale, its patchy or diffuse distribution, as well as its color, represent particularly useful clues for the recognition of the disease. In contrast with psoriasis and other erythematosquamous skin diseases, the scales in dermatitis have a yellow color either alone or in combination with white.[6] The term yellow clod sign has been described in cases of nummular eczema, and refers to the same dermoscopic characteristic (yellow scales).[17] Yellow scale color can be dermoscopically detected not only in cases of acute dermatitis but also in long-standing lesions. Although the dermoscopic pattern of each disease subtype has not been separately investigated, several case studies, including contact dermatitis, nummular eczema,

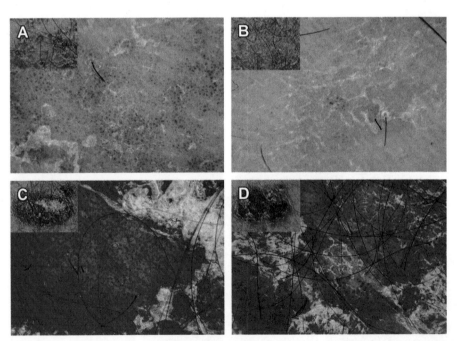

Fig. 3. Dermoscopy of a psoriatic plaque at baseline (*A*) and 1 month after initiation of treatment with a biologic agent (*B*). The involution of the morphologic characteristics of the disease is more evident by dermoscopy, compared with clinical examination alone, suggesting response to treatment. (*D*) The morphologic evolution of the lesion depicted in (*C*), 1 month after treatment initiation. Although the lesion clinically looks similar, dermoscopy reveals significant involution of dotted vessels. The dotted vessels have either disappeared or appear as punctate hemorrhagic spots.

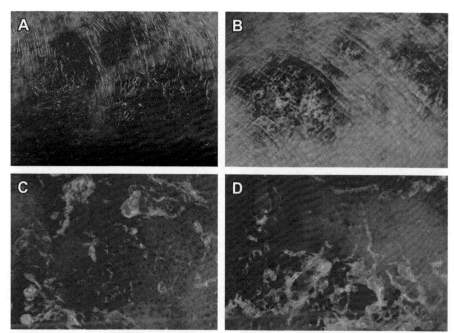

Fig. 4. Psoriasis (*A*) may be clinically indistinguishable from nummular eczema (*B*). Dermoscopy facilitates the differentiation between the two entities, by revealing the characteristic regular arrangement of dot vessels in psoriasis, in conjunction with white scales (*C*). In contrast, dermatitis is typified by yellow scales (and crusts), whereas the dotted vessels are distributed in a patchy pattern (*D*).

generalized dermatitis, chronic dermatitis, seborrheic dermatitis, and other subtypes, report on similar dermoscopic findings (as described earlier).[6,11,18] This is reasonable, because all entities included in the spectrum of dermatitis share common histopathologic characteristics.

LICHEN PLANUS

Although traditionally regarded as a clinical sign, present particularly in mucosal lesions, white crossing streaks (Wickham striae [WS]) are considered the dermoscopic hallmark of lichen planus (**Fig. 5**A).[8,10] WS are a constant dermoscopic finding in the various presentations of lichen planus. Given that WS have not been described in any other disease, the specificity of this dermoscopic criterion for the diagnosis of lichen planus is also considered to be high.[19] Vessels of mixed morphology (dotted and linear), usually distributed at the periphery of the lesion, represent additional dermoscopic findings of the disease.

PITYRIASIS ROSEA

A yellowish background color and peripheral whitish (collarette) scales are the most important dermoscopic features of pityriasis rosea (PR).[6,20,21] In addition, similar to psoriasis and dermatitis,

dotted vessels can be detected dermoscopically in most PR lesions, but the vascular pattern is usually irregular or patchy, lacking the characteristic regular distribution of psoriasis (see **Fig. 5**B).

PITYRIASIS RUBRA PILARIS

Round/oval yellowish areas surrounded by vessels of mixed morphology (ie, linear and dotted) have been reported in a single case of pityriasis rubra pilaris (PRP).[22] Although the dermoscopic pattern of the disease requires further investigation, this initial observation suggests at least that PRP lacks the characteristic pattern of psoriasis, which is the most common differential diagnosis.

POROKERATOSIS

Several studies suggest that the cornoid lamella, which represents the histopathologic hallmark of porokeratosis, is highlighted by dermoscopic examination as a well-defined, thin, white-yellow peripheral annular structure or rim (white track, resembling the outlines of a volcanic crater as observed from a high point).[23–26] The peripheral track may be hyperpigmented in disseminated superficial actinic porokeratosis.[24,27,28] The central part of the lesion(s) may exhibit a brownish pigmentation, dotted or linear vessels, or a structureless whitish area, depending on the disease

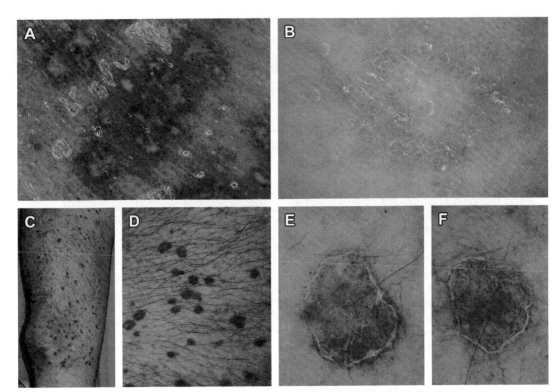

Fig. 5. (*A*) Detection of WS under dermoscopic examination allows a reliable diagnosis of lichen planus. Pityriasis rosea (*B*) is typified by the combination of a yellowish background and peripheral white scales, whereas dotted vessels (not regularly distributed) represent a common additional finding. Clinical evaluation of the eruption shown in (*C, D*) suggested the diagnosis of psoriasis. However, dermoscopy of all lesions revealed the characteristic whitish peripheral rim or white track of porokeratosis, clarifying a difficult clinical diagnosis (*E, F*).

subtype and the stage of progression. The diagnosis of porokeratosis is straightforward using dermoscopy, even in clinically atypical cases (see **Fig. 5**C, D).

GRANULOMATOUS SKIN DISEASES

This group encompasses several distinct inflammatory dermatoses that are histopathologically characterized by granuloma formation in the dermis. To date, the dermoscopic patterns of several of these conditions have been described. Based on the available data, it seems that dermoscopy enables visualization of dermal granulomas, facilitating diagnosis of granulomatous skin diseases.

SARCOIDOSIS, LUPUS VULGARIS, AND CUTANEOUS LEISHMANIASIS

Orange-yellow translucent globular or structureless areas in combination with linear vessels have been reported in cases of sarcoidosis and lupus vulgaris (LV) (**Fig. 6**A, B).[29,30] The former structures have been suggested to correspond with the underlying granulomas. Generalized erythema, yellow tears (follicular plugs), hyperkeratosis, central erosion/ulceration, and vascular structures (including commalike, linear irregular, dotted, and hairpin vessels) were the commonest dermoscopic findings in a series of cases of cutaneous leishmaniasis (CL).[31] Furthermore, at times a translucent orange-yellow color (as is more typical of sarcoidosis) is also present. Although it may currently be difficult to differentiate among these various granulomatous disorders using dermoscopy, the combination of orange-yellow globules or areas and linear vessels generally suggests a granulomatous skin disease.

GRANULOMA ANNULARE AND NECROBIOSIS LIPOIDICA

Granuloma annulare (GA) and necrobiosis lipoidica (NL) are the commonest granulomatous dermatoses. The dermoscopic criteria of the two entities have been described in case reports and recently in a study including a large number of patients (see **Fig. 6**C, D).[32–34] NL has a characteristic and repetitive pattern, typified by a prominent

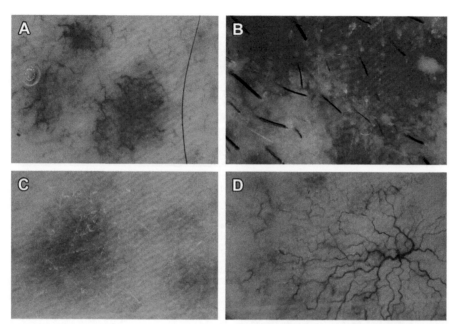

Fig. 6. Sarcoidosis (*A*) and LV (*B*) dermoscopically have orange-yellow areas, combined with linear branching vessels. The dermoscopic pattern of granuloma annulare (*C*) appears unspecific, often comprising dotted vessels and a red background. In contrast, necrobiosis lipoidica (*D*) typically has a prominent network of linear branching vessels on a yellowish background. In general, the combination of yellow color and linear branching vessels under dermoscopy strongly suggests a granulomatous skin disease.

network of linear arborizing vessels and a yellow background color. Ulcerations and yellow crusts represent the most common additional features. Considering that yellow-colored structures and linear vessels also characterize sarcoidosis or LV, the prominent vascular network of NL might represent the most valuable feature for discrimination of NL from the other diseases. In contrast, GA is characterized by a high variability of dermoscopic findings. Vessels may be dotted, short linear, or linear arborizing, whereas background color may present as a combination of red and white, as red only, white only, or occasionally as white and yellow. Pigmented structures may also be detected in a proportion of lesions. Although a predominant and repetitive dermoscopic pattern has not been identified, the observation that GA rarely has features of other granulomatous skin diseases, such as NL or sarcoidosis, might help clinicians rule out the other conditions.[34]

DISCOID LUPUS ERYTHEMATOSUS

A recent study described the dermoscopic criteria observed in different stages of progression of discoid lupus erythematosus (DLE), and investigated their histopathologic correlation.[35] Perifollicular whitish halo, follicular plugging, and white scales were the predominant features of early

lesions, whereas telangiectatic vessels, pigmentation structures, and whitish structureless areas characterized longer-standing lesions (**Fig. 7**A, B). This distinct dermoscopic pattern might be particularly useful for discriminating DLE from diseases sharing similar clinical characteristics, such as lupus pernio (cutaneous sarcoidosis) and LV (cutaneous tuberculosis). As described earlier, lupus pernio and LV lack the predominant follicular abnormalities of DLE, and have a characteristic pattern consisting of orange-yellow areas/globules and linear or branching vessels.[29,30]

ROSACEA

A characteristic dermoscopic vascular pattern of polygonal vessels has recently been described in erythematotelangiectatic rosacea (ER) (see **Fig. 7**C).[36] Intense vasodilatation, which represents a major pathophysiologic alteration of the disease, results in a characteristic morphologic pattern of dermoscopic vascular polygons. Telangiectasias may also be detected on chronically sun-damaged, atrophic facial skin, but they usually lack the characteristic polygonal arrangement. Because this polygonal pattern has not been reported in any other skin disease, it stands as a useful criterion for the diagnosis of ER. In addition to diagnostic purposes, considering that the

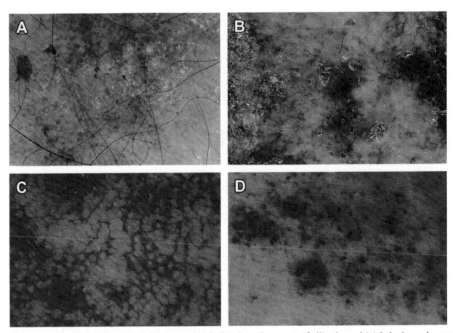

Fig. 7. Dermoscopy of early DLE on the face reveals follicular plugs, perifollicular whitish haloes, hyperkeratosis, and dilated (ie, dotted and coiled) vessels (*A*). In contrast, pigmentation structures, linear telangiectasias, and whitish structureless areas are common findings in longer-standing lesions (*B*). A specific arrangement of linear vessels in polygons typifies erythematotelangiectatic rosacea (*C*). Pigmented purpuric dermatoses are dermoscopically characterized by purpuric dots or globules and orange-brown areas of pigmentation (*D*).

vascular alterations of ER are clearly highlighted by dermoscopy, the technique might also be useful for following up the course of the disease and response to treatments. Additional dermoscopic findings of ER include follicular plugs, white scales, and features related to *Demodex*, namely *Demodex* tails and whitish amorphic follicular material.[37] However, the frequency of *Demodex*-related criteria was low in the largest reported series of cases to date.[36]

In papulopustular rosacea, dermoscopy might highlight clinically invisible pustules, providing a useful clue for differentiation from lupus erythematosus, but this is an initial observation requiring further investigation.

LICHEN SCLEROSUS AND MORPHEA

Dermoscopic characteristics of genital and extragenital lichen sclerosus (LS) in different stages of progression have been investigated.[38–40] White-yellow structureless areas represent the predominant dermoscopic feature of the disease in all locations. Linear vessels are most frequent in genital lesions, whereas early extragenital lesions commonly exhibit keratotic plugs. In addition, lesions of extragenital LS may also be surrounded by an erythematous halo, which represents a

marker of disease activity. In a descriptive study on the dermoscopic features of nontumoral dermatoses, linear vessels within a lilac ring have been reported to occur in morphea.[11] A study investigating the role of dermoscopy in differentiating between the two diseases reported that LS is typified by comedolike openings and whitish patches, whereas morphea exhibits fibrotic beams (correlating histopathologically with dermal sclerosis).[41]

URTICARIA AND URTICARIAL VASCULITIS

A red, reticular network of linear vessels has been described to characterize common urticaria dermoscopically.[42] This network sometimes surrounds areas devoid of vascular structures, which correspond with massive dermal edema. In contrast, urticarial vasculitis displays purpuric dots or globules on an orange-brown background.[43] Although neither the red lines of urticaria nor the purpuric dots of urticarial vasculitis are specific criteria, dermoscopic examination may facilitate the discrimination between the two entities, given that purpuric dots suggest an underlying vasculitis or capillaritis (pigmented purpura).

PIGMENTED PURPURIC DERMATOSES (CAPILLARITIS)

Five distinct entities are traditionally described with the term pigmented purpuric dermatoses (PPD): Schamberg disease, Majocchi purpura, eczematoid purpura of Doucas and Kapetanakis, lichen aureus, and pigmented purpuric lichenoid dermatitis of Gougerot-Blum. PPDs are typified dermoscopically by the combination of purpuric dots or globules and orange-brown areas of pigmentation (see **Fig. 7**D).[44,45] Although rare, a similar dermoscopic pattern has recently been described in patients with mycosis fungoides (MF), supporting previous evidence reporting a degree of clinical and histopathologic overlap between the two entities.[18] Considering the different biological course and management strategies for PPD and MF, lesions with these dermoscopic patterns should be evaluated thoroughly and managed appropriately.

DARIER DISEASE

Dermoscopy has been suggested as a useful additional tool for clinical recognition of Darier disease (DD), highlighting the characteristic pseudocomedones. The vascular pattern was reported as being variable, comprising erythema, dotted vessels, and linear vessels.[46]

MASTOCYTOSIS

Four dermoscopic patterns characterize cutaneous mastocytosis: light brown blot, pigment network, reticular vascular pattern, and yellow-orange blot.[47–49] There is an association between the dermoscopic pattern and the disease subtype. Light brown blot and pigment network were associated with maculopapular mastocytosis, yellow-orange blot with solitary mastocytoma, and a reticular vascular pattern was detected in all cases of telangiectasia macularis eruptiva perstans.[49] In addition, the reticular vascular pattern was associated with an increased risk of need for daily use of antimediator medication. Based on their results, Vano-Galvan and colleagues[49] suggested that, in combination with other variables, dermoscopy could provide additional help in the identification of patients at risk for more severe symptoms.

VASCULITIDES

Although purpura, which represents the hallmark of cutaneous vasculitides, is highlighted by dermoscopy, there is little evidence on the dermoscopic pattern of the diseases included in this group. In 4 reported cases of Henoch-Schönlein purpura, dermoscopy revealed irregularly shaped red patches with blurred borders, whereas reported findings of urticarial vasculitis are described earlier.[50]

Granuloma faciale is a rare, benign, chronic inflammatory skin disease that is classified in the group of vasculitides. It has to be differentiated clinically from sarcoidosis, DLE, LV, lymphoma, or basal cell carcinoma. Dilated follicular openings, perifollicular whitish haloes, pigmentation structures (whitish gray areas, brown dots/globules), follicular keratotic plugs, and elongated or linear branching vessels represent the commonest dermoscopic characteristics of the disease.[36,51,52] Elongated or linear branching vessels might adequately differentiate granuloma faciale from its clinical mimickers, apart from DLE, which can display similar findings.

MF

Although a neoplastic disease, MF is included in this article because it must be differentiated from several inflammatory skin disorders. A recent study investigated the dermoscopic patterns of early stage MF and chronic dermatitis, revealing significant differences between the two diseases.[18] In detail, in contrast with the dotted vessels observed in dermatitis, MF was typified by the combination of short linear vessels and orange-yellow areas (**Fig. 8**). A peculiar vascular structure consisting of a dotted and a linear component (spermatozoonlike structure) was detected in half of the MF cases. Considering that differentiation between the two entities is often problematic, requiring a series of biopsies, this observation is particularly relevant. In the clinical setting, during assessment of a chronic or recurrent eruption previously diagnosed as dermatitis, dermoscopic examination is expected to reveal dotted vessels, occasionally combined with white to yellowish scales.[6] Lesions under long-term treatment with topical steroids may represent an exception to this rule. Instead, when dermoscopy reveals linear vessels, the suspicion of MF increases strongly and, in this case, the patient's management should be adjusted accordingly.

DERMOSCOPY OF INFECTIOUS SKIN DISEASES (ENTOMODERMOSCOPY)

Specific dermoscopic patterns have been described for several infectious skin diseases, including those of viral, fungal, and parasitic origin.[53] The use of the new-generation dermatoscopes that do not require direct contact with the skin minimizes the risk of cross infection

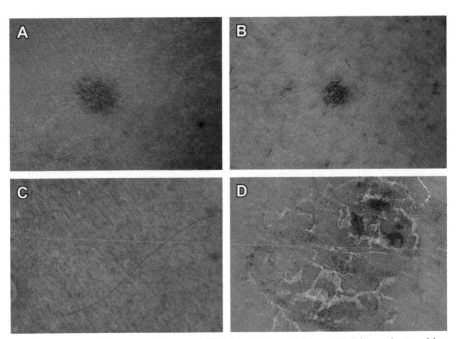

Fig. 8. Clinical differentiation between early stage MF (*A*) and chronic dermatitis (*B*) may be troublesome, often requiring sequential biopsies. Dermoscopy might enhance the clinical differential diagnosis, by revealing short linear vessels in MF (*C*), in contrast with the dotted vessels (in a patchy distribution) and white to yellow scales/crusts that typify dermatitis (*D*).

between patients. Although the risk of bacterial contamination using contact dermoscopy (with disinfection) is reported to be low, viral transmission might still represent a problem.[54]

SCABIES

The typical dermoscopic pattern of scabies was first described by Argenziano and colleagues[55] as consisting of small, dark brown, triangular structures located at the end of whitish structureless lines (curved or wavy), giving an appearance reminiscent of a delta-wing jet with contrail (**Fig. 9**A). On microscopy, the brown triangle corresponds with the pigmented anterior part of the mite, whereas the burrow of the mite correlates dermoscopically with the contrail feature. Since then, the value of dermoscopy in diagnosis of scabies has been extensively investigated in several studies.[7,56–59] The diagnostic accuracy of the technique was reported to be at least equal to traditional ex vivo microscopic examination (ie, skin scraping), whereas additional comparative advantages of dermoscopy include its noninvasiveness and lower requirements in terms of time, costs, and experience.[58,59] Dermoscopy has now replaced ex vivo microscopy as the routine method for diagnosis of scabies in several dermatology centers. In addition to its value for diagnosis, dermoscopy may also be useful in

treatment monitoring, heralding treatment success when dermoscopic jet-with-contrail features can no longer been detected.[60]

TUNGIASIS

Tungiasis is a skin infestation caused by the sand flea *Tunga penetrans* and is mainly endemic in the tropical regions of South and Central America, Africa, Asia, and the Caribbean islands. Because of its low incidence outside endemic areas, its clinical features are less recognized and diagnosis may be delayed. Dermoscopy of the disease typically reveals a white to flesh-colored to light brown nodule with a central targetoid brownish ring, which in turn surrounds a central (often blackish) pore.[61–67]

CUTANEOUS LARVA MIGRANS

Dermoscopy has been shown to facilitate the clinical recognition of larva migrans (creeping eruption), by revealing translucent, brownish, structureless areas in a segmental arrangement, corresponding with the body of the larva.[53,68]

PEDICULOSIS

Dermoscopy allows a rapid and reliable diagnosis of pediculosis by revealing the lice or the nits fixed to the hair shaft (see **Fig. 9**B).[5,69] Nits containing

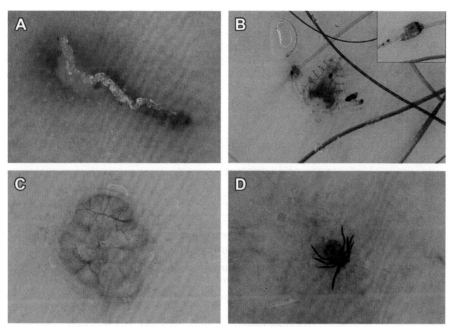

Fig. 9. Entomodermoscopy. Detection of the characteristic jet with contrail of scabies (*A*) permits a reliable clinical diagnosis without the need for microscopic confirmation. Dermoscopy allows a rapid and reliable diagnosis of pediculosis by revealing the lice (*B*) and/or the nits fixed to the hair shaft (*insert*). A central pore or umbilication and polylobular white to yellow amorphous structures, surrounded by linear or branching vessels, compose the stereotypic dermoscopic pattern of molluscum contagiosum (*C*). Dermoscopy highlights tick infestation on the skin (*D*), and can be also used for confirmation of its removal.

vital nymphs dermoscopically display ovoid brown structures, whereas the empty nits are translucent and typically show a plane and fissured free ending. This information is particularly useful for treatment monitoring, because dermoscopic detection of vital nits should lead to a continuation or modification of therapy.[69] In addition, dermoscopy has recently been shown to enable the discrimination between nits and the so-called pseudonits, such as hair casts from the debris of hair spray or gel. Pseudonits are not firmly attached to the hair shaft and appear dermoscopically as amorphous, whitish structures.[70]

TINEA NIGRA

Tinea nigra (TN) is a superficial mold infection that usually develops on the palms or soles as a gradually enlarging, irregular brown to black macule that can mimic melanocytic lesions, including acral melanoma. On dermoscopy, TN shows an overall reticulated pattern, consisting of superficial fine, wispy, light brown strands or pigmented spicules.[71,72] Dermoscopy can distinguish TN from acral melanocytic lesions, which are typified by parallel furrow and parallel ridge patterns.

HUMAN PAPILLOMAVIRUS INFECTIONS

Dermoscopy has been shown to be valuable in the diagnosis and treatment monitoring of human papillomavirus (HPV) infections. Common warts (verruca vulgaris) dermoscopically display multiple densely packed papillae, each containing a central red dot or loop, which is surrounded by a whitish halo. Hemorrhages represent a possible additional feature, appearing as irregularly distributed, small, red to black, tiny dots or streaks.[53,73,74] Dermoscopy of plantar warts typically reveals multiple prominent hemorrhages within a well-defined, yellowish papilliform surface in which skin lines are interrupted. This pattern is particularly useful for their discrimination from callus, which lacks blood spots, but instead displays central reddish to bluish structureless pigmentation.[75–77] Dermoscopy of plane warts typically reveals regularly distributed, tiny red dots on a light brown to yellow background. These findings allow differentiation from acne or folliculitis, which display a central white to yellow pore corresponding with the comedo or pus within the hair follicle opening.[53]

The dermoscopic pattern of genital warts was initially described as a mosaic pattern consisting of a white reticular network surrounding central small islands of unaffected mucosal skin.[53] More recently, a study including a large number of patients identified 4 different dermoscopic patterns that may also coexist in a single wart: unspecific, fingerlike, mosaic, and knoblike patterns.[78] Glomerular, hairpin/dotted, and glomerular/dotted vessel morphologies were detected. The investigators suggested a time-related alteration of dermoscopic characteristics, with early and clinically flat lesions showing a mosaic pattern dermoscopically, whereas more advanced and

Table 1
Dermoscopic criteria of inflammatory skin diseases

Disease	Dermoscopic Criteria
Psoriasis	Dotted vessels with regular distribution, white scales
Dermatitis	Dotted vessels with patchy distribution, yellow crusts/scales
Lichen planus	WS, peripheral dotted/linear vessels
PR	Yellowish background, peripheral white scales, dotted vessels with patchy distribution
PRP	Yellowish areas, dotted and linear vessels with patchy or peripheral distribution
Sarcoidosis	Orange-yellow globules or areas, linear vessels
GA	Dotted, linear, or dotted/linear vessels; white, red, or yellow background
NL	Prominent network of linear arborizing vessels and a yellow background color
DLE	Early lesions: perifollicular whitish halo, follicular plugging, and white scales Late lesions: telangiectasias, pigmentation structures, and whitish structureless areas
Rosacea	Erythematotelangiectatic type: polygonal vessels Papulopustular type: follicular plugs, follicular pustules, polygonal vessels
LS	Genital lesions: white/yellowish structureless areas, linear vessels Extragenital lesions: white/yellowish structureless areas, yellowish keratotic plugs (pseudocomedones)
Morphea	Whitish fibrotic beams, linear vessels
Urticaria	Network of linear vessels surrounding avascular areas
Urticarial vasculitis	Purpuric dots or globules, orange-brown background
PPD	Purpuric dots or globules, orange-brown background
Porokeratosis	White-yellow or brownish peripheral annular structure. In the center, brownish pigmentation, dotted/linear vessels, or structureless whitish areas
DD	Pseudocomedones, erythema, dotted/linear vessels
Mastocytosis	Light brown blot, pigment network, reticular vascular pattern, or yellow-orange blot
Henoch-Schönlein purpura	Irregularly shaped red patches with blurred borders
Granuloma faciale	Dilated follicular openings, perifollicular whitish haloes, pigmentation structures, follicular keratotic plugs, elongated or linear branching vessels
Livedo reticularis	Linear vessels with a regular distribution[11]
Erythema multiforme	Linear vessels peripherally, bluish patches in the center[11]
Sweet syndrome	Structureless bluish patches[11]
MF	Short linear vessels, orange-yellow areas, spermatozoalike structures

raised or papillomatous warts frequently had a fingerlike or knoblike pattern. In summary, dermoscopy might help to differentiate early genital warts from other clinically similar diseases, such as seborrheic keratosis (SK), vestibular papillae (VP), and pearly penile papules (PPP).[78–80] The dermoscopic criteria of SK are well known and were not present in the reported cases. VP dermoscopically display multiple transparent and cylindrical projections with separate bases, containing irregular vascular structures.[79] PPP appear as whitish pink cobblestone or grapelike structures with central delicate vessels.[80]

MOLLUSCUM CONTAGIOSUM

Molluscum contagiosum is caused by a poxvirus infection and has a characteristic dermoscopic pattern that may facilitate its clinical recognition in selected cases. Dermoscopy is especially useful in detecting the infection before the development of numerous lesions, in pediatric dermatology, or in immunosuppressed patients who may display unusual clinical manifestations. A central pore or umbilication in conjunction with polylobular white to yellow amorphous structures surrounded by linear or branched vessels (red corona) is the stereotypic dermoscopic pattern of the disease (see **Fig. 9C**).[81–84]

TICK BITES

Dermoscopy has been reported to highlight tick infestation by enabling the visualization of the tick's anterior legs protruding from the surface of the skin; a brown to gray translucent shield with pigmented streaks corresponds with the tick's body (see **Fig. 9D**). Following the removal of the tick, detection of brown to black to gray areas of pigmentation by dermoscopy indicates incomplete removal.[85,86]

Tables 1 and **2** summarize the commonest dermoscopic criteria of inflammatory and infectious skin diseases, respectively.

Table 2
Dermoscopic criteria of infectious skin diseases

Disease	Dermoscopic Criteria
LV	Orange-yellow globules or areas, linear vessels
Leishmaniasis	Orange-yellow globules or areas, linear vessels, erythema, follicular plugs, hyperkeratosis, central ulceration
Scabies	Jet-with-contrail structure
Tungiasis	White to light brown color, targetoid brownish ring surrounding a black central pore
Cutaneous larva migrans	Translucent brownish structureless areas in a segmental arrangement
Pediculosis	The lice, ovoid brownish structures (nits with vital nymphs), ovoid translucent structures (empty nits)
TN	Reticulated pattern, consisting of superficial fine, wispy, light brown strands or pigmented spicules
HPV infections	Common warts: multiple densely packed papillae with a central red dot or loop, surrounded by a whitish halo. Hemorrhages (small red to black dots or streaks) may also be present Plantar warts: prominent hemorrhages within a well-defined, yellow papilliform surface in which skin lines are interrupted Plane warts: regularly distributed red dots, light brown to yellow background Genital warts: mosaic (early/flat lesions), fingerlike, and knoblike pattern (raised/papillomatous lesions), unspecific pattern
Molluscum contagiosum	Central pore or umbilication, white to yellow amorphous structures, peripheral linear or branching vessels (red corona)
Tick bites	Visualization of the anterior legs protruding from the skin surface, brown to gray translucent shield
Spider leg spines	Small black spines[87]

SUMMARY

In addition to its well-established value in the diagnosis of skin tumors, dermoscopy is increasingly used in other fields of dermatology, expanding its spectrum of application. With novel data being increasingly gathered, the dermatoscope is gradually becoming equivalent to the dermatologist's stethoscope, acquiring an irreplaceable role in clinical diagnosis.

REFERENCES

1. Argenziano G, Puig S, Zalaudek I, et al. Dermoscopy improves accuracy of primary care physicians to triage lesions suggestive of skin cancer. J Clin Oncol 2006;24:1877–82.
2. Argenziano G, Albertini G, Castagnetti F, et al. Early diagnosis of melanoma: what is the impact of dermoscopy? Dermatol Ther 2012;25:403–9.
3. Zalaudek I, Kreusch J, Giacomel J, et al. How to diagnose nonpigmented skin tumors: a review of vascular structures seen with dermoscopy: part II. Nonmelanocytic skin tumors. J Am Acad Dermatol 2010;63:377–86 [quiz: 387–8].
4. Zalaudek I, Argenziano G, Di Stefani A, et al. Dermoscopy in general dermatology. Dermatology 2006;212:7–18.
5. Micali G, Lacarrubba F, Massimino D, et al. Dermatoscopy: alternative uses in daily clinical practice. J Am Acad Dermatol 2011;64:1135–46.
6. Lallas A, Kyrgidis A, Tzellos TG, et al. Accuracy of dermoscopic criteria for the diagnosis of psoriasis, dermatitis, lichen planus and pityriasis rosea. Br J Dermatol 2012;166:1198–205.
7. Dupuy A, Dehen L, Bourrat E, et al. Accuracy of standard dermoscopy for diagnosing scabies. J Am Acad Dermatol 2007;56:53–62.
8. Vázquez-López F, Manjón-Haces JA, Maldonado-Seral C, et al. Dermoscopic features of plaque psoriasis and lichen planus: new observations. Dermatology 2003;207:151–6.
9. Vázquez-López F, Zaballos P, Fueyo-Casado A, et al. A dermoscopy subpattern of plaque-type psoriasis: red globular rings. Arch Dermatol 2007; 143:1612.
10. Zalaudek I, Argenziano G. Dermoscopy subpatterns of inflammatory skin disorders. Arch Dermatol 2006;142:808.
11. Vázquez-López F, Kreusch J, Marghoob AA. Dermoscopic semiology: further insights into vascular features by screening a large spectrum of nontumoral skin lesions. Br J Dermatol 2004;150:226–31.
12. Lallas A, Apalla Z, Tzellos T, et al. Dermoscopy in clinically atypical psoriasis. J Dermatol Case Rep 2012;6. http://dx.doi.org/10.3315/jdcr.2012.1102.
13. De Angelis R, Bugatti L, Del Medico P, et al. Video-capillaroscopic findings in the microcirculation of the psoriatic plaque. Dermatology 2002;204:236–9.
14. Kim GW, Jung HJ, Ko HC, et al. Dermoscopy can be useful in differentiating scalp psoriasis from seborrhoeic dermatitis. Br J Dermatol 2011;164: 652–6.
15. Gniadecki R, Kragballe K, Dam TN, et al. Comparison of drug survival rates for adalimumab, etanercept and infliximab in patients with psoriasis vulgaris. Br J Dermatol 2011;164:1091–6.
16. Vázquez-López F, Marghoob AA. Dermoscopic assessment of long-term topical therapies with potent steroids in chronic psoriasis. J Am Acad Dermatol 2004;51:811–3.
17. Navarini AA, Feldmeyer L, Töndury B, et al. The yellow clod sign. Arch Dermatol 2011;147:1350.
18. Lallas A, Apalla Z, Lefaki I, et al. Dermoscopy of early stage mycosis fungoides. J Eur Acad Dermatol Venereol 2013;27:617–21.
19. Vázquez-López F, Palacios-Garcia L, Gomez-Diez S, et al. Dermoscopy for discriminating between lichenoid sarcoidosis and lichen planus. Arch Dermatol 2011;147:1130.
20. Chuh AA. Collarette scaling in pityriasis rosea demonstrated by digital epiluminescence dermatoscopy. Australas J Dermatol 2001;42:288–90.
21. Chuh AA. The use of digital epiluminescence dermatoscopy to identify peripheral scaling in pityriasis rosea. Comput Med Imaging Graph 2002;26: 129–34.
22. Lallas A, Apalla Z, Karteridou A, et al. Photoletter to the editor: dermoscopy for discriminating between pityriasis rubra pilaris and psoriasis. J Dermatol Case Rep 2013;7:20–2.
23. Delfino M, Argenziano G, Nino M. Dermoscopy for the diagnosis of porokeratosis. J Eur Acad Dermatol Venereol 2004;18:194–5.
24. Zaballos P, Puig S, Malvehy J. Dermoscopy of disseminated superficial actinic porokeratosis. Arch Dermatol 2004;140:1410.
25. Pizzichetta MA, Canzonieri V, Massone C, et al. Clinical and dermoscopic features of porokeratosis of Mibelli. Arch Dermatol 2009;145:91–2.
26. Uhara H, Kamijo F, Okuyama R, et al. Open pores with plugs in porokeratosis clearly visualized with the dermoscopic furrow ink test: report of 3 cases. Arch Dermatol 2011;147:866–8.
27. Oiso N, Kawada A. Dermoscopic features in disseminated superficial actinic porokeratosis. Eur J Dermatol 2011;21:439–40.
28. Panasiti V, Rossi M, Curzio M, et al. Disseminated superficial actinic porokeratosis diagnosed by dermoscopy. Int J Dermatol 2008;47:308–10.
29. Pellicano R, Tiodorovic-Zivkovic D, Gourhant JY, et al. Dermoscopy of cutaneous sarcoidosis. Dermatology 2010;221:51–4.

30. Brasiello M, Zalaudek I, Ferrara G, et al. Lupus vulgaris: a new look at an old symptom- the lupoma observed with dermoscopy. Dermatology 2009; 218:172–4.

31. Llambrich A, Zaballos P, Terrasa F, et al. Dermoscopy of cutaneous leishmaniasis. Br J Dermatol 2009;160:756–61.

32. Micali G, Lacarrubba F. Possible applications of videodermatoscopy beyond pigmented lesions. Int J Dermatol 2003;42:430–3.

33. Bakos RM, Cartell A, Bakos L. Dermatoscopy of early-onset necrobiosis lipoidica. J Am Acad Dermatol 2012;66:e143–4.

34. Lallas A, Zaballos P, Zalaudek I, et al. Dermoscopic patterns of granuloma annulare and necrobiosis lipoidica. Clin Exp Dermatol 2013;38:424–9.

35. Lallas A, Apalla Z, Lefaki I, et al. Dermoscopy of discoid lupus erythematosus. Br J Dermatol 2012; 168:284–8.

36. Lallas A, Argenziano G, Apalla Z, et al. Dermoscopic patterns of common facial inflammatory skin diseases. J Eur Acad Dermatol Venereol 2013. http://dx.doi.org/10.1111/jdv.12146. [Epub ahead of print].

37. Segal R, Mimouni D, Feuerman H, et al. Dermoscopy as a diagnostic tool in demodicidosis. Int J Dermatol 2010;49:1018–23.

38. Larre Borges A, Tiodorovic-Zivkovic D, Lallas A, et al. Clinical, dermoscopic and histopathologic features of genital and extragenital lichen sclerosus. J Eur Acad Dermatol Venereol 2012. http://dx.doi.org/10.1111/j.1468-3083.2012.04595.x. [Epub ahead of print].

39. Garrido-Ríos AA, Alvarez-Garrido H, Sanz-Muñoz C, et al. Dermoscopy of extragenital lichen sclerosus. Arch Dermatol 2009;145:1468.

40. Apalla Z, Lallas A. Dermoscopy of atypical lichen sclerosus involving the tongue. J Dermatol Case Rep 2012;6. http://dx.doi.org/10.3315/jdcr.2012. 1100.

41. Shim WH, Jwa SW, Song M, et al. Diagnostic usefulness of dermatoscopy in differentiating lichen sclerous et atrophicus from morphea. J Am Acad Dermatol 2012;66:690–1.

42. Vázquez-López F, Fueyo A, Sanchez-Martin J, et al. Dermoscopy for the screening of common urticaria and urticaria vasculitis. Arch Dermatol 2008;144: 568.

43. Vázquez-López F, Maldonado-Seral C, Soler-Sánchez T, et al. Surface microscopy for discriminating between common urticaria and urticarial vasculitis. Rheumatology (Oxford) 2003; 42:1079–82.

44. Zaballos P, Puig S, Malvehy J. Dermoscopy of pigmented purpuric dermatoses (lichen aureus): a useful tool for clinical diagnosis. Arch Dermatol 2004;140:1290–1.

45. Zalaudek I, Ferrara G, Brongo S, et al. Atypical clinical presentation of pigmented purpuric dermatosis. J Dtsch Dermatol Ges 2006;4:138–40 [in German].

46. Vázquez-López F, Lopez-Escobar M, Maldonado-Seral C, et al. The handheld dermoscope improves the recognition of giant pseudocomedones in Darier's disease. J Am Acad Dermatol 2004;50:454–5.

47. Arpaia N, Cassano N, Vena GA. Lessons on dermoscopy: pigment network in nonmelanocytic lesions. Dermatol Surg 2004;30:929–30.

48. Akay BN, Kittler H, Sanli H, et al. Dermatoscopic findings of cutaneous mastocytosis. Dermatology 2009;218:226–30.

49. Vano-Galvan S, Alvarez-Twose I, De las Heras E, et al. Dermoscopic features of skin lesions in patients with mastocytosis. Arch Dermatol 2011;147: 932–40.

50. Ohnishi T, Nagayama T, Morita T, et al. Angioma serpiginosum: a report of 2 cases identified using epiluminescence microscopy. Arch Dermatol 1999;135:1366–8.

51. Lallas A, Sidiropoulos T, Lefaki I, et al. Dermoscopy of granuloma faciale. J Dermatol Case Rep 2012;6: 59–60.

52. Caldarola G, Zalaudek I, Argenziano G, et al. Granuloma faciale: a case report on long-term treatment with topical tacrolimus and dermoscopic aspects. Dermatol Ther 2011;24:508–11.

53. Zalaudek I, Giacomel J, Cabo H, et al. Entodermoscopy: a new tool for diagnosing skin infections and infestations. Dermatology 2008;216:14–23.

54. Penso-Assathiany D, Gheit T, Prétet JL, et al. Presence and persistence of human papillomavirus types 1, 2, 3, 4, 27, and 57 on dermoscope before and after examination of plantar warts and after cleaning. J Am Acad Dermatol 2013;68:185–6.

55. Argenziano G, Fabbrocini G, Delfino M. Epiluminescence microscopy. A new approach to in vivo detection of *Sarcoptes scabiei*. Arch Dermatol 1997;133:751–3.

56. Bauer J, Blum A, Sönnichsen K, et al. Nodular scabies detected by computed dermatoscopy. Dermatology 2001;203:190–1.

57. Prins C, Stucki L, French L, et al. Dermoscopy for the in vivo detection of *Sarcoptes scabiei*. Dermatology 2004;208:241–3.

58. Walter B, Heukelbach J, Fengler G, et al. Comparison of dermoscopy, skin scraping, and the adhesive tape test for the diagnosis of scabies in a resource-poor setting. Arch Dermatol 2011;147: 468–73.

59. Park JH, Kim CW, Kim SS. The diagnostic accuracy of dermoscopy for scabies. Ann Dermatol 2012;24: 194.

60. Hamm H, Beiteke U, Höger PH, et al. Treatment of scabies with 5% permethrin cream: results of a

German multicenter study. J Dtsch Dermatol Ges 2006;4:407–13.

61. Bauer J, Forschner A, Garbe C, et al. Dermoscopy of tungiasis. Arch Dermatol 2004;140:761–3.

62. Bauer J, Forschner A, Garbe C, et al. Variability of dermoscopic features of tungiasis. Arch Dermatol 2005;141:643–4.

63. Di Stefani A, Rudolph CM, Hofmann-Wellenhof R, et al. An additional dermoscopic feature of tungiasis. Arch Dermatol 2005;141:1045–6.

64. Cabrera R, Daza F. Tungiasis: eggs seen with dermoscopy. Br J Dermatol 2007;158:635–6.

65. Gibbs SS. The diagnosis and treatment of tungiasis. Br J Dermatol 2008;159:981.

66. Cabrera R, Daza F. Dermoscopy in the diagnosis of tungiasis. Br J Dermatol 2009;160:1136–7.

67. Dunn R, Asher R, Bowling J. Dermoscopy: ex vivo visualization of fleas head and bag of eggs confirms the diagnosis of tungiasis. Australas J Dermatol 2011;53:120–2.

68. Veraldi S, Schianchi R, Carrera C. Epiluminescence microscopy in cutaneous larva migrans. Acta Derm Venereol 2000;80:233.

69. Di Stefani A, Hofmann-Wellenhof R, Zalaudek I. Dermoscopy for diagnosis and treatment monitoring of pediculosis capitis. J Am Acad Dermatol 2006;54:909–11.

70. Zalaudek I, Argenziano G. Dermoscopy of nits and pseudonits. N Engl J Med 2012;367:1741.

71. Piliouras P, Allison S, Rosendahl C, et al. Dermoscopy improves diagnosis of tinea nigra: a study of 50 cases. Australas J Dermatol 2011;52:191–4.

72. Gupta G, Burden AD, Shankland GS, et al. Tinea nigra secondary to *Exophiala werneckii* responding to itraconazole. Br J Dermatol 1997;137:483–4.

73. Tanioka M, Nakagawa Y, Maruta N, et al. Pigmented wart due to human papilloma virus type 60 showing parallel ridge pattern in dermoscopy. Eur J Dermatol 2009;19:643–4.

74. Yoong C, Di Stefani A, Hofmann-Wellenhof R, et al. Unusual clinical and dermoscopic presentation of a wart. Australas J Dermatol 2009;50:228–9.

75. Lee DY, Park JH, Lee JH, et al. The use of dermoscopy for the diagnosis of plantar wart. J Eur Acad Dermatol Venereol 2009;23:726–7.

76. Dalmau J, Abellaneda C, Puig S, et al. Acral melanoma simulating warts: dermoscopic clues to prevent missing a melanoma. Dermatol Surg 2006; 32:1072–8.

77. Bae JM, Kang H, Kim HO, et al. Differential diagnosis of plantar wart from corn, callus and healed wart with the aid of dermoscopy. Br J Dermatol 2009;160:220–2.

78. Dong H, Shu D, Campbell TM, et al. Dermatoscopy of genital warts. J Am Acad Dermatol 2011;64:859–64.

79. Kim SH, Seo SH, Ko HC, et al. The use of dermatoscopy to differentiate vestibular papillae, a normal variant of the female external genitalia, from condyloma acuminata. J Am Acad Dermatol 2009;60: 353–5.

80. Watanabe T, Yoshida Y, Yamamoto O. Differential diagnosis of pearly penile papules and penile condyloma acuminatum by dermoscopy. Eur J Dermatol 2010;20:414–5.

81. Morales A, Puig S, Malvehy J, et al. Dermoscopy of molluscum contagiosum. Arch Dermatol 2005;141: 1644.

82. Zaballos P, Ara M, Puig S, et al. Dermoscopy of molluscum contagiosum: a useful tool for clinical diagnosis in adulthood. J Eur Acad Dermatol Venereol 2006;20:482–3.

83. Ianhez M, Cestari Sda C, Enokihara MY, et al. Dermoscopic patterns of molluscum contagiosum: a study of 211 lesions confirmed by histopathology. An Bras Dermatol 2011;86:74–9.

84. Alfaro-Castellón P, Mejía-Rodríguez SA, Valencia-Herrera A, et al. Dermoscopy distinction of eruptive vellus hair cysts with molluscum contagiosum and acne lesions. Pediatr Dermatol 2012;29:772–3.

85. Oiso N, Kawara S, Yano Y, et al. Diagnostic effectiveness of dermoscopy for tick bite. J Eur Acad Dermatol Venereol 2010;24:231–2.

86. Matsuda M, Oiso N, Yano Y, et al. Dermoscopy for tick bite: reconfirmation of the usefulness for the initial diagnosis. Case Rep Dermatol 2011;3:94–7.

87. Bakos RM, Rezende RL, Bakos L, et al. Spider spines detected by dermoscopy. Arch Dermatol 2006;142:1517–8.

Hair Shafts in Trichoscopy
Clues for Diagnosis of Hair and Scalp Diseases

Lidia Rudnicka, MD, PhD[a,b,c], Adriana Rakowska, MD, PhD[a],
Marta Kerzeja, MD[a], Małgorzata Olszewska, MD, PhD[c,]*

KEYWORDS

- Alopecia areata • Dermoscopy • Dermatoscopy • Flame hairs • Trichoptilosis
- Trichorrhexis nodosa • Trichoscopy • Trichotillomania

KEY POINTS

- Trichoscopy allows analysis of the structure and size of growing hair shafts.
- With trichoscopy is possible to diagnose most genetic hair shaft defects without the need of pulling hairs for light microscopic evaluation.
- Hair shaft structure abnormalities may provide diagnostic clues for multiple causes of hair loss beyond genetic hair shaft disorders.

Trichoscopy is dermoscopy of hair and scalp.[1,2] Among other diagnostic functions, trichoscopy allows analysis of the structure and size of hair shafts. This function has two major applications in clinical practice. First, trichoscopy may replace light microscopy in diagnosing patients with genetic hair shaft defects.[3,4] Second, the structure of hair shafts may provide a clue for diagnosing multiple conditions beyond classic hair shaft abnormalities.[1] In these disorders, changes in hair shaft structure is secondary to an underlying, acquired pathologic process. Examples of such diseases are tinea capitis, alopecia areata, and trichotillomania.[3]

NORMAL HAIRS

A normal terminal hair is uniform in thickness and color throughout its length.[5,6] An individual may have hair shafts that differ from each other by color and by thickness. Presence of diversely pigmented hairs is a normal finding in graying persons. In children and young adults, simultaneous presence of dark and gray hairs is rare and may be indicative of vitiligo, ectodermal dysplasia, or another other cause of premature graying.[7]

The thickness of normal hairs is usually more than 55 μm. Hair shaft thickness may be roughly estimated with a handheld dermoscope (thin, normal, thick). Some digital dermoscopes (videodermoscopy) allow detailed assessment of hair shaft thickness in micrometers.[1] Precise measurement of hair shaft thickness is not essential for clinical diagnosis, but may be useful for monitoring treatment efficacy,[8] especially in clinical trials.[1]

Terminal hairs may have a medulla that is continuous, interrupted, fragmented, or absent.[9] The impression of a fragmented medulla results from a thick medulla separated by thin medulla that is not visible by trichoscopy. The thickness

Authors have no conflict of interest.
a Department of Dermatology, CSK MSW, Woloska 137, Warsaw 02-507, Poland; b Department of Neuropeptides, Mossakowski Medical Research Centre, Polish Academy of Sciences, Pawinskiego 5, Warsaw 02-106, Poland; c Department of Dermatology, Medical University of Warsaw, Koszykowa 82A, Warsaw 02-008, Poland
* Corresponding author. Department of Dermatology, Medical University of Warsaw, Koszykowa 82A, Warsaw 02-008, Poland.
E-mail address: malgorzata.olszewska@wum.edu.pl

Dermatol Clin 31 (2013) 695–708
http://dx.doi.org/10.1016/j.det.2013.06.007
0733-8635/13/$ – see front matter © 2013 Published by Elsevier Inc.

or presence of a medulla has no influence on hair strength.[9]

Up to 10% of normal human scalp hairs are vellus hairs.[5,6] These are hairs that are less than 3 mm long and less than 30 μm thick. An increased proportion of vellus hairs may be present in androgenetic alopecia and in long-lasting alopecia areata. Vellus hairs are more visible in patients with dark skin phototypes.[1] They have to be differentiated from short, healthy regrowing hairs (**Table 1**). Variants of normal hairs are presented in **Fig. 1**.

CLASSIFICATION OF HAIR SHAFT ABNORMALITIES IN TRICHOSCOPY

The authors propose a classification of hair shaft features observed in trichoscopy (**Fig. 2**). The proposed classification adopts a structure-based approach, also observed in light microscopy,[10] wherever applicable. It distinguishes the following groups of hair shaft abnormalities observed by trichoscopy: (1) hair shafts with fractures, (2) hair narrowings, (3) hairs with node-like structures, (4) curls and twists, (5) bands, and (6) short hairs. We consider hairs as short hairs when the entire hair shaft is visible in one field of view of a dermoscope (10- to 20-fold magnification). These hairs are usually less than 10 mm long.

Many types of hair shaft abnormalities may provide clues for differential diagnosis of inherited and acquired causes of hair loss (**Table 2**). Examples of hair shaft abnormalities are presented in **Fig. 3**.

COMMON HAIR SHAFT ABNORMALITIES IN TRICHOSCOPY
Exclamation Mark Hairs

Exclamation mark hairs (exclamation point hairs) are hairs with thin proximal ends and significantly thicker distal ends. Often, the proximal end is hypopigmented, whereas the distal end appears hyperpigmented.[11] Exclamation mark hairs, which are 1 to 3 cm long, may be observed with the naked eye and are a well-known feature of alopecia areata.[12–14] With a dermoscope, it is possible to observe exclamation mark hairs that are significantly shorter, usually 1 to 5 mm.[15] Thus, some investigators call them micro-exclamation mark hairs.[11]

Exclamation mark hairs are observed in trichoscopy in 30% to 44% of patients with alopecia areata.[16] Lacarrubba and colleagues[17] and Inui and colleagues[18] identified exclamation mark hairs as markers of disease activity in these patients. It was suggested that presence of exclamation mark hairs may be a positive predictive marker for response to intralesional triamcinolone treatment[19] and that the presence of exclamation mark hairs withdraws after successful therapy of alopecia areata.[20]

Exclamation mark hairs may also be observed in other hair diseases, such as trichotillomania,[3,21,22] chemotherapy-induced alopecia,[23] and anagen effluvium in the course of severe intoxication.[24]

Tapered Hairs

Tapered hairs are very elongated exclamation mark hairs.[25,26] In these hairs, the proximal end is thinned and the distal end is outside of the field of view of the dermoscope. Occasionally, these are full-length terminal hairs. Hair coudability is sometimes used to describe this phenomenon. The interesting story behind the term hair coudability was recently described by Shuster.[23] The clinical associations of tapered hairs are analogous to those of exclamation mark hairs. However, in tapered hairs the hair shaft thickens slowly over time, corresponding to a less prominent activity of disease in alopecia areata. Tapered hairs may be also observed in patients with malnutrition, blood loss, and chronic intoxication.[1]

Pohl-Pinkus Constrictions and Monilethrix-like Hairs

The phenomenon widely known as Pohl-Pinkus constriction was first described by the German dermatologist Joseph Pohl-Pincus (with a c, not a k) in 1885. The mistake in the name was made for the first time in 1906, repeated by many other authors since then, and is now the accepted term.

The term refers to zones of decreased hair thickness within the hair shaft. These constrictions occur most commonly when the metabolic and mitotic activity of the follicle are rapidly and repeatedly suppressed by an external or internal factor. Various chronic, acquired, and congenital

Table 1
Trichoscopy of new regrowing hairs versus vellus hairs

New Regrowing Hairs	Vellus Hairs
Short (usually 3–5 mm)	Very short (below 3 mm)
Thin (below 50 μm)	Very thin (below 30 μm)
Normally pigmented	Hypopigmented
Upright position	Wavy shape
Firm appearance	Weak appearance
Pointed distal end	Blurred distal end

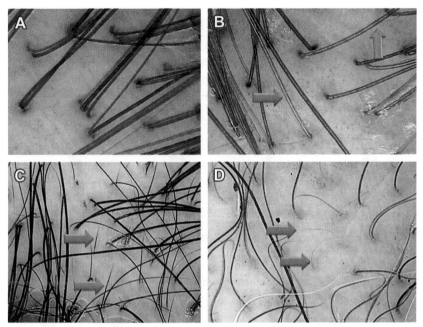

Fig. 1. Variants of normal hair shafts in trichoscopy: normal terminal hairs (*A*), hairs with a continuous medulla (*blue arrow*) and fragmented medulla (*orange arrow*, *B*), upright regrowing hairs (*blue arrows*, *C*) and vellus hairs (*blue arrows*, *D*).

diseases have been associated with Pohl-Pinkus constrictions. This abnormality was observed in alopecia areata, chemotherapy-induced alopecia, cicatricial alopecias, following severe general infections, after major blood loss, in severe nutrient deficiencies, after interferon alpha 2c therapy, and in localized hereditary hypotrichosis.[1] Hairs with multiple Pohl-Pinkus constrictions have a monilethrix-like appearance and they should be differentiated from true monilethrix. Mane and colleagues[27] were the first to show that Pohl-Pinkus constrictions may be observed well by trichoscopy, without the need to pull hair for light microscopic examination.

Comma Hairs and Corkscrew Hairs

Slowinska and colleagues[28] described comma hairs (short, bent, C-shaped hairs), as a feature of tinea capitis. These findings were confirmed in later studies.[29–33] Comma hairs seem to be specific dermoscopic findings of dermatophyte infection of the scalp, regardless of the etiologic agent. We have not observed comma hairs in a patient with a scalp infection caused by *Alternaria*, a genus of the ascomycete fungi.[34] Usually multiple comma hairs may be observed in a field of view of a dermoscope. A single hair that bends to form a C-like shape is not sufficient for a suspicion of tinea capitis.

Comma hairs with multiple twists form corkscrew-like structures. These corkscrew hairs have been initially described in African American patients with tinea capitis,[30] but also may be observed in white patients. They disappear on successful therapy of the dermatophyte infection.[35]

These corkscrew hairs should not be confused with corkscrew hairs observed by light microscopy in children with ectodermal dysplasia[36–38] and deficiency of vitamin C.[39,40]

Trichorrhexis Nodosa

In trichorrhexis nodosa, a short segment of hair shaft splits longitudinally into numerous small fibers in one or more areas. The outer fibers bulge out and cause a segmental increase in hair diameter. Macroscopically these segments may reassemble nodules located along the hair shaft. Hairs eventually break at these points leaving brush-like ends.[41]

There are several inherited and acquired conditions associated with increased tendency to develop trichorrhexis nodosa. These include syndromes with mental retardation (eg, Pollitt syndrome),[42] diarrhea (eg, tricho-hepato-enteric syndrome),[43] argininosuccinic aciduria,[44] Kabuki syndrome,[45] Menkes disease,[46] ectodermal dysplasias,[47,48] biotin deficiency,[41] and several other conditions.[1] This abnormality may also be induced by physical or chemical trauma and can be

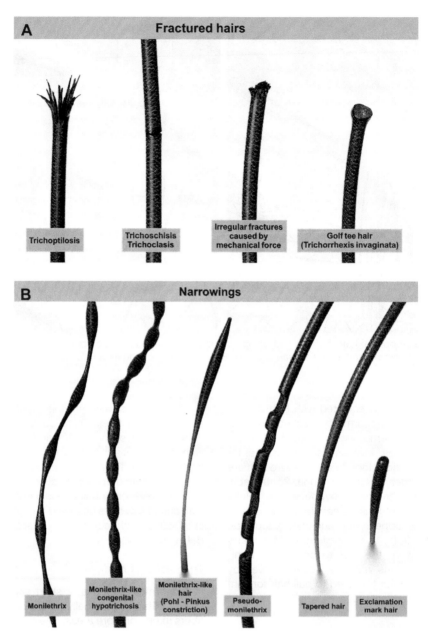

Fig. 2. Classification of hair shaft abnormalities in trichoscopy: fractured hair shafts (*A*), hair narrowings (*B*), hairs with node-like structures (*C*), hairs with curls and twists (*D*), hairs with bands (*E*), short hairs (*F*). (*Courtesy of* Dr Wawrzyniec Podrzucki; *adapted from* Rudnicka L, Olszewska M, Rakowska A. Atlas of trichoscopy: dermoscopy in hair and scalp disease. London: Springer; 2012; with permission.)

reproduced in vitro.[49] Trichorrhexis nodosa also may be associated with severe pruritus in the affected areas and may clear with control of the pruritus, indicating that the condition may be self-induced by scratching.[49] Hair shaft injury observed in trichoscopy of patients with scalp dysesthesia may be considered a model of trichorrhexis nodosa (and trichoptilosis) caused by mechanical trauma.

In patients with trichorrhexis nodosa, trichoscopy may give a slightly different appearance depending on presence or absence of immersion fluid. In presence of immersion fluid, trichoscopy may show nodular thickenings along the hairs shaft. When this thickening is not intensely pigmented, this may appear as almost a gap in a pigmented hair shaft. At the site of these nodular thickenings, hairs bend with a rounded edge.

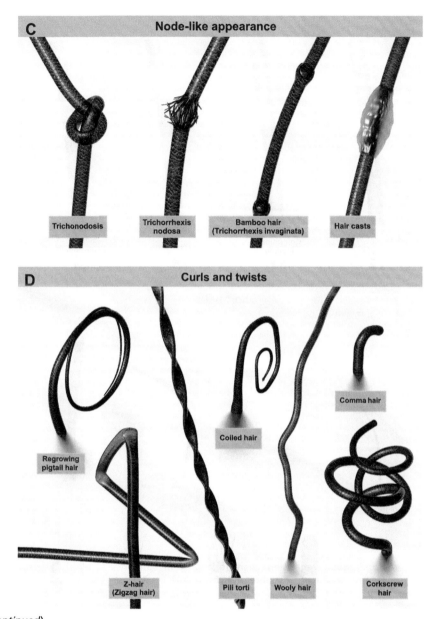

C   Node-like appearance

Trichonodosis | Trichorrhexis nodosa | Bamboo hair (Trichorrhexis invaginata) | Hair casts

D   Curls and twists

Regrowing pigtail hair | Z-hair (Zigzag hair) | Coiled hair | Pili torti | Wooly hair | Comma hair | Corkscrew hair

Fig. 2. *(continued)*

When a hair shaft breaks at the level of the nodule, it leaves a slightly thickened, rounded hair shaft end.

Occasionally, with dry trichoscopy (without immersion fluid), whitish contours of the splitting fibers may be visible. At high magnifications, trichoscopy shows the numerous small fibers that produce a picture resembling two brooms or brushes aligned in opposition. Broken hairs leave brush-like ends with numerous small fibers at the distal end of the hair shaft.

Trichoptilosis (Split Ends)

The term trichoptilosis refers to longitudinal splitting of the distal end of hair shaft. This feature is not pathognomonic for any type of alopecia. It may be observed in healthy individuals. However, in healthy individuals, trichoptilosis is most commonly observed in distal ends of long hair shafts. When trichoptilosis is present in short hair shafts (shorter than one field of view of a dermoscope), it may be a manifestation of several diseases that cause defects in hair shaft structure.[1]

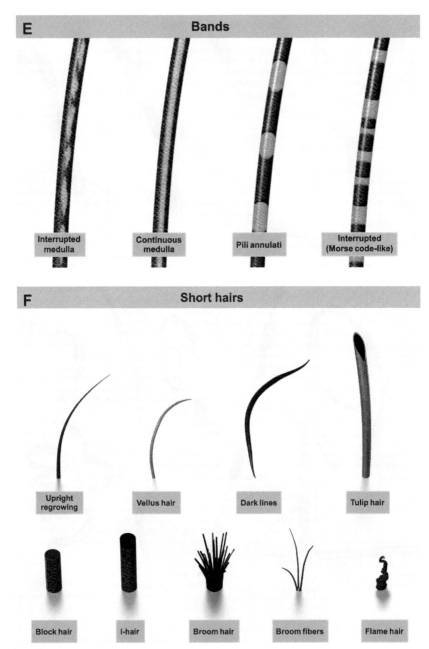

Fig. 2. (*continued*)

Broken Hairs

Broken hairs are hairs with irregular fractures that are most commonly caused by mechanical force. These are short hairs with hair shafts that appear normal except for irregular, ragged, distal ends. This type of abnormality is observed in 100% of patients with active trichotillomania.[50,51] They are also occasionally present in traction alopecia,

alopecia areata, and tinea capitis. Typically, in trichotillomania, hairs are broken at different levels above the scalp. Thus, there is a high variability in their length. In alopecia areata, hairs tend to be broken at a similar levels and their length reflects the time between the last episode of high disease activity and the moment of examination.

Table 2
Classification of hair shaft abnormalities in trichoscopy

Hair Shafts in Trichoscopy	Description	Most Common Clinical Association
Normal hairs		
Normal hairs	Hairs, uniform in shape and color	Normal
Fractured hairs		
Trichoptilosis	Longitudinal splitting of the distal end of hair shaft	Unspecific manifestation of a defect in hair shaft structure
Trichoschisis or trichoclasis	A clean transverse fracture across the hair shaft	Trichothiodystrophy, secondary to conditions that weaken the hair shaft
Broken (fractured) hairs	Irregular transverse fracture across the hair shaft	Trichotillomania, traction alopecia, alopecia areata, tinea capitis
Golf tee hairs	A hair with a concave distal end	Specific for Netherton syndrome
Narrowings		
Monilethrix	Hair with regularly distributed nodes and narrowings. The nodes correspond to normal hair shaft thickness; the internodes are the narrowings	Specific for monilethrix
Monilethrix-like congenital hypotrichosis	As in monilethrix, but the spaces between narrowings are extremely short	Specific for monilethrix-like congenital hypotrichosis
Monilethrix-like hairs (Pohl-Pinkus constriction)	Hair with irregularly distributed narrowings (Pohl-Pinkus constrictions)	Alopecia areata, chemotherapy-induced alopecia, bleeding, malnutrition. Artificial: monilethrix-like effect from hair styling gel or immersion fluid
Pseudomonilethrix	Differs from monilethrix—nodes appear thicker than the normal hair shaft and internodes have the thickness of the normal hair	Controversial
Exclamation mark hairs	Hairs with a thin, usually hypopigmented proximal end and thicker, pigmented distal end	Alopecia areata, chemotherapy-induced alopecia, intoxication, trichotillomania
Tapered hairs	Long exclamation mark hairs, the distal end is outside the field of view of a dermoscope	Alopecia areata, cicatricial alopecia, trichotillomania, bleeding, malnutrition, chronic intoxication
Node-like appearance		
Trichonodosis (hair knotting)	A single or double knot in the hair shaft	No clinical significance
Trichorrhexis nodosa	A hair shaft with a restricted area where the shaft splits longitudinally into numerous small fibers. The outer fibers bulge out, causing a segmental increase in hair diameter	Multiple acquired and inherited diseases, commonly due to mechanical or chemical trauma

(continued on next page)

Table 2
(continued)

Hair Shafts in Trichoscopy	Description	Most Common Clinical Association
Trichorrhexis invaginata (bamboo hairs)	The hair shaft telescopes into itself The proximal part of the abnormality is concave and the distal end is convex (bulging), producing an impression of nodular swelling along the hair shaft	Specific for Netherton syndrome
Hair casts (peripilar keratin casts)	Firm, white, tubular masses that encircle the hair shafts	A nonspecific finding, commonly associated with scaling or epidermal detachment Traction alopecia
Curls and twists		
Pigtail hairs	Short, regularly coiled hairs with tapered ends	Alopecia areata
Coiled hairs	Irregularly coiled hairs with a jagged end When not fully coiled, they may have a hook-like appearance	Trichotillomania
Comma hairs	Short, comma-like (C-shaped) hairs, homogeneous in thickness and pigmentation	Tinea capitis
Corkscrew hairs	Hairs with multiple twists and coils, forming corkscrew-like structures	Tinea capitis
Zigzag hairs	Hairs, bent at sharp angles, form zigzag structures	Tinea capitis, alopecia areata
Pili torti	Hairs that are flattened and twisted on their own axis at irregular intervals, usually through an angle of 180°	Associated with multiple inherited and acquired hair diseases
Wooly hairs	Hair shafts with waves at very short intervals, giving a crawling snake appearance	Inherited syndromes
Bands		
Continuous medulla	Longitudinal white band along the midpart of the hair shaft that covers less than 50% of the hair shaft thickness	Normal
Interrupted medulla	Interrupted longitudinal white band along the midpart of the hair shaft The band covers less than 50% of the hair shaft thickness	Normal
Pili annulati	Hair shafts with transverse light, blurry, whitish bands covering (nearly) the width of a hair	Inherited hair shaft abnormality; possible association with alopecia areata
Interrupted (Morse Code-like) hairs	Hairs with multiple thin white bands across the hair shaft	Tinea capitis

(continued on next page)

Table 2
(continued)

Hair Shafts in Trichoscopy	Description	Most Common Clinical Association
Short hairs		
Upright regrowing	New, healthy, regrowing hairs that have a tapered end and a straight-up position	Normal If abundant, may reflect a regrowth phase of telogen effluvium
Vellus hairs	Short, thin, hypopigmented, delicate, nonmedullated hairs, usually somewhat wavy in shape	Normal If abundant, may reflect androgenetic alopecia
Dark lines	Thin, short, intensely pigmented hairs, appearing tapered at both sides	Noncicatricial alopecia
Tulip hairs	Short hairs with a tulip leaf-like hyperpigmentation at the distal end	Trichotillomania
Block hairs	Very short hairs with a transverse horizontal distal end	Noncicatricial alopecia associated with shaft hair fragility
i-Hairs	i-Hairs are block hairs with an accented dark distal end	Noncicatricial alopecia associated with high shaft hair fragility (eg, tinea capitis)
Broom hairs	Few or more linear, short hairs emerging from one follicular opening	Observed in diverse entities, both cicatricial and noncicatricial
Broom fibers	Few or more linear, short, dark fibers (significantly thinner than terminal hairs) emerging from one follicular opening	Observed in diverse entities, both cicatricial and noncicatricial
Flame hairs	Hair residues, semitransparent, wavy, and cone-shaped, resembling a fire flame	Trichotillomania

RARE HAIR SHAFT ABNORMALITIES IN TRICHOSCOPY

Trichoclasis and Trichoschisis

Trichoclasis (trichoclasia) and trichoschisis are clean transverse fractures across the hair shaft. There is some confusion in the literature about the exact meaning of these terms. Most investigators use the term trichoclasis to describe hair fractures induced by chemical or physical trauma that develop secondary to conditions that weaken the hair.[52,53] Trichoclasis have been described in otherwise healthy individuals (idiopathic trichoclasis)[54] and in patients with alopecia areata.[55] In trichoclasis, the hair may be bound only by an intact cuticle, which results in the appearance of a greenstick fracture.

Trichoschisis is a complete, clean transverse fracture across the hair shaft. It is most commonly associated with trichothiodystrophy.[56]

Bamboo Hairs and Golf Tee Hairs (Trichorrhexis Invaginata)

Trichorrhexis invaginata (bamboo hair), is an abnormality of the hair in which the hair shaft telescopes into itself (invaginates) at several points along the shaft.[57] In low magnification trichoscopy, this appears as multiple small nodules spaced along the shaft at irregular intervals. High-magnification trichoscopy shows an invagination of the distal portion of the hair shaft into its proximal portion forming a ball-in-cup appearance that is considered pathognomonic of Netherton syndrome. Occasionally, ragged, cupped proximal hair ends may be seen where the distal end has fractured. This abnormality is often referred to as golf tee hairs.[58–60] Bamboo and golf tee hairs are easiest to find by trichoscopy of the eyebrow area,[4,59,61] because their density (the number of lesions per millimeter of hair shaft)

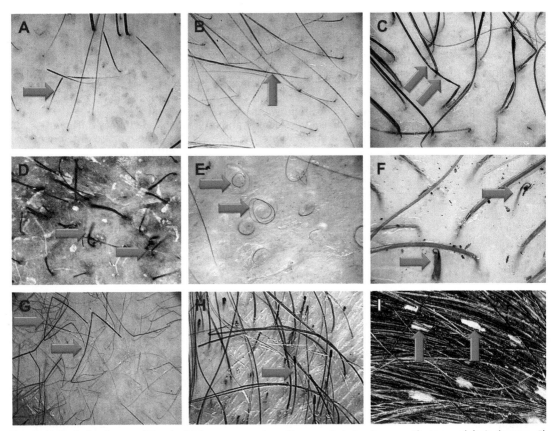

Fig. 3. Hair shaft abnormalities in trichoscopy: exclamation mark hairs (*arrow, A*), tapered hair (*arrow, B*), Pohl-Pinkus constrictions (*arrows, C*), comma hairs (*arrows, D*), pigtail hairs (*arrows, E*), coiled hairs (*arrows, F*), zigzag hairs (*arrows, G*), tulip hairs (*arrow, H*), hair casts (*arrows, I*).

is higher in the eyebrow area compared with the scalp in patients with Netherton syndrome.[62] Eyelashes may also exhibit trichoscopy features of trichorrhexis invaginata.[63]

Monilethrix, Monilethrix-like, Congenital Hypotrichosis, and Pseudomonilethrix

Monilethrix is an autosomal dominant hair disorder characterized by regular, periodic thinning of hair shafts. Nodosities correspond to the normal hair caliber, whereas the defect is in the constricted sections.[64] The interval between constrictions is constant in an individual patient. Trichoscopy shows abnormalities in terminal and vellus hairs of the scalp.[65] Hairs are bent regularly at multiple locations and have a tendency to fracture at constriction sites.[66–69] An additional finding in these patients is the presence of horny follicular papules, observed most commonly in association with the affected hairs.

In monilethrix-like congenital hypotrichosis, the spaces between narrowings are significantly shorter and more superficial compared with true monilethrix. They may be barely visible by trichoscopy on thicker hairs.

Pseudomonilethrix is characterized by irregular, square, flattening of hair shafts. It remains controversial whether pseudomonilethrix is a true disease[70] or an artifact produced by either procedure of preparing hairs for microscopic examination or by excessive use of cosmetic hair care products.[71]

Pseudomonilethrix has to be clearly distinguished from monilethrix-like hairs that show the same type of ovoid constrictions as in monilethrix but with no regularity characteristic as in true monilethrix.[1]

Trichonodosis

Trichonodosis (hair knotting) is an acquired, transient condition in which a knot occurs in the hair shaft, either spontaneously or as an effect of scratching or hair styling procedures. It is observed most commonly in patients with short, curly hair. Trichonodosis is usually an incidental finding of no clinical significance.[1]

Hair Cast

Hair casts (peripilar keratin casts) are firm, white, freely movable tubular masses that encircle the hair shafts. They were historically called also pseudonits because on macroscopic evaluation they may resemble nits. This is a nonspecific feature that may be associated with several diseases of intense scaling, such as psoriasis, seborrheic dermatitis, or lichen planopilaris.[68,72,73] Trichoscopy examination may also identify hair casts associated with epidermal detachment in traction alopecia[74] and in diseases with acantholysis, such as pemphigus vulgaris.[75] Hair cosmetics may be another cause of hair casts.[76] Idiopathic hair casts are occasionally present in healthy individuals.[1]

Pigtail Hairs

Pigtail hairs are short, regrowing, regularly coiled hairs with tapered ends. They are usually circular or oval and have a pigtail-like appearance. Pigtail hairs are a rare finding, associated with hair regrowth in patients with acute, diffuse hair loss, such as in alopecia areata or chemotherapy-induced alopecia.[76] These regrowing hairs with a tendency to curl appear in trichoscopy as pigtail hairs. Solitary, regrowing pigtail hairs may also be observed at the hair-bearing margin of cicatricial alopecia.[1]

Coiled Hairs and Hook Hairs

The term coiled hairs was first coined by Ross and colleagues[51] and was identified as a characteristic feature of trichotillomania. These hairs differ from pigtail hairs by their irregular structure and a ragged distal end.[1]

These hairs result from hair pulling tension force. After fracturing, the remaining, proximal part of the hair coils irregularly at the site of fracture. The appearance of the coiled hair depends on tension, pulling direction, length of the remaining hair, and hair growth after the moment of pulling. In patients with multiple coiled hairs, this will result in a different appearance of each coiled hair.

Coiled hairs are present in 40% of patients with trichotillomania and very rarely (<1%) may be observed in other conditions associated with hair loss.[50]

Hairs that are only partly coiled may have a hook-like (or question mark-like) appearance. These hairs are also called also hook hair.[1]

Zigzag Hairs

Zigzag hairs are hairs with numerous bends at sharp angles. These hairs are observed rarely in trichoscopy examinations. They are observed in tinea capitis, alopecia areata, trichorrhexis nodosa, and in other diseases associated with focal weakening of the hair shaft.[3]

Pili Torti

In pili torti, trichoscopy shows twists of hair shafts along the long axis, usually through an angle of 180°. Images taken at a low magnification may demonstrate the hair shafts slightly bent at different angles at irregular intervals. The abnormality is best observed in dry trichoscopy and at high magnification.[67] Pili torti is a common, nonspecific symptom associated with many types of hair loss, both inherited and acquired.[1]

Wooly Hair

In woolly hair, trichoscopy demonstrates intensely wavy hair with a crawling snake appearance and broken hair shafts. Trichoscopy is not decisive for diagnosis; however, the typical wavy appearance of hairs may indicate the need for detailed clinical evaluation.[67,77] The condition is classified into three variants: woolly hair nevus, autosomal dominant woolly hair, and autosomal recessive woolly hair.[78,79] Woolly hair may be a manifestation of various inherited syndromes.[57,80]

Pili Annulati

In pili annulati, trichoscopy shows hair shafts with alternating white and dark bands. The white bands are subtle, cloudy, and shorter than the remaining, dark portion of the hair shaft. They cover between 50% and 100% of the width of a hair shaft.[67,81] About 20% to 80% of hairs are affected and the bands tend to disappear distally.[3,82] Pili annulati should not be misdiagnosed in patients with fragmented medulla or inaccurate hair colorization. In pseudopili annulati,[83] trichoscopy will show no white bands, but only twisted hairs.[1]

Pili annulati is an autosomal dominant disorder, usually not associated with other abnormalities.[57] However, few cases of pili annulati associated with alopecia areata were reported.[84] Some investigators indicate that coexistence of pili annulati and alopecia areata is a coincidence rather than a true pathogenetic association.[82]

Interrupted (Morse Code) Hairs

Interrupted hairs (Morse code hairs) were first observed by the authors' group[3] in children with tinea capitis caused by Microsporum canis. These are hairs with multiple thin white bands across the hair shafts. The frequency and specificity of this finding remains to be investigated.

Dark Lines

Dark lines are to hairs that are thin, short, and intensely pigmented. They may be darker than the natural hair color of the patient. These hairs appear tapered at both ends, frequently making it difficult to distinguish the distal end from the proximal end. They are present in noncicatricial alopecia, most commonly in alopecia areata incognita.[1]

Tulip Hairs

Tulip hairs have a tulip leaf-like hyperpigmentation at the distal end. This appearance of the distal end is believed to result from a diagonal fracture of the hair shaft. The tulip hairs tend to be slightly thinner at the base. They are characteristic but not pathognomonic for trichotillomania.[3] They may be present in patients with alopecia areata.[50]

Blocks and i-Hairs

Blocks hairs are very short hairs with a horizontal distal end. i-Hairs are block hairs with accented dark distal ends. Both types of hairs are observed in noncicatricial alopecia associated with high shaft hair fragility, especially in tinea capitis.[50]

Broom Hairs and Broom Fibers

The term broom hair was suggested for all abnormalities associated with multiple short hairs emerging from one follicular opening in patients with otherwise long hairs.[3] Broom hairs differ from tufted hairs in they are short (<1 cm) and not associated with clinically or trichoscopically apparent folliculitis. Broom fibers refers to an analogous situation, but differs because the emerging fibers are not full-thickness hairs but thin hair-like fibers. Both broom hairs and broom fibers may be observed in diverse conditions associated with cicatricial and noncicatricial alopecia.[1]

Flame Hairs

Flame-like hairs are residues from recently pulled hairs and are most commonly observed in active trichotillomania.[3] They are present in 25% of patients with active trichotillomania.[50] Flame hairs have not been observed in other diseases.

SUMMARY

Trichoscopy allows evaluation of the hair shaft structure, scalp surface, follicular openings, and superficial blood vessels. This article has summarized how evaluation of hair shaft structure alone may provide clues for differential diagnosis of hair loss.

REFERENCES

1. Rudnicka L, Olszewska M, Rakowska A. Atlas of trichoscopy: dermoscopy in hair and scalp disease. London: Springer; 2012.
2. Rudnicka L, Olszewska M, Rakowska A, et al. Trichoscopy: a new method for diagnosing hair loss. J Drugs Dermatol 2008;7:651–4.
3. Rudnicka L, Olszewska M, Rakowska A, et al. Trichoscopy update 2011. J Dermatol Case Rep 2011;5:82–8.
4. Olszewska M, Rudnicka L, Rakowska A, et al. Trichoscopy. Arch Dermatol 2008;144:1007.
5. Rakowska A. Trichoscopy (hair and scalp videodermoscopy) in the healthy female. Method standardization and norms for measurable parameters. J Dermatol Case Rep 2009;3:14–9.
6. Vogt A, McElwee KJ, Blume-Peytavi U. Biology of the hair follicle. In: Blume-Peytavi U, Tosti A, Whiting D, et al, editors. Hair; from basic science to clinical application. Berlin: Springer-Verlag; 2008. p. 1–22. ISBN: 3540469087.
7. Trueb RM. Pharmacologic interventions in aging hair. Clin Interv Aging 2006;1:121–9.
8. Olszewska M, Rudnicka L. Effective treatment of female androgenic alopecia with dutasteride. J Drugs Dermatol 2005;4:637–40.
9. Wagner R, Joekes I. Hair medulla morphology and mechanical properties. J Cosmet Sci 2007;58:359–68.
10. Adya KA, Inamadar AC, Palit A, et al. Light microscopy of the hair: a simple tool to "untangle" hair disorders. Int J Trichology 2011;3:46–56.
11. Rudnicka L, Rakowska A, Olszewska M. Trichoscopy: how it may help the clinician. Dermatol Clin 2013;31:29–41.
12. Alkhalifah A. Alopecia areata update. Dermatol Clin 2013;31:93–108.
13. Jackson AJ, Price VH. How to diagnose hair loss. Dermatol Clin 2013;31:21–8.
14. Alkhalifah A, Alsantali A, Wang E, et al. Alopecia areata update: part I. Clinical picture, histopathology, and pathogenesis. J Am Acad Dermatol 2010;62:177–88 [quiz: 89–90].
15. Inui S. Trichoscopy for common hair loss diseases: algorithmic method for diagnosis. J Dermatol 2011; 38:71–5.
16. Rudnicka L, Olszewska M, Rakowska A, et al. Alopecia areata. In: Rudnicka L, Olszewska M, Rakowska A, editors. Atlas of trichoscopy dermoscopy in hair and scalp disease. London: Springer; 2013.
17. Lacarrubba F, Dall'Oglio F, Rita Nasca M, et al. Videodermatoscopy enhances diagnostic capability in some forms of hair loss. Am J Clin Dermatol 2004;5:205–8.
18. Inui S, Nakajima T, Nakagawa K, et al. Clinical significance of dermoscopy in alopecia areata:

analysis of 300 cases. Int J Dermatol 2008;47: 688–93.

19. Chang KH, Rojhirunsakool S, Goldberg LJ. Treatment of severe alopecia areata with intralesional steroid injections. J Drugs Dermatol 2009; 8:909–12.

20. Ganzetti G, Campanati A, Simonetti O, et al. Videocapillaroscopic pattern of alopecia areata before and after diphenylciclopropenone treatment. Int J Immunopathol Pharmacol 2011;24:1087–91.

21. Ihm CW, Han JH. Diagnostic value of exclamation mark hairs. Dermatology 1993;186:99–102.

22. Peralta L, Morais P. Photoletter to the editor: the Friar Tuck sign in trichotillomania. J Dermatol Case Rep 2012;6:63–4.

23. Pirmez R, Pineiro-Maceira J, Sodre CT. Exclamation marks and other trichoscopic signs of chemotherapy-induced alopecia. Australas J Dermatol 2013;54(2):129–32.

24. Feldman J, Levisohn DR. Acute alopecia: clue to thallium toxicity. Pediatr Dermatol 1993;10:29–31.

25. Shuster S. The coudability sign of alopecia areata: the real story. Clin Exp Dermatol 2011;36:554–5.

26. Inui S, Nakajima T, Itami S. Coudability hairs: a revisited sign of alopecia areata assessed by trichoscopy. Clin Exp Dermatol 2010;35:361–5.

27. Mane M, Nath AK, Thappa DM. Utility of dermoscopy in alopecia areata. Indian J Dermatol 2011; 56:407–11.

28. Slowinska M, Rudnicka L, Schwartz RA, et al. Comma hairs: a dermatoscopic marker for tinea capitis: a rapid diagnostic method. J Am Acad Dermatol 2008;59:S77–9.

29. Sandoval AB, Ortiz JA, Rodriguez JM, et al. Dermoscopic pattern in tinea capitis. Rev Iberoam Micol 2010;27:151–2.

30. Hughes R, Chiaverini C, Bahadoran P, et al. Corkscrew hair: a new dermoscopic sign for diagnosis of tinea capitis in black children. Arch Dermatol 2011;147:355–6.

31. Hernandez-Bel P, Malvehy J, Crocker A, et al. Comma hairs: a new dermoscopic marker for tinea capitis. Actas Dermosifiliogr 2012;103:836–7.

32. Mapelli ET, Gualandri L, Cerri A, et al. Comma hairs in tinea capitis: a useful dermatoscopic sign for diagnosis of tinea capitis. Pediatr Dermatol 2012; 29(2):223–4.

33. Tangjaturonrusamee C, Piraccini BM, Vincenzi C, et al. Tinea capitis mimicking folliculitis decalvans. Mycoses 2011;54:87–8.

34. Rudnicka L, Łukomska M. Alternaria scalp infection in a patient with alopecia areata. Coexistence or causative relationship? J Dermatol Case Rep 2012;6:120–4.

35. Vazquez-Lopez F, Palacios-Garcia L, Argenziano G. Dermoscopic corkscrew hairs dissolve after successful therapy of Trichophyton violaceum tinea

capitis: a case report. Australas J Dermatol 2012; 53:118–9.

36. Abramovits-Ackerman W, Bustos T, Simosa-Leon V, et al. Cutaneous findings in a new syndrome of autosomal recessive ectodermal dysplasia with corkscrew hairs. J Am Acad Dermatol 1992;27: 917–21.

37. Trueb R, Burg G, Bottani A, et al. Ectodermal dysplasia with corkscrew hairs: observation of probable autosomal dominant tricho-odonto-onychodysplasia with syndactyly. J Am Acad Dermatol 1994;30:289–90.

38. Argenziano G, Monsurro MR, Pazienza R, et al. A case of probable autosomal recessive ectodermal dysplasia with corkscrew hairs and mental retardation in a family with tuberous sclerosis. J Am Acad Dermatol 1998;38:344–8.

39. Ben-Zvi GT, Tidman MJ. Be vigilant for scurvy in high-risk groups. Practitioner 2012;256:23–5, 3.

40. Maltos AL, Silva LL, Bernardes Junior AG, et al. Scurvy in a patient with AIDS: case report. Rev Soc Bras Med Trop 2011;44:122–3.

41. Bartels NG, Blume-Peytavi U. Hair loss in children. In: Blume-Peytavi U, Tosti A, Whiting D, et al, editors. Hair growth and disorders. Leipzig (Germany): Springer; 2008. p. 293–4.

42. Pollitt RJ, Jenner FA, Davies M. Sibs with mental and physical retardation and trichorrhexis nodosa with abnormal amino acid composition of the hair. Arch Dis Child 1968;43:211–6.

43. Fabre A, Andre N, Breton A, et al. Intractable diarrhea with "phenotypic anomalies" and tricho-hepato-enteric syndrome: two names for the same disorder. Am J Med Genet A 2007;143:584–8.

44. Erez A, Nagamani SC, Lee B. Argininosuccinate lyase deficiency-argininosuccinic aciduria and beyond. Am J Med Genet C Semin Med Genet 2011;157:45–53.

45. Abdel-Salam GM, Afifi HH, Eid MM, et al. Ectodermal abnormalities in patients with kabuki syndrome. Pediatr Dermatol 2011;28(5):507–11.

46. Wang XH, Lu JL, Zhang LP, et al. Clinical and laboratory features of the Menkes disease. Zhonghua Er Ke Za Zhi 2009;47:604–7.

47. Kelly SC, Ratajczak P, Keller M, et al. A novel GJA 1 mutation in oculo-dento-digital dysplasia with curly hair and hyperkeratosis. Eur J Dermatol 2006;16: 241–5.

48. Rouse C, Siegfried E, Breer W, et al. Hair and sweat glands in families with hypohidrotic ectodermal dysplasia: further characterization. Arch Dermatol 2004;140:850–5.

49. Chernosky ME, Owens DW. Trichorrhexis nodosa. Clinical and investigative studies. Arch Dermatol 1966;94:577–85.

50. Rakowska A, Slowinska M, Olszewska M, et al. New trichoscopy findings in trichotillomania: flame

hairs, v-sign, hook hairs, hair powder, tulip hairs. Acta Derm Venereol, in press.

51. Ross EK, Vincenzi C, Tosti A. Videodermoscopy in the evaluation of hair and scalp disorders. J Am Acad Dermatol 2006;55:799–806.

52. Whiting DA. Structural abnormalities of the hair shaft. J Am Acad Dermatol 1987;16:1–25.

53. Whiting DA, Dy LC. Office diagnosis of hair shaft defects. Semin Cutan Med Surg 2006;25:24–34.

54. Levin MM, Evstaf'ev VV, Gronskii KT, et al. Idiopathic trichoclasia. Vestn Dermatol Venerol 1982;(9):61–2.

55. Wolowa F, Stachow A. Treatment of alopecia areata with zinc sulfate. Z Hautkr 1980;55:1125–34.

56. Ferrando J, Mir-Bonafe JM, Cepeda-Valdes R, et al. Further insights in trichothiodistrophy: a clinical, microscopic, and ultrastructural study of 20 cases and literature review. Int J Trichology 2012;4:158–63.

57. Rogers M. Hair shaft abnormalities: part II. Australas J Dermatol 1996;37:1–11.

58. de Berker DA, Paige DG, Ferguson DJ, et al. Golf tee hairs in Netherton disease. Pediatr Dermatol 1995;12:7–11.

59. Rakowska A, Kowalska-Oledzka E, Slowinska M, et al. Hair shaft videodermoscopy in Netherton syndrome. Pediatr Dermatol 2009;26:320–2.

60. Burk C, Hu S, Lee C, et al. Netherton syndrome and trichorrhexis invaginata—a novel diagnostic approach. Pediatr Dermatol 2008;25:287–8.

61. Goujon E, Beer F, Fraitag S, et al. 'Matchstick' eyebrow hairs: a dermoscopic clue to the diagnosis of Netherton syndrome. J Eur Acad Dermatol Venereol 2010;24:740–1.

62. Powell J. Increasing the likelihood of early diagnosis of Netherton syndrome by simple examination of eyebrow hairs. Arch Dermatol 2000;136:423–4.

63. Neri I, Balestri R, Starace M, et al. Videodermoscopy of eyelashes in Netherton syndrome. J Eur Acad Dermatol Venereol 2011;25(11):1360–1.

64. Neila Iglesias J, Rodriguez Pichardo A, Garcia Bravo B, et al. Masquerading of trichotillomania in a family with monilethrix. Eur J Dermatol 2011; 21:133.

65. Miteva M, Tosti A. Dermatoscopy of hair shaft disorders. J Am Acad Dermatol 2013;68:473–81.

66. Rakowska A, Slowinska M, Czuwara J, et al. Dermoscopy as a tool for rapid diagnosis of monilethrix. J Drugs Dermatol 2007;6:222–4.

67. Rakowska A, Slowinska M, Kowalska-Oledzka E, et al. Trichoscopy in genetic hair shaft abnormalities. J Dermatol Case Rep 2008;2:14–20.

68. Wallace MP, de Berker DA. Hair diagnoses and signs: the use of dermatoscopy. Clin Exp Dermatol 2010;35:41–6.

69. Jain N, Khopkar U. Monilethrix in pattern distribution in siblings: diagnosis by trichoscopy. Int J Trichology 2010;2:56–9.

70. Zitelli JA. Pseudomonilethrix. An artifact. Arch Dermatol 1986;122:688–90.

71. Itin PH, Schiller P, Mathys D, et al. Cosmetically induced hair beads. J Am Acad Dermatol 1997; 36:260–1.

72. Wang E, Lee JS, Hee TH. Is Propionibacterium acnes associated with hair casts and alopecia? Int J Trichology 2012;4:93–7.

73. Franca K, Villa RT, Silva IR, et al. Hair casts or pseudonits. Int J Trichology 2011;3:121–2.

74. Tosti A, Miteva M, Torres F, et al. Hair casts are a dermoscopic clue for the diagnosis of traction alopecia. Br J Dermatol 2010;163:1353–5.

75. Pirmez R. Acantholytic hair casts: a dermoscopic sign of pemphigus vulgaris of the scalp. Int J Trichology 2012;4:172–3.

76. Ena P, Mazzarello V, Chiarolini F. Hair casts due to a deodorant spray. Australas J Dermatol 2005;46: 274–7.

77. Patil S, Marwah M, Nadkarni N, et al. The medusa head: dermoscopic diagnosis of woolly hair syndrome. Int J Trichology 2012;4:184–5.

78. Hutchinson PE, Cairns RJ, Wells RS. Woolly hair. Clinical and general aspects. Trans St Johns Hosp Dermatol Soc 1974;60:160–77.

79. Venugopal V, Karthikeyan S, Gnanaraj P, et al. Woolly hair nevus: a rare entity. Int J Trichology 2012;4:42–3.

80. Al-Owain M, Wakil S, Shareef F, et al. Novel homozygous mutation in DSP causing skin fragility-woolly hair syndrome: report of a large family and review of the desmoplakin-related phenotypes. Clin Genet 2011;80:50–8.

81. Haliasos EC, Kerner M, Jaimes-Lopez N, et al. Dermoscopy for the pediatric dermatologist part I: dermoscopy of pediatric infectious and inflammatory skin lesions and hair disorders. Pediatr Dermatol 2013;30:163–71.

82. Giehl KA, Ferguson DJ, Dawber RP, et al. Update on detection, morphology and fragility in pili annulati in three kindreds. J Eur Acad Dermatol Venereol 2004;18:654–8.

83. Lee SS, Lee YS, Giam YC. Pseudopili annulati in a dark-haired individual: a light and electron microscopic study. Pediatr Dermatol 2001;18: 27–30.

84. Castelli E, Fiorella S, Caputo V. Pili annulati coincident with alopecia areata, autoimmune thyroid disease, and primary IgA deficiency: case report and considerations on the literature. Case Rep Dermatol 2012;4:250–5.

Index

Note: Page numbers of article titles are in **boldface** type.

Dermatol Clin 31 (2013) 709–715
http://dx.doi.org/10.1016/S0733-8635(13)00082-X
0733-8635/13/$ – see front matter © 2013 Elsevier Inc. All rights reserved.

United States Postal Service

Statement of Ownership, Management, and Circulation
(All Periodicals Publications Except Requestor Publications)

1. Publication Title
Dermatologic Clinics

2. Publication Number
0 0 0 - 7 0 5

3. Filing Date
9/14/13

4. Issue Frequency
Jan, Apr, Jul, Oct

5. Number of Issues Published Annually
4

6. Annual Subscription Price
$346.00

7. Complete Mailing Address of Known Office of Publication (Not printer) (Street, city, county, state, and ZIP+4®)

Elsevier Inc.
360 Park Avenue South
New York, NY 10010-1710

Contact Person
Stephen R. Bushing

Telephone (Include area code)
215-239-3688

8. Complete Mailing Address of Headquarters or General Business Office of Publisher (Not printer)

Elsevier Inc., 360 Park Avenue South, New York, NY 10010-1710

9. Full Names and Complete Mailing Addresses of Publisher, Editor, and Managing Editor (Do not leave blank)

Publisher (Name and complete mailing address)

Linda Belfus, Elsevier, Inc., 1600 John F. Kennedy Blvd. Suite 1800, Philadelphia, PA 19103-2899

Editor (Name and complete mailing address)

Stephanie Donley, Elsevier, Inc., 1600 John F. Kennedy Blvd. Suite 1800, Philadelphia, PA 19103-2899

Managing Editor (Name and complete mailing address)

Adrianne Brigido, Elsevier, Inc., 1600 John F. Kennedy Blvd. Suite 1800, Philadelphia, PA 19103-2899

10. Owner (Do not leave blank. If the publication is owned by a corporation, give the name and address of the corporation immediately followed by the names and addresses of all stockholders owning or holding 1 percent or more of the total amount of stock. If not owned by a corporation, give the names and addresses of the individual owners. If owned by a partnership or other unincorporated firm, give its name and address as well as those of each individual owner. If the publication is published by a nonprofit organization, give its name and address.)

Full Name	Complete Mailing Address
Wholly owned subsidiary of	1600 John F. Kennedy Blvd., Ste. 1800
Reed/Elsevier, US holdings	Philadelphia, PA 19103-2899

11. Known Bondholders, Mortgagees, and Other Security Holders Owning or Holding 1 Percent or More of Total Amount of Bonds, Mortgages, or Other Securities. If none, check box ☑ None

Full Name	Complete Mailing Address
N/A	

12. Tax Status (For completion by nonprofit organizations authorized to mail at nonprofit rates) (Check one)
The purpose, function, and nonprofit status of this organization and the exempt status for federal income tax purposes:
☐ Has Not Changed During Preceding 12 Months
☐ Has Changed During Preceding 12 Months (Publisher must submit explanation of change with this statement)

PS Form 3526, September 2007 (Page 1 of 3 (Instructions Page 3)) PSN 7530-01-000-9931 PRIVACY NOTICE: See our Privacy policy in www.usps.com

---

13. Publication Title
Dermatologic Clinics of North America

14. Issue Date for Circulation Data Below
April 2013

15. Extent and Nature of Circulation

		Average No. Copies Each Issue During Preceding 12 Months	No. Copies of Single Issue Published Nearest to Filing Date
a. Total Number of Copies (Net press run)		571	597
b. Paid Circulation (By Mail and Outside the Mail)	(1) Mailed Outside-County Paid Subscriptions Stated on PS Form 3541. (Include paid distribution above nominal rate, advertiser's proof copies, and exchange copies)	193	164
	(2) Mailed In-County Paid Subscriptions Stated on PS Form 3541 (Include paid distribution above nominal rate, advertiser's proof copies, and exchange copies)		
	(3) Paid Distribution Outside the Mails Including Sales Through Dealers and Carriers, Street Vendors, Counter Sales, and Other Paid Distribution Outside USPS®	105	81
	(4) Paid Distribution by Other Classes Mailed Through the USPS (e.g. First-Class Mail®)		
c. Total Paid Distribution (Sum of 15b (1), (2), (3), and (4))		298	245
d. Free or Nominal Rate Distribution (By Mail and Outside the Mail)	(1) Free or Nominal Rate Outside-County Copies Included on PS Form 3541	49	79
	(2) Free or Nominal Rate In-County Copies Included on PS Form 3541		
	(3) Free or Nominal Rate Copies Mailed at Other Classes Through the USPS (e.g. First-Class Mail)		
	(4) Free or Nominal Rate Distribution Outside the Mail (Carriers or other means)		
e. Total Free or Nominal Rate Distribution (Sum of 15d (1), (2), (3) and (4))		49	79
f. Total Distribution (Sum of 15c and 15e)		347	324
g. Copies not Distributed (See instructions to publishers #4 (page 83))		224	273
h. Total (Sum of 15f and g)		571	597
i. Percent Paid (15c divided by 15f times 100)		85.88%	75.62%

16. Publication of Statement of Ownership
☐ If the publication is a general publication, publication of this statement is required. Will be printed in the October 2013 issue of this publication. ☐ Publication not required.

17. Signature and Title of Editor, Publisher, Business Manager, or Owner

Stephen R. Bushing - Inventory Distribution Coordinator

Date September 14, 2013

I certify that all information furnished on this form is true and complete. I understand that anyone who furnishes false or misleading information on this form or who omits material or information requested on the form may be subject to criminal sanctions (including fines and imprisonment) and/or civil sanctions (including civil penalties).

PS Form 3526, September 2007 (Page 2 of 3)

Moving?

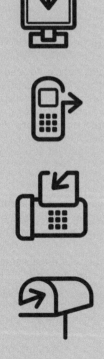

Make sure your subscription moves with you!

To notify us of your new address, find your **Clinics Account Number** (located on your mailing label above your name), and contact customer service at:

Email: journalscustomerservice-usa@elsevier.com

800-654-2452 (subscribers in the U.S. & Canada)
314-447-8871 (subscribers outside of the U.S. & Canada)

Fax number: 314-447-8029

Elsevier Health Sciences Division
Subscription Customer Service
3251 Riverport Lane
Maryland Heights, MO 63043

*To ensure uninterrupted delivery of your subscription, please notify us at least 4 weeks in advance of move.

Printed and bound by CPI Group (UK) Ltd, Croydon, CR0 4YY

03/10/2024

01040370-0001